1989
YEAR BOOK OF
INFECTIOUS DISEASES®

The 1989 Year Book® Series

Year Book of Anesthesia®: Drs. Miller, Kirby, Ostheimer, Roizen, and Stoelting

Year Book of Cardiology®: Drs. Schlant, Collins, Engle, Frye, Kaplan, and O'Rourke

Year Book of Critical Care Medicine®: Drs. Rogers and Parrillo

Year Book of Dentistry®: Drs. Rose, Hendler, Johnson, Jordan, Moyers, and Silverman

Year Book of Dermatology®: Drs. Sober and Fitzpatrick

Year Book of Diagnostic Radiology®: Drs. Bragg, Hendee, Keats, Kirkpatrick, Miller, Osborn, and Thompson

Year Book of Digestive Diseases®: Drs. Greenberger and Moody

Year Book of Drug Therapy®: Drs. Hollister and Lasagna

Year Book of Emergency Medicine®: Dr. Wagner

Year Book of Endocrinology®: Drs. Bagdade, Braverman, Halter, Horton, Korenman, Kornel, Metz, Molitch, Morley, Rogol, Ryan, Sherwin, and Vaitukaitis

Year Book of Family Practice®: Drs. Rakel, Avant, Driscoll, Prichard, and Smith

Year Book of Geriatrics and Gerontology: Drs. Beck, Abrass, Burton, Cummings, Makinodan, and Small

Year Book of Hand Surgery®: Drs. Dobyns, Chase, and Amadio

Year Book of Hematology®: Drs. Spivak, Bell, Ness, Quesenberry, and Wiernik

Year Book of Infectious Diseases®: Drs. Wolff, Barza, Keusch, Klempner, and Snydman

Year Book of Infertility: Drs. Mishell, Lobo, and Paulsen

Year Book of Medicine®: Drs. Rogers, Des Prez, Cline, Braunwald, Greenberger, Wilson, Epstein, and Malawista

Year Book of Neurology and Neurosurgery®: Drs. DeJong, Currier, and Crowell

Year Book of Nuclear Medicine®: Drs. Hoffer, Gore, Gottschalk, Sostman, Zaret, and Zubal

Year Book of Obstetrics and Gynecology®: Drs. Mishell, Kirschbaum, and Morrow

Year Book of Oncology®: Drs. Young, Coleman, Longo, Ozols, Simone, and Steele

Year Book of Ophthalmology®: Dr. Laibson

Year Book of Orthopedics®: Dr. Sledge

Year Book of Otolaryngology–Head and Neck Surgery®: Drs. Bailey and Paparella

Year Book of Pathology and Clinical Pathology®: Drs. Brinkhous, Dalldorf, Grisham, Langdell, and McLendon

Year Book of Pediatrics®: Drs. Oski and Stockman

Year Book of Perinatal/Neonatal Medicine: Drs. Klaus and Fanaroff

Year Book of Plastic, Reconstructive, and Aesthetic Surgery®: Drs. Miller, Bennett, Haynes, Hoehn, McKinney, and Whitaker

Year Book of Podiatric Medicine and Surgery®: Dr. Jay

Year Book of Psychiatry and Applied Mental Health®: Drs. Talbott, Frances, Freedman, Meltzer, Schowalter, and Weiner

Year Book of Pulmonary Disease®: Drs. Green, Ball, Michael, Peters, Terry, Tockman, and Wise

Year Book of Rehabilitation®: Drs. Kaplan, Frank, Gordon, Lieberman, Magnuson, Molnar, Payton, and Sarno

Year Book of Sports Medicine®: Drs. Shepard, Sutton, and Torg, Col. Anderson, and Mr. George

Year Book of Surgery®: Drs. Schwartz, Jonasson, Peacock, Shires, Spencer, and Thompson

Year Book of Urology®: Drs. Gillenwater and Howards

Year Book of Vascular Surgery®: Drs. Bergan and Yao

Editor
Sheldon M. Wolff, M.D.
Endicott Professor and Chairman, Department of Medicine, Tufts University School of Medicine; Physician-in-Chief, New England Medical Center, Boston

Associate Editors
Michael J. Barza, M.D.
Professor of Medicine, Tufts University School of Medicine; Attending Physician, Division of Geographic Medicine and Infectious Diseases, Department of Medicine, New England Medical Center, Boston
Gerald T. Keusch, M.D.
Professor of Medicine, Tufts University School of Medicine; Chief, Division of Geographic Medicine and Infectious Diseases, Department of Medicine, New England Medical Center, Boston
Mark S. Klempner, M.D.
Associate Professor of Medicine, Tufts University School of Medicine; Division of Geographic Medicine and Infectious Diseases, Department of Medicine, New England Medical Center, Boston
David R. Snydman, M.D.
Associate Professor of Medicine and Pathology, Tufts University School of Medicine; Hospital Epidemiologist and Director, Clinical Microbiology, New England Medical Center, Boston

The Year Book of INFECTIOUS DISEASES®

1989

Editor
Sheldon M. Wolff, M.D.

Associate Editors
Michael J. Barza, M.D.
Gerald T. Keusch, M.D.
Mark S. Klempner, M.D.
David R. Snydman, M.D.

Year Book Medical Publishers, Inc.
Chicago • London • Boca Raton

Copyright © 1989 by YEAR BOOK MEDICAL PUBLISHERS, INC.

All rights reserved. No part of this publication may be reproduced, stored in a retrieval system, or transmitted, in any form or by any means, electronic, mechanical, photocopying, recording, or otherwise, without prior written permission from the publishers.

Printed in U.S.A.

International Standard Book Number: 0-8151-9379-3

International Standard Serial Number: 0743-9261

Editorial Director, Year Book Publishing: Nancy Gorham
Sponsoring Editor: Leslie Borns
Manager, Medical Information Services: Laura J. Shedore
Assistant Director, Manuscript Services: Frances M. Perveiler
Assistant Managing Editor, Year Book Editing Services: Wayne Larsen
Project Manager: Max F. Perez
Proofroom Manager: Shirley E. Taylor

Table of Contents

The material covered in this volume represents literature reviewed up to February 1988.

JOURNALS REPRESENTED ix
INTRODUCTION xi

1. Bacterial Infections 1
    Sepsis and Endocarditis 1
    Respiratory Tract 6
    Gastrointestinal Tract 11
    Genitourinary Tract 20
    Skin, Soft Tissue, Bone, and Joint 27
    Bacterial Vaccines 35
    Antimicrobial Therapy 46
    Miscellaneous Topics 58

2. Viral Infections 73
    Hepatitis Viruses 73
    Herpes Viruses 80
    Other Viruses 90

3. Fungal Infections 99

4. Parasitic Infections 111
    Helminths 111
    Protozoa 112

5. Mycobacterial Infections 131

6. Infections in the Compromised Host 135

7. Human Immunodeficiency Virus (HIV) Infection 147
    Epidemiology 147
    Diagnostic Tests 161
    Clinical Manifestations 166
    Therapy 174

8. Sexually Transmitted Diseases 185

9. Nosocomial Infections 189

10. Pediatric Infections 207
    Perinatal Infections 207
    Respiratory Tract 208
    Central Nervous System 213
    Miscellaneous Topics 215

11. Miscellaneous Topics 225
    Subject Index 239
    Author Index 255

Journals Represented

Year Book Medical Publishers subscribes to and surveys more than 700 U.S. and foreign medical and allied health journals. From these journals, the Editors select the articles to be abstracted. Journals represented in this YEAR BOOK are listed below.

Acta Medica Scandinavica
American Journal of Epidemiology
American Journal of Medicine
American Journal of Obstetrics and Gynecology
American Journal of Public Health
American Review of Respiratory Disease
Annals of Internal Medicine
Antimicrobial Agents and Chemotherapy
Archives of Dermatology
Archives of Internal Medicine
Archives of Otolaryngology–Head and Neck Surgery
Archives of Surgery
British Dental Journal
British Medical Journal
Chest
Clinical Orthopaedics and Related Research
Clinical Pediatrics
Diagnostic Microbiology and Infectious Disease
Infection and Immunity
International Journal of Leprosy and Other Mycobacterial Diseases
International Orthopaedics
Journal of the American Academy of Dermatology
Journal of the American Medical Association
Journal of Antimicrobial Chemotherapy
Journal of Bone and Joint Surgery (American vol.)
Journal of Clinical Investigation
Journal of Clinical Microbiology
Journal of Clinical Pathology
Journal of Experimental Medicine
Journal of Infectious Diseases
Journal of Laboratory and Clinical Medicine
Journal of Pediatric Orthopedics
Journal of Pediatric Surgery
Journal of Pediatrics
Klinische Wochenschrift
Lancet
Medical Journal of Australia
Medicine
Nature
Neurology
New England Journal of Medicine
Ophthalmology
Pathology
Pediatric Infectious Disease Journal
Pediatric Research
Pediatrics

Quarterly Journal of Medicine
Science
Spine
Surgery
Transplantation

Introduction

It is exciting and interesting to have the opportunity to review the literature in infectious diseases for an entire year. The quality and quantity of the papers in our discipline continue to grow and increase in importance. During the past year many exciting papers were published, and it is unfortunate that we cannot include all the worthwhile material in this YEAR BOOK.

The long and difficult task of finding a satisfactory therapy for the human immunodeficiency virus and its consequences has begun. The papers on azidothymidine (AZT) therapy summarized in this volume will be marked as important milestones in the treatment of human immunodeficiency virus infection. Unfortunately, AZT is not curative and is toxic, and therefore better agents must be developed. In this volume new and exciting information on bacterial vaccines against typhoid fever and synthetic vaccines against malaria is summarized. Innovative work on immunoglobulins from milk to protect against oral challenge with *Escherichia coli* could open a whole new area of human immunopharmacology. Other new and interesting topics covered in this volume include the use of immune globulin to prevent cytomegalovirus infection in transplant patients. These are just some of the many interesting observations covered.

Once again, I want to express my appreciation to my associate editors who did more than their share of the work to prepare this volume.

Sheldon M. Wolff, M.D.

1 Bacterial Infections

Sepsis and Endocarditis

A Controlled Clinical Trial of High-Dose Methylprednisolone in the Treatment of Severe Sepsis and Septic Shock
Bone RC, Fisher CJ Jr, Clemmer TP, Slotman GJ, Metz CA, Balk RA, the Methylprednisolone Severe Sepsis Study Group
N Engl J Med 317.:653–658, Sept 10, 1987   1–1

The use of high-dose corticosteroids in the treatment of severe sepsis and septic shock continues to be controversial. In a prospective, randomized, double-blind, placebo-controlled trial, 382 patients with severe sepsis and septic shock received either high-dose methylprednisolone sodium succinate, 30 mg/kg body weight, or placebo in 4 infusions starting within 2 hours of diagnosis. Diagnosis was based on the clinical suspicion of infection plus the presence of fever or hypothermia (rectal temperature > 38.3C [101F] or < 35.6C [96F]), tachypnea (>20 breaths per minute), tachycardia (>90 beats per minute), and presence of one of the following indicators of organ dysfunction: change in mental status, hypoxemia, elevated lactate levels, or oliguria.

There were no significant differences between treatment groups in the prevention of shock, the reversal of shock, or overall mortality at 14 days. Patients who had renal insufficiency (serum creatinine level >2 mg/dl) initially and were treated with methylprednisolone had significantly higher incidences of shock development and mortality and tended to have decreased shock reversal. Although the incidence of secondary infection did not differ between groups, patients treated with steroids had significantly more deaths related to secondary infection. The use of high-dose corticosteroids provides no benefit in the treatment of severe sepsis and septic shock.

Effect of High-Dose Glucocorticoid Therapy on Mortality in Patients With Clinical Signs of Systemic Sepsis
VA Systemic Sepsis Cooperative Study Group (VA Med Ctr, West Haven, Conn)
N Engl J Med 317:659–665, Sept 10, 1987   1–2

Although improvements have steadily been made in antibiotic therapy and intensive care, mortality from fulminant sepsis remains unacceptably high. Of the many adjunctive therapies proposed, none is as controversial as glucocorticoids. Studies with animals have shown that these drugs decrease morbidity and mortality; however, results from human studies are less convincing. To clarify the role of adjunctive glucocorticoid therapy in patients treated as early as possible after systemic sepsis is recognized, a multicenter, randomized, double-blind, placebo-controlled trial of early short-term, high-dose methylprednisolone sodium succinate was conducted.

The 223 patients studied had clinical signs of systemic sepsis and normal sensoriums. One hundred twelve received glucocorticoid, and 111 received placebo. Antibiotics and intravenous fluids were also administered. Glucocorticoid or placebo was given intravenously by a bolus in a dose of 30 mg/kg body weight over 15 minutes. This was followed by infusion of 5 mg/kg/hour for 9 hours. The average time between diagnosis of sepsis and the initiation of infusion was 2.8 hours.

The 14-day mortality was not significantly different between the two groups: 21.6% in the placebo group and 20.5% in the glucocorticoid group. Mortality was also not significantly different between those receiving placebo and those receiving glucocorticoid in subgroups with evidence of sepsis, gram-negative bacteremia, gram-positive bacteremia, or all gram-negative infections. Resolution of secondary infection in 14 days was significantly higher in patients taking placebo than in those taking glucocorticoid: 12 of 23 patients and 3 of 16 patients, respectively. However, mortality was similar in both treatment groups for those with unresolved infection.

It is concluded that early high-dose glucocorticoid therapy does not reduce mortality significantly among patients with systemic sepsis and normal sensoriums. Therefore, it should not be used as adjunctive therapy.

▶ Whether or not to use adrenal corticosteroids for sepsis and septic shock has been a subject of controversy for more than 25 years. Animal experiments demonstrated efficacy, but most human studies did not (with one notable exception; see *Ann Surg* 184:333, 1976). These two well-controlled and carefully performed studies (Abstracts 1–1 and 1–2) should end the controversy and put an end to the use of these agents in sepsis and septic shock.—S.M. Wolff, M.D.

Native Valve Endocarditis due to Coagulase-Negative Staphylococci: Clinical and Microbiologic Features
Caputo GM, Archer GL, Calderwood SB, DiNubile MJ, Karchmer AW (New England Deaconess Hosp, Boston; Massachusetts Gen Hosp, Boston; Harvard Med School; Med College of Virginia Hosp, Virginia Commonwealth Univ)
Am J Med 83:619–625, October 1987   1–3

Coagulase-negative staphylococci, while the most frequent isolate from patients with prosthetic valve endocarditis, rarely cause native valve endocarditis. Of 21 patients with this disease, 14 had preexisting valvular or congenital heart disease. The 17 men and 4 women had a mean age of 53 years. Only 2 patients acquired endocarditis while hospitalized.

The clinical features were similar to those of infective endocarditis caused by other bacteria: fever and weight loss were the most frequent symptoms. Eight patients had symptoms of congestive heart failure. Laboratory changes also resembled those of subacute endocarditis due to other organisms. Two thirds of the patients had at least one of the following: systemic embolization, congestive heart failure, or new conduction system abnormalities. Appropriate antibiotic therapy led to a cure in 81% of patients. The organisms were highly susceptible to rifampin, gentamicin, vancomycin, and teicoplanin. Seven of 9 patients undergoing valve replacement during active endocarditis were cured, as were 10 of 12 medically treated patients.

Some patients with native valve endocarditis due to coagulase-negative staphylococcus have destructive infection leading to major complications. Combination treatment may be more effective than single-drug therapy. Because of aminoglycoside toxicity, however, combination therapy might best be reserved for infection due to more resistant organisms or patients who respond suboptimally to single-drug therapy.

▶ The authors emphasize that the rate of methicillin resistance among coagulase-negative staphylococci in this group of patients with native valve endocarditis is much lower than would be expected in patients with prosthetic valve endocarditis in whom the infection would generally be nosocomially acquired. The distribution of species of coagulase-negative staphylococci also differs between native and prosthetic valve endocarditis. Thus, only 8 of 16 strains causing native valve endocarditis in this study were identified as *Staphylococcus epidermidis,* whereas in a previous study of prosthetic valve endocarditis, 53 of 55 coagulase-negative staphylococcal infections were caused by *S. epidermidis.* This difference may help to explain why treatment with a beta-lactam antibiotic produced a better result in this group of patients than in patients with prosthetic valve endocarditis; of course, the presence of the foreign body in the latter group no doubt contributes to the poor outcome. The authors remind us that routine susceptibility tests of coagulase-negative staphylococci may overestimate susceptibility to beta-lactam antibiotics, especially cephalosporins.—M.J. Barza, M.D.

Prophylaxis of Dental Bacteremia With Oral Amoxicillin in Children
Roberts GJ, Radford P, Holt R (Guy's Hosp, London; Queen Mary's Hosp for Children, Carshalton, England)
Br Dent J 162:179–182, March 7, 1987   1–4

Bacteremia following dental treatment may be hazardous for patients with heart disease. The efficacy of amoxicillin in preventing dental bacteremia was studied in patients younger than 16 years who required extensive conservative work and the removal of at least one tooth. Study patients received 50 mg/kg amoxicillin along with diazepam 2 hours before operation. Forty-seven of 94 patients took oral amoxicillin.

All five positive cultures obtained 2 minutes after nasal intubation were in control patients or refusers (Table 1). The organisms were typical of those colonizing the upper respiratory tract (Table 2). All but 3 of 21

TABLE 1.—Detected Bacteremia

Group	Number	Positive blood culture Pre-intubation	Post-intubation	Post-extraction
Control	47	0	3*	18‡
Oral amoxycillin	47	0	–†	1§
Refusers	6	0	2	2
Cardiac patients				
Oral amoxycillin	6	0	–	–
IV amoxycillin	2	0	–	–

*vs. † $\chi^2 = .26 < P\ .30$.; ‡ vs. § $\chi^2 = 38.38 < P\ .001$.
(Courtesy of Roberts GJ, Radford P, Holt R: Br Dent J 162:179–182, March 7, 1987.)

TABLE 2.—Microorganisms Isolated From Blood Samples

	Number of positive cultures	Antibiotic sensitivity Ampicillin/amoxycillin	Erythromycin	Cephradine
Post-intubation				
Control group				
Bacteroides sp.	10	S	S	S
Staphylococcus albus	220	R	S	R
Anaerobic streptococci	10	S	PR	PR
Refuser group				
Staphylococcus albus	100	R	S	S
Anaerobic streptococci	10	S	S	S
Post-extraction				
Control group				
viridans streptococci	3	S	S	S
Staphylococcus albus	5	S	S	S
Bacteroides sp.	10	S	S	S
viridans streptococci	60	S	S	S
Non-haemolytic streptococci	150	S	S	S
viridans streptococci	10	S	S	S
Neisseria pharyngis	24	S	S	S
viridans streptococci	140	S	S	S
viridans streptococci	200	S	S	S
viridans streptococci	450	S	S	S
Staphylococcus albus	500	R	S	R
viridans streptococci	45	S	S	S
Anaerobic streptococci	10	S	PR	S
Anaerobic streptococci	10	S	PR	R
Anaerobic streptococci	10	S	R	S
viridans streptococci	140	S	S	S
Anaerobic streptococci	10	S	S	S
Non-haemolytic streptococci	500	S	S	S
Amoxycillin group				
Veillonella sp.	300	R	PR	PR
Refuser group				
Anaerobic streptococci	600	S	S	S
Staphylococcus albus	50	R	S	S

Note: S, sensitive; PR, partially resistant; R, resistant.
(Courtesy of Roberts GJ, Radford P, Holt R: Br Dent J 162:179–182, March 7, 1987.)

positive postextraction blood samples were from control patients, and 2 others were from refusers. Only 1 positive postextraction sample was from an amoxicillin-treated patient.

Oral amoxicillin is an active prophylactic agent against odontogenic bacteremia. An oral dose of 50 mg/kg is safe when given 2 hours before general anesthesia.

▶ The results of this study are neither earthshaking nor surprising. They simply lend credence to the use of oral amoxicillin prophylaxis for children with cardiac diseases who are about to have dental work under general anesthesia.—G.T. Keusch, M.D.

Shigella **Bacteremia in Adults: A Report of Five Cases and Review of the Literature**
Morduchowicz G, Huminer D, Siegman-Igra Y, Drucker M, Block CS, Pitlik SD (Tel Aviv Univ, Israel)
Arch Intern Med 147:2034–2037, November 1987   1–5

Shigella bacteremia has been described in neonates and children but occurs infrequently in adults. The authors encountered 5 adults with shigellemia seen at 2 centers in a 4-year period. These patients and the 22 previously reported were reviewed.

Most of the adults with shigellemia were women, and they usually were elderly. Three patients presented from nursing homes in a malnourished state. Diarrhea, fever, and signs of dehydration were noted. The diarrhea usually was mucoid, bloody, or greenish. Two patients were apathetic or confused, and 1 was hypotensive. Hypokalemia and hyponatremia were noted in 3 cases each, and hypoalbuminemia, in 2. All isolates were sensitive to chloramphenicol in vitro. Patients received antibiotics intravenously and hydration parenterally, but nevertheless, 2 died.

Shigella flexneri was responsible for 11 infections, and *S. sonnei*, for 9. Only 1 adult was infected by *S. dysenteriae*, in contrast to the frequent isolation of this organism in children. It is possible that *Shigella* bacteremia is underdiagnosed because of failure to obtain blood cultures, inhibition of circulating organisms by humoral factors or leukocytes, or previous antibiotic treatment. Shigellemia carries a high mortality, suggesting that blood cultures be obtained in febrile adults with diarrhea, especially older and immunocompromised patients.

▶ Shigellemia is not rare, just uncommon, in part because early blood cultures are not usually done. Complement resistant *S. dysenteriae* 1 or *S. flexneri* strains predominate. *Shigella sonnei,* the most common isolate in the United States, is generally serum sensitive, hence less frequently found in the blood. Bacteremia with *flexneri* and *dysenteriae* 1 strains is predictive of risk of mortality in Bangladeshi patients, reflecting their young age (< 1 year of age), severity of underlying malnutrition, and extent of mucosal damage due to the infection.—G.T. Keusch, M.D.

Respiratory Tract

Community-Acquired Pneumonia in Adults in British Hospitals in 1982–1983: A Survey of Aetiology, Mortality, Prognostic Factors and Outcome
Harrison BDW, Farr BM, Pugh S, Selkon JB, Prescott RJ, Connolly CK (Research Committee of the British Thoracic Society and the Public Health Lab Service)
Q J Med 62:195–220, March 1987

Community-acquired pneumonia remains a significant health problem. A prospective study of community-acquired pneumonia was undertaken in 453 British adults to determine prognostic factors, ascertain long-term outcome, and evaluate diagnostic tools.

Microbiologic diagnosis was established in 67% of the cases. *Streptococcus pneumoniae* was identified in 34%, *Mycoplasma pneumoniae* comprised 18%, and influenza A virus comprised 7% of the cases. In the group in which no organism was identified, evidence supported the diagnosis of *S. pneumoniae*. The most useful initial tests were cultures of blood and sputum, tests for sputum pneumococcal antigen and serum mycoplasma specific immunoglobulin IgM.

Of the 453 patients, 26 died. Age, absence of chest pain, absence of vomiting, digoxin therapy, tachypnea, diastolic hypotension, confusion, leukopenia, leukocytosis, and elevated levels of urea in the blood were significantly correlated with death by multivariate analysis. Patients with 2 of the following 3 characteristics had a 21-fold increased risk of death: admission respiratory rate greater than or equal to 30 per minute, admission diastolic blood pressure less than 60 mm Hg, and admission blood urea greater than 7 mmole/L. Mortality was not related to etiology, except in cases of combined *Staphylococcus aureus* and influenza A infection.

Assisted ventilation was used in 22 patients. Of these patients, 14 survived. The hospital stay averaged 10.8 days for survivors. After 6 weeks, 79% were able to return to normal activities and 55% demonstrated resolution of pneumonia signs by radiography.

It is recommended that antibiotic therapy begin rapidly and cover *S. pneumoniae*. Oxygen therapy should be used to maintain a PaO_2 greater than 60 mm Hg. Poor prognosis is indicated by age greater than 60 years, high respiratory rate, low diastolic blood pressure, elevated levels of urea in the blood, low arterial oxygen tension, very high or very low white blood cell count, or low serum albumin. Sputum and blood culture, Gram's stain of sputum, sputum and urine examination for pneumococcal antigen, and serum analysis for mycoplasma-specific IgM are valuable in the diagnosis of patients with pneumonia. Intensive care may be needed for several weeks, but by 6 weeks following admission, 79% of these patients are fit for normal activity.

Adult Supraglottitis: A Prospective Analysis
Shapiro J, Eavey RD, Sullivan Baker A (Massachusetts Eye and Ear Infirmary, Boston; Massachusetts Gen Hosp, Boston; Harvard Med School)
JAMA 259:563–567, Jan 22–29, 1988

In children, epiglottitis is an infection caused by *Hemophilus influenzae* type b that can quickly lead to sepsis and asphyxial death. The course is similar for many adults; however, only a minority of adult cases of epiglottitis appear to be caused by *H. influenzae*. The authors undertook a prospective study to evaluate epiglottitis in adults.

Eight adults with supraglottitis underwent full ear, nose, and throat examination. Bacterial cultures taken from the nasopharynx, oropharynx, vallecula, and blood were obtained from all patients, and from the preepiglottic space in 2 patients. Each patient also underwent a daily laryngeal examination.

Multiple sites in the larynx and oropharynx were inflamed, but the epiglottis was often not the most involved area and was normal in one patient. *Hemophilus influenzae* was not found in any patient, nor did any patient suffer respiratory compromise.

The findings would indicate that *epiglottitis* is an erroneous term for this disorder. The non-*H. influenzae* adult type of supraglottitis appears to follow a less pernicious course than the classic infection. Further investigation for a possible viral cause in adult supraglottitis seems appropriate.

▶ The central point of this study is that what in the adult may appear to be simple epiglottitis often, in fact, involves supraglottic structures more than the epiglottis. In contrast to epiglottitis, this infection is not usually caused by *H. influenzae* and generally has a more benign course than epiglottitis in children. Indeed, a bacterial cause could not be shown for the infections in this study, and the authors suggest that the infection may be viral. Nevertheless, they recommend that, pending the results of blood and nasopharyngeal cultures, empiric antibiotic treatment should be given, for example, a combination of ampicillin and chloramphenicol or a broad-spectrum cephalosporin.—M.J. Barza, M.D.

Colistin Inhalation Therapy in Cystic Fibrosis Patients With Chronic *Pseudomonas aeruginosa* Lung Infection
Jensen T, Pedersen SS, Garne S, Heilmann C, Høiby N, Koch C (Rigshospitalet, Statens Seruminstitut, Copenhagen)
J Antimicrob Chemother 19:831–838, June 1987

It is common for cystic fibrosis patients to develop chronic lower airway infections with *Pseudomonas aeruginosa*. These infections are considered to be the most important factor in determining their prognoses. Colistin has good activity against *P. aeruginosa*. A placebo-controlled trial of colistin inhalation was conducted with 40 cystic fibrosis patients who had chronic bronchopulmonary *P. aeruginosa* infection, which had a mean duration of 6.7 years.

Colistin treatment consisted of inhalation of 1 million units of colistin twice daily for 3 months. Significantly more patients in the colistin group completed the study than in the placebo group. The colistin group had significantly better clinical symptom scores, maintenance of pulmonary function, and inflammatory parameters. Resistance to colistin did not develop in any patient.

Colistin inhalation was safe and effective against *P. aeruginosa* infections in cystic fibrosis patients. Therefore, colistin inhalation therapy is recommended as a supplement to intravenously given antipseudomonas therapy for cystic fibrosis patients with chronic *P. aeruginosa* infections.

▶ The authors carefully hedge their advice by recommending colistin inhalation therapy as a supplement to intravenous antipseudomonal therapy only for patients with cystic fibrosis who have chronic *Pseudomonas aeruginosa* lung infection and deteriorating pulmonary function. I would underline their advice to monitor the flora of the sputum in patients receiving colistin because *Pseudomonas cepacia,* which commonly causes infection in these patients, is resistant to colistin.—M.J. Barza, M.D.

***Bordetella pertussis* Infection: A Cause of Persistent Cough in Adults**
Robertson PW, Goldberg H, Jarvie BH, Smith DD, Whybin LR (The Prince of Wales Hosp, Randwick, Australia)
Med J Aust 146:522–525, May 18, 1987

In this study, a sensitive and specific enzyme-linked immunosorbent assay (ELISA) test was used to determine titers of *Bordetella pertussis* specific immunoglobulin IgA in 13 patients with confirmed whooping cough and in an age-matched control group. The assay was then used to determine the incidence of elevated specific-IgA levels in 218 adult patients who presented with persistent cough of greater than 1 month's duration.

All 13 patients with whooping cough had elevated levels of *B. pertussis*-IgA (table). Of the 218 patients with persistent cough, 25.7% had elevated levels of IgA to *B. pertussis,* suggesting recent infection.

This confirms that the *B. pertussis*-IgA ELISA is a sensitive diagnostic test for *B. pertussis* infections. Infection with *B. pertussis* may be a common cause of persistent cough in adults and should be considered in the diagnosis of persistent cough among adult patients.

▶ This is a provocative study. However, I am disturbed by the titer of *B. pertussis* specific antibody in patients with persistent cough revealing a progressive decline in the number of patients with increasingly higher titers, rather than showing a bimodal distribution as I would have expected if only a small proportion of adults had active infection. Notwithstanding the author's statement regarding the specificity of this assay, one wonders whether this is not a

Bordetella pertussis-specific IgA Enzyme-Linked Immunosorbent Assay Levels Expressed as Optical Densities

	Optical density										
	<0.1	0.1	0.2	0.3	0.4	0.5	0.6	0.7	0.8	0.9	≥1.0
Number of patients											
Patients with whooping cough (n = 13)	—	—	—	—	3	2	2	1	3	—	2
Healthy age-matched control subjects (n = 13)	4	6	1	2	—	—	—	—	—	—	—
Blood donors (n = 234)	108	89	26	8	1	1	—	1	—	—	—
Patients with persistent cough (n = 218)	64	50	28	25	16	5	9	6	3	7	5

(Courtesy of Robertson PW, Goldberg H, Jarvie BH, et al: *Med J Aust* 146:522–525, May 18, 1987.)

manifestation of cross-reactive antibody to other gram-negative microorganisms that might be present in the respiratory tract or elsewhere.—M.J. Barza, M.D.

Lung Bullae With Air-Fluid Levels
Peters JI, Kubitschek KR, Gotlieb MS, Awe RJ (Univ of Texas Health Sciences Center at San Antonio; Baylor College of Medicine, Houston)
Am J Med 82:759–763, April 1987

Fluid accumulation in a preexisting emphysematous bulla may be incorrectly interpreted as a lung abscess. The findings for 14 patients with bullous disease and 1 or more air-fluid levels were reviewed. Patients with a history of tuberculosis or active tuberculous disease were excluded. The 13 men and 1 woman had a mean age of 47 years. All patients had smoked, and chest x-rays had demonstrated bullous emphysema involving the upper lobes in all cases but 1. Three patients had aspirated, and 5 others had risk factors for aspiration.

Twelve patients were symptomatic at presentation, usually with cough and pleuritic pain. Few physical findings related to the acute pulmonary process were apparent. Sputum cultures yielded no pathogens, and blood cultures in 5 patients were negative. Five patients had pulmonary infiltration associated with the bullae containing fluid. Fiberoptic bronchoscopy was noncontributory. Symptoms resolved, and radiographic clearing occurred in about 12 weeks on average, independently of which antibiotic was given.

This benign disorder is clearly distinct from bacterial lung abscess. Fluid likely accumulates within a bulla because of pneumonitis from adjacent air spaces or secondary to a local inflammatory response within the bulla. Invasive procedures generally should be avoided, for a benign course can be expected with oral antibiotic therapy. One of the patients improved without treatment, but patients with symptoms of acute inflammatory disease probably benefit from antibiotic administration.

▶ This paper clearly documents that prolonged oral penicillin or tetracycline is more than adequate therapy for patients who have bullous emphysema and develop air fluid levels in a preexisting bullous lesion. The problem, however, is separating patients with infected bullae from those who have bacterial lung abscesses. The authors offer several points that are useful in making this distinction. For patients with infected bullae, these include a chest x-ray that demonstrates preexisting bullous disease, a sharp inner margin of the wall of the cavity, minimal involvement of the lung immediately surrounding the cavity, fairly rapid changes in the quantity of intrabullous fluid by chest x-ray without expectoration of putrid sputum, and clinically mild illness in most patients. Other helpful criteria are a relatively lower peak temperature, a duration of fever usually less than 2 days compared to 7 days in patients with a bacterial lung abscess, a lower peripheral leukocyte count with a mean of less than 10,000, and the complete absence of putrid sputum.

In one large series of lung abscesses, 62% of the patients with bacterial lung abscesses had putrid sputum (Bartlett JG, Feingold SM: Am Rev Respir Dis 110:56-75, 1974), and in this series, no patients had foul-smelling sputum. If the overall clinical picture is consistent with an infected bullous lesion, then one should anticipate a benign course simply treated with oral antibiotics over a prolonged period. The authors also comment on whether bronchoscopy should be performed. Since many of these patients with bullous disease have an extensive smoking history and despite the fact that bronchoscopy did not alter the diagnosis or therapy in the patients in this study, this procedure may still be necessary for selected patients to exclude an endobronchial lesion.—M.S. Klempner, M.D.

Gastrointestinal Tract

Protection by Milk Immunoglobulin Concentrate Against Oral Challenge With Enterotoxigenic *Escherichia coli*
Tacket CO, Losonsky G, Link H, Hoang Y, Guesry P, Hilpert H, Levine MM (Univ of Maryland School of Medicine; Nestle Research Ctr, Lausanne, Switzerland)
N Engl J Med 318:1240-1243, May 12, 1988

Because diarrhea is so frequent among travelers to less developed countries, any prophylactic agent should have few or no side effects. Use of a bovine milk immunoglobulin (Ig) has been proposed, since human breast milk containing secretory Ig protects infants against diarrhea. A double-blind, controlled trial evaluated bovine milk Ig having specific activity against enterotoxigenic *Escherichia coli*. Volunteer subjects were challenged orally with *E. coli* strain H10407. Ten of 20 healthy adults received Ig against *E. coli*, while 10 received Ig concentrate against rotavirus.

No subject given Ig against *E. coli* had diarrhea after bacterial challenge, but 9 of the 10 control subjects did. There were no side effects from the immunoglobulin concentrate, but several subjects had a transient moderate rise in serum hepatic transaminase levels. The rate of seroconversion and the peak geometric mean titer of anti-078 were higher in control subjects. Rates of seroconversion against heat-labile enterotoxin were the same in the study subjects and the controls.

These encouraging results justify further studies exploring the spectrum of activity of milk immunoglobulin concentrate and the proper dose when used to prevent traveler's diarrhea from enterotoxigenic *E. coli*. This preparation provides passive immunity and allows the development of some active immunity after infection with enterotoxigenic *E. coli*.

▶ If you don't like Pepto-Bismol, it may be possible in the future to chug a bovine Ig preparation for passive immunity to traveler's diarrhea. This paper is an early study in the course of developing such preventive modalities and demonstrates a high degree of efficacy under controlled conditions. The Ig was obtained by immunization of cows with a number of enterotoxic *E. coli* (ETEC) serotypes, and it resulted in antibody to the somatic O antigens, to LT toxin, and to CFA-I and CS-3 colonization factors. The deck was stacked in favor of the Ig preparation, which was given 3 times a day for 7 days, by challenging 2 hours after dose number 7. Protection was complete, and this bodes well for a high degree of efficacy with a more "real-life" test.

The conundrum will be for the developing world, where frequent diarrhea is a critical factor in pathogenesis of malnutrition (see Keusch and Scrimshaw: *Rev Infect Dis* 8:273–287, 1986). The infants of the poor, who need such protection, can neither afford nor safeguard infant formula, which is a likely vehicle for protective Ig's. If this approach is to be more than just an alternative to Pepto-Bismol for the more affluent, it will be necessary for some appropriate technology to be developed for the third world that is both affordable and feasible. Still, the approach is worth pursuing for ETEC and for other infectious enteritis disease agents in order to establish its utility (see, for example, Brussow H et al: *Bovine milk immunoglobulins for passive immunity to infantile rotavirus gastroenteritis. J Clin Microbiol* 25:982–986, 1987). Then we can figure out how to make use of the stuff.—G.T. Keusch, M.D.

A Severe Outbreak of *Escherichia coli* O157:H7: Associated Hemorrhagic Colitis in a Nursing Home

Carter AO, Borczyk AA, Carlson JAK, Harvey B, Hockin JC, Karmali MA, Krishnan C, Korn DA, Lior H (Dept of Natl Health and Welfare, Ottawa; Ontario Ministry of Health, Toronto; Univ of Toronto; Hosp for Sick Children, Toronto; Univ Hosp, London, Ont; et al)
N Engl J Med 317:1496–1500, Dec 10, 1987

The verotoxin-producing *Escherichia coli*, including the serotype O157:H7, has been linked to two syndromes: hemorrhagic colitis and hemolytic uremic syndrome. The clinical and epidemiologic features of a large outbreak of verotoxin-producing *E. coli* O157:H7 infection in a nursing home in southwestern Ontario are presented. This outbreak was unusual because of an extremely high level of morbidity, including hemolytic uremic syndrome, and mortality among elderly residents and a very high attack rate among the staff.

In September 1985, an outbreak of *E. coli* O157:H7 enteritis affected 55 of 169 residents (mean age, 83.5 ± 10.8 years) and 18 of 137 staff members at a nursing home. The epidemic curve was biphasic, with a primary wave suggesting a common-source outbreak, probably a contaminated sandwich meal, and a secondary wave compatible with person-to-person transmission of infection. The incubation period for the elderly residents ranged from 4 to 9 days (mean, 5.7 ± 1.2), and that of the staff ranged from 3 to 8 days (mean, 5.0 ± 1.7). Most of the affected residents had watery diarrhea initially, with stools becoming grossly bloody at a mean 0.6 days (range 0 to 5) later. Fever was not prominent.

Older age and previous gastrectomy increased the risk of infection, while antibiotic therapy during exposure was associated with acquiring a secondary infection. Hemolytic uremic syndrome, as evidenced by thrombocytopenia, microangiopathic hemolytic anemia, and acute renal failure, occurred in 12 residents (22%), 11 of whom died. Overall, 19 (35%) of the affected residents died, 17 (31%) from causes attributable to their infection. There were no complications or deaths among the affected staff members. All isolates belonged to phage type 2.

This outbreak of verotoxin-producing *E. coli* O157:H7 infection is unusual because of the extremely high level of morbidity, including hemolytic uremic syndrome (HUS), and mortality in elderly residents and a very high attack rate in the staff. These emphasize the need for proper food hygiene, rapid identification of outbreaks, and prompt institution of infection-control techniques among the institutionalized elderly.

▶ This is a clear-cut paper describing severe disease due to *E. coli* O157:H7, with high morbidity, frequent complication by HUS, and high mortality in the elderly. Having said this I would like to discuss nomenclature a bit. The Canadians and the British call the *E. coli* shigella-like cytotoxin "verotoxin" whereas in this country it is generally called "Shiga-like toxin," because of its similarity to the toxin produced by Shiga's bacillus, *Shigella dysenteriae* I. Verotoxin, so called because it was first described as an *E. coli* toxin lethal to Vero cells, is a misnomer. It is neither made by Vero cells nor is it specific for Vero cells. Shiga-like toxin I (neutralized by anti-Shiga toxin) is probably identical to Shiga toxin and should be called Shiga toxin because of the historical precedence of the name. Shiga-like toxin-2 (not neutralized by anti-Shiga toxin) is acceptable at present and is generally designated *SLT-2*. This term is preferable to *Verotoxin type-2* (VT-2) for the reasons noted already. However, as a good friend and famous toxinologist has stated publicly, it should probably be called Shiga-toxin-like-toxin-2, though I can see that *STLT-2* would be easily confused with *ST/LT* (heat-stable and heat labile) enterotoxin-producing *E. coli*.

Recently, a group in Britain may have solved the problem when they put in print (Wallis et al: *J Med Microbiol* 21:19–23, 1986) what a number of us have only dared to think or at best show in slides. Shiga-toxin was designated ShiT, in order to distinguish it from ST, the *E. coli* heat stable toxin. I suppose the non-cross-reactive toxin could then be called ShiT-LT. Whatever they are called, these toxins are highly active inhibitors of protein synthesis, although their role in disease pathogenesis remains unproven.— G.T. Keusch, M.D.

Massive Outbreak of Antimicrobial-Resistant Salmonellosis Traced to Pasteurized Milk
Ryan CA, Nickels MK, Hargrett-Bean NT, Potter ME, Endo T, Mayer L, Langkop CW, Gibson C, McDonald RC, Kenney RT, Puhr ND, McDonnell PJ, Martin RJ, Cohen ML, Blake PA (Ctrs for Disease Control, Atlanta; Illinois Dept of Public Health, Springfield)
JAMA 258:3269–3274, Dec 11, 1987

State and federal health agencies began an investigation in March 1985 of 2 waves of antimicrobial-resistant *Salmonella typhimurium* infections in Illinois. A report was compiled to present the epidemiologic and labo-

Relationship Between Use of Antimicrobials in Month Before Illness and Average Daily Consumption of Implicated Brands of Milk*

	Took No Antibiotics		Took "Resistant"† Antibiotics		
	Cups	No.	Cups	No.	P‡
Ill	3.6	38	2.4	16	.010
Well	1.9	76	1.6	5	.184
P‡	.000039		.034		...

*By case and case family members (case-control study 3). No. indicates number of persons in the cell.
†Resistant antibiotics are antibiotics to which the outbreak strain of *Salmonella typhimurium* was resistant.
‡By *t* test for clustered samples.
(Courtesy of Ryan CA, Nickels MK, Hargrett-Bean NT, et al: *JAMA* 258:3269–3274, Dec 11, 1987.)

ratory studies used, to examine the risk factors associated with symptomatic infection, and to describe the emergence of this unusual epidemic strain.

The 2 waves of infection totaled more than 16,000 culture-confirmed cases. Two surveys conducted to determine the number of people actually affected by these outbreaks yielded estimates of 168,791 and 197,581 persons, making this the largest outbreak of salmonellosis ever identified in the United States. The infections were traced to 2 brands of pasteurized 2% milk produced by a single dairy plant in northern Illinois. Salmonellosis was associated with the taking of antimicrobials before the onset of illness; the usual number of cups of milk drunk was less for ill persons who had taken antimicrobials in the month before illness than for ill persons who had not taken antimicrobials (table).

The epidemic strain was easily identified because it had a rare antimicrobial resistance pattern and a very unusual plasmid profile. Examination of stored isolates showed that it had caused clusters of salmonellosis during the previous 10 months that might have been related to the same plant, suggesting that the strain had persisted in the plant and repeatedly contaminated milk after pasteurization.

A massive outbreak of antimicrobial-resistant *Salmonella typhimurium* infections totaling more than 16,000 culture-confirmed cases were traced to two brands of pasteurized milk produced in a dairy plant in northern Illinois. Infection was associated with consumption of antimicrobials before the onset of illness.

▶ At last a human study to confirm the results in mice from 25 years ago that antibiotic administration increases the risk of intestinal salmonellosis. Two-percent milk was the vehicle, and in spite of pasteurization, repeated contamination of the product occurred. Although the point in processing where the contamination occurred was not identified, the plant in question pasteurized the milk early on, before separation, blending of skim and whole milk to make

2% milk, and packaging, leaving a number of places where this could happen.— G.T. Keusch, M.D.

Campylobacter pylori Detected Noninvasively by the ^{13}C-Urea Breath Test
Graham DY, Klein PD, Evans DJ Jr, Evans DG, Alpert LC, Opekun AR, Boutton TW (VA Med Ctr, USDA/ARS Children's Nutrition Research Ctr, Baylor College of Medicine, Houston)
Lancet 1:1174–1177, May 23, 1987

Although *Campylobacter pylori* colonization of the stomach has been linked to the development of gastric ulcers, nonulcer dyspepsia, and gastritis, the role of *C. pylori* in these disorders remains unclear. Because *C. pylori* has high endogenous urease activity, a simple, noninvasive breath test was developed to identify *C. pylori* infection; the test is based on the use of ^{13}C-labeled urea.

The study population comprised 54 volunteers (30 men) aged 20–57 years and 11 male ulcer patients aged 34–64 years. Six volunteers had dyspepsia. Both groups were given a nutrient-dense test meal to delay gastric emptying, followed by an oral solution containing ^{13}C-labeled urea. Breath samples, obtained every 10 minutes for 180 minutes, were analyzed for excess $^{13}CO_2$ by mass spectrometry. The test was validated in 26 individuals who underwent endoscopic biopsy of the antral mucosa for culture and histologic examination.

Individuals with *C. pylori* infection had excess $^{13}CO_2$ within 20 minutes; this continued at a constant rate for more than 100 minutes, whereas normal individuals had little or no change in respiratory $^{13}CO_2$ until after 120 minutes, when urea reached the colon and was hydrolyzed by colonic bacteria (Fig 1–1). The reproducibility of the urea breath test

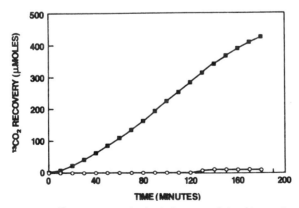

Fig 1–1.—Recovery of $^{13}CO_2$ in a normal individual *(open circles)* and in a patient with a positive culture for *C. pyloris* in a gastric specimen *(solid squares)* after administration of a test meal followed by ^{13}C-urea, 5 mg/kg. (Courtesy of Graham DY, Klein PD, Evans DJ Jr, et al: *Lancet* 1:1174–1177, May 23, 1987.)

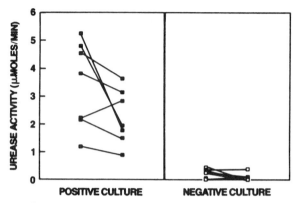

Fig 1–2.—Reproducibility of urea breath test in 7 individuals with positive breath tests *(solid squares)* and in 7 with negative breath tests *(open squares)*. (Courtesy of Graham DY, Klein PD, Evans DJ Jr, et al: *Lancet* 1:1174–1177, May 23, 1987.)

was verified in 11 persons with and without *C. pylori* colonization (Fig 1–2). The density of *C. pylori* colonies in culture specimens and in antral biopsy specimens was directly related to the findings of the urea breath test (Fig 1–3). This is a simple, noninvasive, reproducible test to establish the presence of *C. pylori* infection of the stomach.

▶ This is a nice clinical adaptation of a microbial property useful for identification of the bug in the lab. Unfortunately, I would hardly call a ^{13}C breath test "simple," as mass spec is not your everyday house-officer lab procedure (not even in the clinical pathology lab). Can we send samples to the USDA Center at Baylor?—G.T. Keusch, M.D.

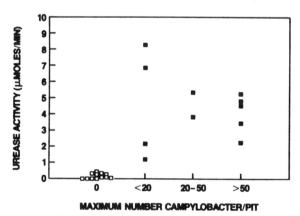

Fig 1–3.—Relationship between urease activity as determined by the urea breath test and the numbers of *C. pylori* found per gastric pit by histologic examination of gastric antral biopsy specimens. (Courtesy of Graham DY, Klein PD, Evans DJ Jr, et al: *Lancet* 1:1174–1177, May 23, 1987.)

Prospective Study of Enteric *Campylobacter* Infections in Children From Birth to 6 Months in the Central African Republic
Georges-Courbot MC, Beraud-Cassel AM, Gouandjika I, Georges AJ (Institut Pasteur, Bangui, Central African Republic)
J Clin Microbiol 25:836–839, May 1987
1–15

The role of *Campylobacter* species in the etiology of diarrhea is not well understood. *Campylobacter* infections were surveyed twice weekly in stools from 127 children from birth to 6 months of age in Bangui, Central African Republic.

During this period, 82 such infections were detected. However, only 15.9% of the infected children had diarrhea. In eight of the 13 symptomatic infections, another enteropathogen was also detected. Of the 127 children, 53 had at least one *Campylobacter* infection before the age of 6 months. In children younger than 1 month of age, the infection was always asymptomatic. After 1 month of age, isolation of *Campylobacter* was significantly more frequent among those with diarrhea (Table 1). The rate of infection was higher among those who were exclusively breast-fed than among those who also received formula (Table 2).

Campylobacter species are frequently isolated from the stools of infants in the Central African Republic. This infection can occur very early but is asymptomatic in most cases.

▶ This is another study suggesting that enteric *Campylobacter* infection in youngsters in developing countries is generally asymptomatic. Similar data have been obtained in Bangladesh (see Glass et al: *J Infect Dis* 148:292–296, 1983). This suggests a developmentally regulated susceptibility to disease, for example, the possibility that a maturational event in the gut epithelial cell surface is necessary for *Campylobacter* to cause diarrhea.

Data already suggest that developmentally regulated epithelial cell changes may govern the susceptibility of humans to EPEC and Shigella, to name a few examples. The possibility that this is also true for *Campylobacter* is consistent with the epidemiology of the disease in the United States, where it affects primarily young adults. This is presumably because young children in the U.S. are

TABLE 1.—Rate of Isolation of Enteric *Campylobacter* Species From Diarrheic and Control Routinely Cultured Children

Age (mo)	Diarrheic stools		Routinely cultured stools	
	Total no.	No. positive (%)	Total no.	No. positive (%)
0–1	19	0 (0.0)	993	23 (2.3)
2–3*	118	10 (8.5)	1,906	23 (1.2)
3–6*	138	21 (15.2)	2,882	82 (2.8)
Total*	275	31 (11.3)	5,781	128 (2.2)

*Chi-square analysis: $P < .001$.
(Courtesy of Georges-Courbot MC, Beraud-Cassel AM, Gouandjika I, et al: *J Clin Microbiol* 25:836–839, May 1987.)

TABLE 2.—Number of *Campylobacter* Infections According to Type of Feeding

Group	No. of children	No. of infections (%) All	Diarrheic
0–1 mo			
Breast fed	95	10 (10.5)	0 (0.0)
Breast and bottle fed	32	1 (3.1)	0 (0.0)
2–3 mo			
Breast fed	83	12 (14.5)	3 (3.6)
Breast and bottle fed	44	2 (4.5)	1 (2.3)
4–6 mo			
Breast fed	6	6 (100.0)	2 (33.3)
Breast and bottle fed	121	51 (42.1)	7 (5.8)

(Courtesy of Georges-Courbot MC, Beraud-Cassel AM, Gouandjika I, et al: *J Clin Microbiol* 25:836–839, May 1987.)

not exposed early in life when they are naturally protected but are able to develop protective immune responses that prevent later symptomatic disease after reexposure. If this is true, then a live oral vaccine for infants may be the way to go for preventive strategies for this organism.—G.T. Keusch, M.D.

Prevention of Travelers' Diarrhea by the Tablet Formulation of Bismuth Subsalicylate
DuPont HL, Ericsson CD, Johnson PC, Bitsura JAM, DuPont MW, de la Cabada FJ (Univ of Texas Health Science Ctr at Houston; Hosp Gen de Occidente, Guadalajara, Mexico)
JAMA 257:1347–1350, March 13, 1987

Bismuth subsalicylate in tablet form (Pepto-Bismol) was tested as a diarrhea preventive in a group of 182 U.S. students who attended summer classes in Mexico. Within 48 hours of arrival, the students were randomly assigned to receive either 2 tablets (n = 55) or 1 tablet (n = 66) of bismuth subsalicylate, or a placebo (n = 61), taken 4 times daily for 3 weeks. Ten of 182 students did not complete the 21-day study.

Of the remaining 172 students, 7 of 51 (14%) in the high-dose group; 15 of 63 (24%) in the low-dose group; and 23 of 58 (40%) in the placebo group developed diarrhea (Fig 1–4). Diarrhea caused by enterotoxigenic *Escherichia coli* was found in 1 student in the high-dose group, in none in the low-dose group, and in 7 students in the placebo group. Two tablets of bismuth subsalicylate taken four times daily is a safe and effective prevention against travelers' diarrhea.

▶ We have been waiting for this paper ever since the luggage of Mexico-bound American tourists began to clink from the Pepto-Bismol bottles within. Now, DuPont et al. have lightened our load with the convincing demon-

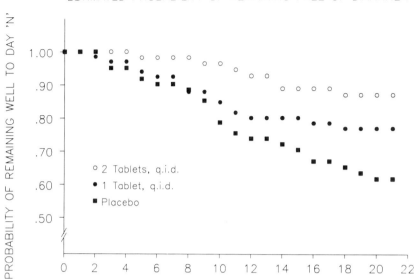

Fig 1–4.—Estimated probability of remaining free of diarrhea throughout 21-day study; *qid*, 4 times daily. Statistical significance of difference between 2 survival patterns was assessed by log-rank method ($P < .05$). (Courtesy of DuPont HL, Ericsson CD, Johnson PC, et al: *JAMA* 257:1347–1350, March 13, 1987.)

stration that tablets of bismuth subsalicylate offer 40% (1 tablet q.i.d.) to 65% (2 tablets q.i.d.) protection from diarrhea, and near complete protection from toxigenic *E. coli*, for at least 3 weeks of exposure. This is a much better recommendation for prophylaxis than are antibiotics, and travelers to Mexico (and elsewhere) ought to be so advised.—G.T. Keusch, M.D.

Isolation of Enterotoxigenic *Bacteroides fragilis* From Humans With Diarrhea

Myers LL, Shoop DS, Stackhouse LL, Newman FS, Flaherty RJ, Letson GW, Sack RB (Montana State Univ; Montana Dept of Livestock, Helena; Med Associates, Bozeman, Mont; Johns Hopkins Univ, Balitmore)
J Clin Microbiol 25:2330–2333, December 1987   1–17

Bacteroides fragilis is a gram-negative, non-spore-forming, anaerobic obligate in the intestinal tract of humans and animals. A recent study indicates that enterotoxigenic *B. fragilis* can also be isolated from diarrheic persons and that human isolates of enterotoxigenic *B. fragilis* are virulent in an adult rabbit model.

Enterotoxigenic *B. fragilis* was isolated from stool specimens of 8 of 44 diarrheic patients, aged 4 months to 69 years. The clinical course was characterized by watery diarrhea—usually 1 to 4 weeks in duration—

and often with mild to moderate intestinal cramping in adults and hyperthermia, vomiting, and blood in the stools of diarrheic infants. No recognized enteric pathogens were detected in 7 of 8 diarrheic patients with enterotoxigenic B. fragilis. The bacterium elaborated a heat-labile enterotoxin in concentrated broth that supported bacterial growth. Enterotoxin activity was also detected in the eluant buffer following gel filtration of broth retentates on Sephadex G-75.

Fifteen adult rabbits with ligated ceca received intraileal injections of 5×10^9 colony-forming units (CFU) of enterotoxigenic B. fragilis. All developed fatal enteric disease characterized by mucoid, often hemorrhagic, diarrhea. In contrast, 8 rabbits given nonenterotoxigenic B. fragilis remained clinically normal. The bacterium colonized the caudal small intestine and the colon and caused moderate to severe necrotizing colitis. As few as 5×10^3 CFU of enterotoxigenic B. fragilis caused fatal enteric disease in the rabbit model.

Enterotoxigenic B. fragilis, which can be isolated from the intestinal tract of diarrheic humans, is enteropathogenic in adult rabbits with ligated ceca. Further studies are warranted to determine the role of enterotoxigenic B. fragilis in the enteric disease complex.

Genitourinary Tract

Prospective Randomized Comparison of Therapy and No Therapy for Asymptomatic Bacteriuria in Institutionalized Elderly Women
Nicolle LE, Mayhew WJ, Bryan L (Univ of Calgary, Alberta)
Am J Med 83:27–33, July 1987

The validity of nontreatment of asymptomatic bacteriuria in the elderly population has been questioned because of reports of increased mortality among bacteriuric (compared with nonbacteriuric) ambulant elderly. A study was conducted in which 50 elderly institutionalized women with asymptomatic bacteriuria were randomly assigned either to receive antimicrobial therapy for all episodes of bacteriuria identified on monthly culture or to receive no therapy unless symptoms developed. The mean age of patients was 83.4 ± 8.8 years. The total follow-up period was 261 patient-months for the no-therapy group and 259 patient-months for the therapy group. Trimethoprim/sulfamethoxazole was used in 75% of all antimicrobial courses.

Despite a significantly lower monthly prevalence of bacteriuria in the therapy group—a mean $31\% \pm 15\%$ lower than that of the no-therapy group—bacteriuria-free periods lasting 6 months or longer were documented for only 5 (24%) patients in the therapy group. Residents in the no-therapy group tended to have persistent infections (71%) with the same organism(s), whereas those in the therapy group more frequently had reinfections (1.67 vs. 0.87 per patient-year). Antimicrobial therapy was associated with significantly more adverse drug reactions (0.51 vs. 0.46 per patient-year) and isolation of increasingly resistant organisms in recurrent infection when compared with no therapy. The genitouri-

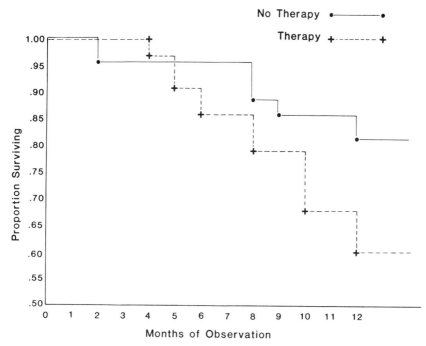

Fig 1–5.—Survival for women with asymptomatic bacteriuria either treated or nontreated. (Courtesy of Nicolle LE, Mayhew WJ, Bryan L: *Am J Med* 83:27–33, July 1987.)

nary morbidity or mortality did not differ significantly between groups (Fig 1–5).

Antimicrobial therapy for asymptomatic bacteriuria in institutionalized elderly women apparently offers no short-term benefits and may even cause some harmful effects. These results support current recommendations of no therapy for asymptomatic bacteriuria in institutionalized elderly women.

▶ Asymptomatic bacteriuria is common among elderly patients, occurring in at least 10% of men and women older than 65 years of age. In one study of elderly institutionalized patients, two thirds of the asymptomatic infections were shown to involve the kidney (Nicolle LE et al: *J Infect Dis* 157:65–70, 1988). Whether or not asymptomatic bacteriuria in the elderly has clinical consequences has remained controversial. As many studies have argued against significant consequences such as hypertension, renal impairment, and reduced life span as have argued for such an effect.

The results of this study of *institutionalized* elderly women showed no benefit of treatment of asymptomatic bacteriuria. The study of Boscia et al. (*JAMA* 257:1067–1071, 1987) by contrast, showed that in elderly, *ambulatory* women with asymptomatic bacteriuria, a short course of treatment resulted in temporary sterilization of the urine and a slight reduction in symptomatic urinary tract infections (UTI) (8% incidence of UTI in treated patients vs. 16% in untreated controls) over a 6-month period of follow-up, a benefit which many would regard as questionable. In summary, there seems to be little benefit from treatment of asymptomatic bacteriuria in elderly institutionalized patients and a questionable one from the treatment of such infections in elderly, ambulatory patients.—M.J.Barza, M.D.

Periurethral Enterobacterial Carriage Preceding Urinary Infection
Brumfitt W, Gargan RA, Hamilton-Miller JMT (Royal Free Hosp and School of Medicine, London)
Lancet 1:824–826, Apr 11, 1987

It is not known whether periurethral carriage of gram-negative bacilli (GNB) is a necessary precursor to bladder bacteriuria. Some investigators believe that bacteriuria is inevitably preceded by carriage of the same strain of GNB, while others conclude that significant bacteriuria is usually preceded by carriage (which may be intermittent) of the same strain. Still other investigators judge that the presence of GNB in the periurethral area is not the principal determining factor in the pathogenesis of recurrent urinary infections. The periurethral flora of women with recurrent urinary infections was analyzed.

The periurethral enterobacterial flora were identified before infective episodes in 56 women with recurrent urinary infections. There were 91 episodes of infection, and colonization by aerobic gram-negative bacilli was noted in 60. Nevertheless, in only 31 (34%) episodes were the colonizing and infecting strains the same; in 31 episodes there was no colonization of the perineum, and in 29 there was heterologous colonization (table). In a second group of 54 women investigated during an enterobacterial infection of the urine, colonization with the infecting organism was noted in 55 (86%) of 64 episodes; in 2 women there was no colonization, and in 7 women (11%) there was heterologous colonization.

It is concluded that women with recurrent urinary infections are un-

Periurethral Carriage of Gram-Negative Bacilli (GNB) Before Infection

No of wk before infection (days)	No of episodes	GNB	Carrier state Homologous	Heterologous	Nil
1 (1–7)	20	90%	9	9	2
2 (8–14)	10	70%	6	1	3
3 (15–21)	13	61·5%	6	2	5
4 (22–28)	12	50%	2	4	6
5–12 (29–84)	36	58%	8	13	15
Total (1–12 wk)	91	66%	31	29	31

(Courtesy of Brumfitt W, Gargan RA, Hamilton-Miller JMT: Lancet 1:824–826, Apr 11, 1987.)

usually susceptible to perineal and periurethral colonization with gram-negative bacteria, for their infections often are not caused by the colonizing enterobacteria.

▶ This study deals with an old controversy regarding the pathogenesis of urinary tract infections (UTI) in women, that is, whether UTI is generally preceded by periurethral colonization by the infecting strain. Given the appealing logic of that hypothesis, it is disquieting that several studies have failed to support it. In fact, the results of this study are not as much in conflict with the hypothesis as it might appear. In patients in whom cultures were taken at the time of the UTI, there was colonization with the homologous strain in 86%. Among patients who were studied prospectively and in whom cultures were taken within 7 days of infection, the cultures showed gram-negative bacilli in the introitus in 90%. In half of these colonized patients, the same strain was found in the urine and in the introitus.—M.J. Barza, M.D.

The Association of Bacteriuria With Resident Characteristics and Survival in Elderly Institutionalized Men
Nicolle LE, Henderson E, Bjornson J, McIntyre M, Harding GKM, MacDonell JA
(Univ of Manitoba; Univ of Calgary, Alberta)
Ann Intern Med 106:682–686, May 1987

Asymptomatic bacteriuria in an elderly population has been associated with lowered survival. It is most prevalent in nursing home residents, in whom bacteriuria increases with the degree of functional impairment. Resident characteristics were examined in relation to bacteriuria in a series of 91 elderly men living in a skilled nursing facility. Organic brain syndrome and cerebrovascular disease predominated. The subjects were generally highly functionally impaired.

One fourth of the residents had continuous bacteriuria, and one third had intermittent bacteriuria. These groups did not differ significantly in age, number of diagnoses, or number of drugs used. Those with bacteriuria were more often confused or demented, however, and more frequently exhibited incontinence of urine or feces. Survival was similar for all groups. One of 5 patients with sepsis had a positive urine culture and no other apparent focus of infection at the time of death. Another, who died with pneumonia, had a urinary tract infection that may have contributed to death.

Bacteriuria was associated with greater functional impairment but not with increased mortality in this population of elderly institutionalized men. There appears to be an association between bacteriuria and mortality, but it is masked by significant associated medical problems in an institutionalized population.

Acute Renal Infection in Women: Treatment With Trimethoprim-Sulfamethoxazole or Ampicillin for Two or Six Weeks: A Randomized Trial

Stamm WE, McKevitt M, Counts GW (Univ of Washington School of Medicine)
Ann Intern Med 106:341–345, March 1987

Although it is generally presumed that acute renal infections require longer courses of antimicrobial therapy than acute cystitis, few controlled trials have been done to confirm this premise. In a randomized trial, the efficacy of regimens lasting 2 or 6 weeks was compared in outpatients with acute uncomplicated renal infections. Ampicillin and trimethoprim-sulfamethoxazole were the drugs used.

The study was done of 98 women (median age 21 years) who were randomly assigned to 4 treatment groups after they had been diagnosed with acute renal infections. The treatment regimens consisted of oral administration of 160–800 mg of trimethoprim-sulfamethoxazole for either 2 or 6 weeks or 500 mg of ampicillin every 6 hours for 2 or 6 weeks.

Of 98 initial participants in the study, 38 were subsequently excluded from the final analysis. The remaining 60 women had renal infections (fever and flank tenderness or a positive test for antibody-coated bacteriuria) with susceptible strains; they complied with the drug regimens, and they completed the required follow-up.

All 60 patients were clinically improved after 7 days of treatment. Twelve of 27 women treated with ampicillin—but only 4 of 33 women

Comparison of Cure Rates in Women Treated For Acute Renal Infection With 2- and 6-Week Regimens of Ampicillin or Trimethoprim-Sulfamethoxazole

Regimen	Patients Cured of Those Treated*	95% Confidence Interval†	p Value
	$n(\%)$		
Two weeks			
Ampicillin	11/17 (65)		
Trimethoprim-sulfamethoxazole	19/21 (90)	−0.01 to 0.51	0.11
Six weeks			
Ampicillin	4/10 (40)		
Trimethoprim-sulfamethoxazole	10/12 (83)	0.06 to 0.80	0.07
Total			
Ampicillin	15/27 (56)		
Trimethoprim-sulfamethoxazole	29/33 (88)	0.10 to 0.54	0.008

*Cure is defined as eradication of the initially infecting strain and absence of recurrent infection in the 6-week follow-up period.
†95% confidence intervals for the difference between cure rates.
(Courtesy of Stamm WE, McKevitt M, Counts GW: Ann Intern Med 106:341–345, March 1987.)

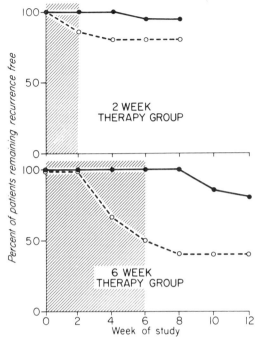

Fig 1-6.—Percentage of patients who remained recurrence-free by week of study. *Shaded areas* indicate period of drug administration. Patients were treated with trimethoprim-sulfamethoxazole *(solid line)* or ampicillin *(broken line)*. (Courtesy of Stamm WE, McKevitt M, Counts GW: Ann Intern Med 106:341–345, March 1987.)

treated with trimethoprim-sulfamethoxazole—experienced recurrences of infection (table). There was no significant difference in recurrence rates between the 2-week and the 6-week regimens. Significantly more repeat infections with drug-resistant strains occurred in the ampicillin-treated groups than in the trimethoprim-sulfamethoxazole-treated groups (Fig 1–6). Side effects occurred significantly more frequently in the 6-week treatment groups than in the 2-week treatment groups.

It is concluded that a 2-week regimen is as effective as a 6-week regimen for the management of outpatients with uncomplicated, acute renal infections and that trimethoprim-sulfamethoxazole is to be preferred over ampicillin.

▶ A well-done study such as this, which helps to address the issue of the optimal duration of treatment of pyelonephritis, will be appreciated by clinicians. The results of this trial show that women with acute pyelonephritis without underlying structural abnormality of the urinary tract, do not gain additional benefit from treatment given for longer than 2 weeks. The superiority of trimethoprim-sulfamethoxazole over ampicillin is not easy to explain given that all eligible patients were required to have infecting organisms susceptible to both agents. The authors suggest that the administration of ampicillin selected for ampicillin-resistant strains in the fecal flora; however, why these resistant strains caused infections so soon after treatment with ampicillin was begun is unclear to me.—M.J. Barza, M.D.

Renal Infection in Autosomal Dominant Polycystic Kidney Disease
Schwab SJ, Bander SJ, Klahr S (Washington Univ School of Medicine, Duke Univ School of Medicine)
Am J Med 82:714–718, April 1987

Patients with autosomal dominant polycystic kidney disease suffer frequent upper urinary tract infections that are difficult to treat. A prospective 3-year trial was conducted to examine the diagnosis and treatment of renal infections in patients with this disorder.

During the study period, 26 upper urinary tract infections—15 cyst and 11 parenchymal infections—occurred in 21 patients. Thirteen of 15 cyst infections (87%), and 10 of 11 parenchymal infections (91%) occurred in women. Gram-negative enteric organisms were isolated in 25 of 26 episodes. Eleven of the 26 infections (mean age, 43.2 years) responded to initial antibiotic therapy. All 11 episodes had been caused by *Escherichia coli*, as confirmed by urinary cultures. All of the parenchymal—but only one of the cyst infections—responded to intravenous (IV) therapy with ampicillin and an aminoglycoside. Fifteen infections did not respond to initial antibiotic therapy, although the isolated organisms had shown sensitivity to antibiotics in vitro.

All 15 refractory renal infections were associated with the development of a new discrete area of palpable tenderness in the involved polycystic kidney, a finding not present in any of the patients who responded to conventional treatment with antibiotics. The refractory infections did respond to treatment with lipid-soluble antibiotics, such as chloramphenicol or trimethoprim/sulfamethoxazole, if the isolated organism was susceptible. Because of the overwhelming female predilection of upper tract renal infections in these patients, it is likely that they arise from retrograde infection from the urinary bladder.

Isolation of Glycine Betaine and Proline Betaine From Human Urine: Assessment of Their Role as Osmoprotective Agents for Bacteria and the Kidney
Chambers ST, Kunin CM (Ohio State Univ)
J Clin Invest 79:731–737, March 1987

Despite the high osmolality and low pH of human urine, it is a good growth medium for enteric bacteria. Human urine is osmoprotective for enteric bacteria. It was shown previously that choline and glycine betaine, present in the urine, are osmoprotective. However, the presence of these compounds is insufficient to explain the effect. Therefore, urine was analyzed in a search for further protective molecules.

The active material in human urine was soluble in methanol and was precipitated by ammonium reineckate at acid pH. Gel filtration and high-pressure liquid chromatography were used to isolate proline betaine. Proline betaine was identified by nuclear magnetic resonance, mass spectrum scanning, and chemical synthesis.

Prior to the isolation and identification of proline betaine, the compound had not been observed in vertebrates. The presence in human urine of the osmoprotective agents, glycine and proline betaine, may reflect an osmoprotective role in the kidney. The protective effect for bacteria may be fortuitous.

Skin, Soft Tissue, Bone, and Joint

Evaluation of Musculoskeletal Sepsis With Indium-111 White Blood Cell Imaging
Ouzounian TJ, Thompson L, Grogan TJ, Webber MM, Amstutz HC (Univ of California, Los Angeles, School of Medicine)
Clin Orthop 221:304–311, August 1987   1–24

The diagnosis of musculoskeletal sepsis is a challenge. This report describes 55 Indium 111 white blood cell (WBC) images performed in 39 patients to evaluate musculoskeletal sepsis.

There were 40 negative and 15 positive Indium 111 WBC images. These were correlated with cultures, pathology, and clinical findings and compared to Tc-99m imaging. Of the 55 scans, 13 were true-positive, 39 were true-negative, two were false-positive, and one was false-negative.

The sensitivity of Indium 111 WBC imaging was 93%, and the specificity was 95%. Indium 111 WBC imaging is useful for the evaluation of musculoskeletal sepsis.

▶ There are excellent theoretical reasons why indium 111 white cell imaging should be a superior method for the detection of localized infection. Of the many soluble agents that have been tried for labeling leukocytes, indium 111 oxine is by far the best agent. With current labeling techniques, 75%–90% of the indium 111 is leukocyte-bound and the labeled leukocytes retain normal function. Moreover, indium 111 WBC uptake in abscesses has been shown to be 35–117 times the peripheral blood uptake compared with 1–8 times for gallium-67 citrate. Unlike gallium, indium 111 labeled leukocytes do not have any affinity for tumors.

Recent experience with indium 111 WBC imaging in evaluating patients with suspected infection after arthroplasty has been encouraging. Like this study, it has shown great sensitivity and specificity for the detection of the genuinely infected joint. The false-positive result in this series was for a patient with rheumatoid arthritis, which is a known cause of positive scans. The false-negative scan was in a patient on chronic antibiotics who had a positive aspiration for pathology but had a negative culture. Previous studies that have used only culture results as criteria for infection may have considered this a true-negative result.

Since technetium and gallium scanning are usually not helpful in suspected sepsis of the postarthroplasty patient, I think this and recent studies make the indium 111 scan the imaging method of choice. What is less clear is whether this will obviate the need to explore or aspirate the persistently painful joint in these patients.—M.S. Klempner, M.D.

Multicenter Collaborative Evaluation of a Standardized Serum Bactericidal Test as a Predictor of Therapeutic Efficacy in Acute and Chronic Osteomyelitis

Weinstein MP, Stratton CW, Hawley HB, Ackley A, Reller LB (Univ of Medicine and Dentistry of New Jersey—Robert Wood Johnson Med School; Vanderbilt Univ School of Medicine; Wright State Univ School of Medicine; Univ of Colorado School of Medicine)
Am J Med 83:218–222, August 1987

Chronic osteomyelitis is associated with frequent relapses of infection. Thus, it would be useful to have available a test that could predict the ultimate therapeutic success or failure of antimicrobial treatment early in the course. To this end, a prospective multicenter collaborative study was carried out to determine whether a standardized serum bactericidal test could predict the outcome of infection.

All centers used a microdilution test method that defined important test variables, including inoculum size, culture medium, dilution technique, incubation time, method of subculture, and bactericidal endpoint. Thirty patients had 30 episodes of acute osteomyelitis, and 13 patients had 18 episodes of chronic osteomyelitis. Osteomyelitis was confirmed by positive results of bone culture or blood culture, as well as by radiographic findings.

In patients with acute osteomyelitis, peak serum bactericidal titers had no predictive value. However, trough titers of 1:2 or higher accurately predicted cure, whereas lower trough titers accurately predicted failure (Fig 1–7). In patients with chronic osteomyelitis, peak serum bactericidal titers of 1:16 or higher and trough titers of 1:4 or higher accurately predicted cure; a lower peak bactericidal titer and a trough titer of less than 1:2 accurately predicted failure (Fig 1–8).

This standardized serum bactericidal test provides valid prognostic data for patients with osteomyelitis. In patients with acute osteomyelitis, serum bactericidal titers should be maintained at 1:2 or higher at all

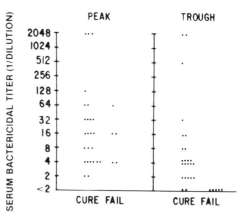

Fig 1–7.—Relationship of outcome of acute osteomyelitis to serum bactericidal test results. (Courtesy of Weinstein MP, Stratton CW, Hawley HB, et al: Am J Med 83:218–222, 1987.)

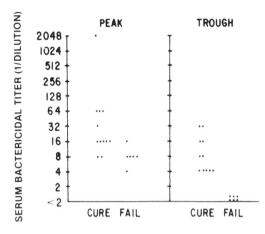

Fig 1–8.—Relationship of outcome of chronic osteomyelitis to serum bactericidal test results. (Courtesy of Weinstein MP, Stratton CW, Hawley HB, et al: *Am J Med* 83:218–222, 1987.)

times, and in patients with chronic osteomyelitis, at 1:4 or higher at all times.

▶ This was a carefully done study with great attention paid to the details of performing the serum bactericidal assay. Unlike the authors' previous study (e.g., Weinstein MP, Stratton CW, Ackley A, et al: *Am J Med* 78:262–269, Feb 1985), which emphasized the predicted value of peaked serum bactericidal levels in predicting the outcome of endocarditis, this study found that maintaining appropriate trough levels was an accurate predictor of the therapeutic outcome in treating osteomyelitis. Their suggestion that patients with acute osteomyelitis have serum bactericidal titers of 1:2 or greater at all times and that patients with chronic osteomyelitis have serum bactericidal levels of 1:4 or greater at all times seems prudent. A review of this topic has recently appeared (Wolfson JS, Swartz MN: *N Engl J Med* 312:968–975, April 11, 1985).—M.S. Klempner, M.D.

Pressure Sores and Underlying Bone Infection
Sugarman B (VA Med Ctr, Houston; Baylor College of Medicine; Michigan State Univ)
Arch Intern Med 147:553–555, March 1987   1–26

Pressure sores are a serious complication of bedridden patients. Infection is usually not present in the bone beneath the sore. However, radiographic and nuclear imaging and soft-tissue cultures are usually abnormal in the area of the pressure sore, suggesting osteomyelitis when it is not present. The optimal method of determining infection in the bone beneath a pressure sore was examined in this long-term, controlled trial.

Hospitalized patients with pressure sores, 385 of them with spinal cord injuries and 17 others, were evaluated over a 4.5-year period. Radiographic studies, Tc-99m bone scans, gallium 67 citrate scans, and bone biopsies were done. In a second group of 41 patients, management was

Evaluation of Bone Beneath Pressure Sores With Biopsy Specimen

Bone Histology	Sores Clinically Infected, No. (%)[†]	Depth of Sore[*]	Months Sore Present[‡]	Routine Studies Suggestive of Osteomyelitis Beneath Sores				
				Plain Radiographs	Bone Scan	Gallium Scan	Computed Tomographic Scan	Positive Bone Cultures[§]
Normal bone Group A (n = 26)	4/26 (15)	B = 5 D = 11 S = 10	<1:2 1-3:9 >3:15	11/23	9/22	11/14	1/1	14/25[∥]
Group B (n = 8)	2/8 (25)	B = 4 D = 3 S = 1	<1:3 1-3:5 >3:0	2/7	3/6	4/5	0/1	2/8[∥]
Pressure-related changes Group A (n = 55)	13/55 (24)	B = 7 D = 34 S = 14	<1:12 1-3:31 >3:12	28/42	39/47	12/18	2/5	29/55[∥]
Group B (n = 23)	5/23 (22)	B = 7 D = 5 S = 11	<1:7 1-3:12 >3:4	13/22	14/20	8/13	1/2	8/23[∥]
Osteomyelitis Group A (n = 31)	6/31 (19)	B = 6 D = 24 S = 1	<1:3 1-3:18 >3:10	16/25	28/28	18/19	2/3	30/30
Group B (n = 10)	3/10 (30)	B = 3 D = 2 S = 5	<1:3 1-3:6 >3:1	3/9	9/9	7/7	0/0	10/10

[*]At time of evaluation: B = bone visible, D = deep tissues exposed, and S = more superficial.
[†]Percent of total number of sores clinically appearing to be infected (i.e., grossly purulent drainage, advancing erythematous border, or systemic signs of infection attributed to pressure sore) by infectious diseases consultant during evaluation before biopsy.
[‡]Length of time sore known to be present before evaluation for osteomyelitis, in months/number of sores.
[§]Any growth on agar or in broth.
[∥]$P < .02$ for group B compared with group A (as a whole) by binomial distribution analysis.
(Courtesy of Sugarman B: Arch Intern Med 147:553–555, March 1987.)

more aggressive, with débridement and treatment with iodophors added to the above tests.

Pressure sores developed in 56% of the spinal cord patients. Results of bone biopsy are shown in the table. Clinical evaluation, depth, and duration of the pressure sore were not useful in determining which sores had bone infections. Normal bone scans were uniformly correct in identifying patients without osteomyelitis, but abnormal diagnostic studies were not useful. Pressure sore cultures were always positive. A false-positive rate of 54% was observed for bone cultures. In the more aggressively managed group (débridement), the rate was 32%.

All patients with bone infection responded to antibiotic therapy with increased healing and in 16 cases with complete sore closure. The other cases required surgery. Patients without bone infection responded to relief of pressure and to surgery; antibiotic therapy was not necessary.

Bone biopsy is usually required to determine whether infection is present in the bone beneath a pressure sore and to identify the organisms responsible. Aggressive débridement is simple to perform and significantly decreases the problem of false-positive bone cultures. The use of this procedure should increase.

▶ The extensive experience of this single author deserves serious attention. He has developed a systematic approach to this very common problem. Clinical evaluation as to the depth and duration of these sores was generally not helpful to determine which had underlying bone infection. Bone scans were of extremely high sensitivity but low specificity. In none of 30 patients with a normal bone scan did the biopsy show an underlying bone infection. Cultures of the pressure sores were all positive. However, bone biopsy cultures revealed fewer or different organisms in the bone three quarters of the time. False-positive bone cultures were common in both groups.

The author suggests an approach to nonhealing pressure sores that includes an initial bone scan. If this is negative, then the evaluation can be discontinued with confidence that osteomyelitis is not present. However, if the sore extends to the bone, the bone scan will most likely be positive and loses its predicted value. Bone biopsy is then generally necessary to determine whether or not osteomyelitis is present beneath nonhealing pressure sores. This also provides the only accurate method of identifying the offending organism.—M.S. Klempner, M.D.

Duration of Antimicrobial Therapy for Acute Suppurative Osteoarticular Infections
Syrogiannopoulos GA, Nelson JD (Univ of Texas Health Science Ctr at Dallas, Southwestern Med School)

Current management of acute suppurative osteoarticular infections includes surgical drainage and antibiotic therapy for a minimal duration of 4–5 weeks. From 1974 to 1983, 274 children with acute suppurative osteoarticular infections were treated with a sequential intravenous-oral antibiotic regimen for a shorter duration than was usually recommended, provided that the patient's clinical response was good and that the erythrocyte sedimentation rate (ESR) returned to normal. The results are presented.

For acute suppurative arthritis caused by staphylococci, streptococci, *Hemophilus influenzae* type b, gram-negative cocci, or other gram-negative bacteria, the median duration of antibiotic therapy was 23, 16, 16, 15, and 22 days, respectively. The median duration of antibiotic treatment for acute osteomyelitis due to staphylococci, streptococci, *H. influenzae*, or other gram-negative bacteria was 24, 23, 17, and 22.5 days, respectively. Osteoarthritis was treated usually for a month. Children with staphylococcal arthritis and osteomyelitis were generally treated the longest periods. A total of 180 patients received large doses of oral antimicrobials after clinical stabilization with intravenous therapy; the median duration of intravenous therapy was about 1 week (range, up to 7 weeks). Needle aspiration for diagnostic purposes was undertaken in 99% of patients. Incision and drainage were performed in 35%, 71%, and 63% of patients with acute suppurative arthritis, osteomyelitis, and osteoarthritis, respectively. Recurrence occurred in 4 patients with acute osteomyelitis and in none of those with suppurative arthritis.

Satisfactory results can be achieved with shorter courses of antibiotic therapy for acute suppurative osteoarticular infections. A minimum of 3 weeks' antibiotic therapy is recommended for acute hematogenous suppurative osteoarticular infections due to staphylococci and gram-negative bacilli, and 10–14 days, for those due to streptococci, meningococci, and *Hemophilus*, provided prompt resolution of systemic and local signs and restoration of ESR are achieved. Serum bactericidal activity, on the day after start of oral antibiotic therapy, should be at least $1/8$ when the pathogen is a gram-negative *Bacillus*, *Staphylococcus*, or *H. influenzae* and at least $1/32$ with *Streptococcus*. Adequate serum bactericidal activity should be maintained during the course of therapy, and patients' compliance must be stressed.

▶ In their conclusions the authors emphasize 2 points that bear stressing. First, the durations of therapy reported by them to be effective should be considered a minimum and should be applied only to patients who have prompt resolution of local and systemic features of infection together with a fall in the ESR to normal. Second, oral antibiotic treatment should be monitored by demonstration of an adequate titer of bactericidal activity in the serum.—M.J. Barza, M.D.

Oral Antimicrobial Therapy for Adults With Osteomyelitis or Septic Arthritis

Black J, Hunt TL, Godley PJ, Matthew E (Univ of Texas at Austin, Central Texas Med Found, Austin)
J Infect Dis 155:968–972, May 1987

The standard treatment for osteomyelitis and septic arthritis is 4 to 6 weeks of parenteral antibiotics administered in the hospital setting. To determine the efficacy of orally administered antibiotic therapy in outpatients, 18 adults with osteomyelitis and 3 with septic arthritis were treated with high-dose orally given antibiotics. Serum bactericidal titers were monitored to provide guidelines for dosage. The patients were followed for a minimum of 6 months.

The patients had an average of 3.6 days of parenteral therapy, followed by an average of 43 days of orally given antibiotic therapy. Following therapy, 18 of the 21 patients did not have recurrences. Three patients had recurrences, of which two were accompanied by sequestra. There were no serious side effects of the high-dose antibiotic therapy. The mean time of hospitalization was 13.4 days. The average duration of outpatient therapy was 31.9 days.

These data suggest that orally administered high-dose antibiotic therapy is a reasonable alternative to parenteral therapy for adult patients with osteomyelitis or septic arthritis. This approach is not only cost-effective but is more convenient and comfortable for the compliant patient.

▶ This study, like others evaluating oral treatment for osteomyelitis, was retrospective and noncomparative; thus, there was no comparison group given intravenous treatment. Although there have been a number of previous reports of the treatment of osteomyelitis and septic arthritis by the oral route in children, this is the first such study in adults. The authors suggest that drug dosages should be adjusted to maintain serum bactericidal titers of at least 1:8 but point out that they have no data to substantiate this preference.—M.J. Barza, M.D.

Amikacin Alone and in Combination With Trimethoprim-Sulfamethoxazole in the Treatment of Actinomycotic Mycetoma
Welsh O, Sauceda E, Gonzalez J, Ocampo J (Universidad Autónoma de Nuevo León, Monterrey, Mexico)

Mycetoma is the most frequent deep mycosis in Mexico and is a potentially disabling disorder. Amikacin, a semisynthetic aminoglycoside, is active in vitro against various strains of *Nocardia*. Amikacin was used alone and in conjunction with trimethoprim-sulfamethoxazole (TMP-SMX) in 15 patients with actinomycotic mycetoma. The patients had responded poorly to conventional treatment or were at risk of dissemination. Two patients received amikacin alone. Amikacin was given intramuscularly in a dose of 15 mg/kg daily for 3-week cycles. The daily doses of TMP and SMX were 7 and 35 mg/kg, respectively.

Combined treatment with amikacin and TMP-SMX was very effective in producing remission, even in previously treated patients. No side effects resulted from amikacin therapy. Two patients with gastritis from TMP-SMX responded to antacids.

Mycetoma responds consistently and rapidly to combined treatment with amikacin and TMP-SMX. As in tuberculosis and leprosy, diseases caused by phylogenetically related organisms, simultaneous treatment with different medications achieves better results in a shorter time.

Epidemic Septic Arthritis Caused by *Serratia marcescens* and Associated With a Benzalkonium Chloride Antiseptic
Nakashima AK, McCarthy MA, Martone WJ, Anderson RL (Ctrs for Disease Control, Atlanta; Pennsylvania State Dept of Health, Harrisburg)
J Clin Microbiol 25:1014–1018, June 1987

Nosocomial epidemics of infections resulting from *Serratia* species have been traced to multiple sources, including contaminated solutions and disinfectants, intravenous (IV) fluids, and arterial-pressure monitors. Septic arthritis from *Serratia* species is rare; when it was diagnosed in 10 patients, intrinsic contamination of a product used for joint injections in the office of 3 orthopedic surgeons was suspected. Nevertheless, this product was distributed widely, and the outbreak of the infection was restricted to 1 geographic location. The results of the outbreak investigation are reported.

From June 1981 to January 1982, 47 patients had cultures positive for *Serratia* species. From June to September 1981, 19 had such positive cultures, but none were from joint fluids. By contrast, from October 1981 to January 1982, 28 patients had positive cultures; and 11 (39%) of the cultures were from joint fluids. Knee or shoulder joints were involved. Ten patients developed severe pain up to 24 hours after their last joint injection. All had diagnostic arthrocentesis 3 to 24 days after the injection. Cultures were positive for *S. marcescens* in 9 patients and for other *Serratia* species in 2.

Ten patients were hospitalized. Studies showed that infections were associated with previous joint infections of methylprednisolone and lidocaine. All patients had been treated by two orthopedic surgeons who shared an office. Environmental cultures revealed that a canister of cotton balls soaked in aqueous benzalkonium chloride and two multiple-dose vials of methylprednisolone had been contaminated by the epidemic strain of *S. marcescens*. It was postulated that the canister may have served as a reservoir for contamination of sterile solutions and equipment used for joint injections, of skin at the injection site, and of the hands of personnel. After the use of aqueous benzalkonium was discontinued, no further cases occurred. Use of aqueous quaternary ammonium compounds should be approached carefully, as intrinsic and extrinsic contamination of these solutions has been well documented in the past and has been of concern for many years.

▶ There are a few lessons to be relearned in this study: (1) Disinfection is not an absolute safeguard against infection and is simply one of many components of sterile technique (it is necessary but not sufficient). (2) Disinfectants can become contaminated and serve as a reservoir for outbreaks of infection. (3) Injections are more likely to transmit infection than is aspiration for diagnosis or treatment. Clustering of somewhat unusual infections is a signal to review the procedure under question and to directly evaluate every step as a possible source.—G.T. Keusch, M.D.

Bacterial Vaccines

Protective Secretory Immunoglobulin A Antibodies in Humans Following Oral Immunization With *Streptococcus mutans*
Gregory RL, Filler SJ (Emory Univ School of Dentistry; Inst of Dental Research and School of Dentistry, Univ of Alabama in Birmingham)
Infect Immun 55:2409–2415, October 1987
1–31

Streptococcus mutans is the chief etiologic agent in human dental caries. Ingestion of bacterial antigen has produced high levels of specific secretory immunoglobulin A (sIgA) antibody in mucosal secretions of experimental animals and has protected against challenge with virulent bacteria. The authors found that ingestion of a vaccine of killed *S. mutans* induces high antibody levels and lowers the number of organisms in dental plaque and saliva.

Daily ingestion for 10 consecutive days of a vaccine of killed *S. mutans* from the same subjects induced higher levels of specific secretory IgA in parotid saliva and tears of 4 healthy men and in the saliva, tears, colostrum, and milk of a pregnant woman. Levels of IgA antibody in secretions remained elevated for longer than 50 days. A second series of immunizations over 1 week led to even higher antibody levels, which peaked earlier and lasted longer than after primary immunization. Serum antibody did not increase. Each series of immunizations lowered numbers of viable *S. mutans* in dental plaque and whole saliva. The proportion of organisms in plaque correlated with the salivary level of IgA antibody to *S. mutans*.

Oral administration of a killed *S. mutans* vaccine induces high levels of secretory IgA antibody and lowers the number of viable organisms in dental plaque. This may be an effective approach to immunizing against dental caries in humans. Heart-reactive antibody was not induced in this study, despite suggestions that antibodies to *S. mutans* components may cross-react with human heart and kidney tissues.

► A vaccine for dental caries? Possibly. Are dentists on the way out? I doubt it. At least it seems no more likely than the speculation that penicillin would be the end of the specialty of infectious diseases!—G.T. Keusch, M.D.

Immunogenicity of *Haemophilus influenzae* Type b Capsular Polysaccharide Vaccines in 18-Month-Old Infants

Hendley JO, Wenzel JG, Ashe KM, Samuelson JS (Univ of Virginia School of Medicine, Connaught Labs, Inc, Swiftwater, Pa)
Pediatrics 80:351–354, September 1987

Protection against *Hemophilus influenzae* type b corresponds to the presence of serum antibody to polyribosyl ribitol phosphate (PRP). A vaccine containing PRP or PRP conjugated to diphtheria toxoid was administered at the same time as, but in a different site from, the routine diphtheria-tetanus-pertussis (DTP) booster in 94 healthy infants at 17–22 months of age.

Systematic reaction to vaccination resembled that for DTP alone. Minor local reactions to the *H. influenzae* injections occurred in 13%–14% of both groups. Only 43% of the nonimmune PRP recipients achieved an antibody titer greater than 0.15 µg/ml in the PRP group. In the PRP-diphtheria toxoid group, 81% of the nonimmune recipients had titers of greater than 0.15 µg/ml following vaccination (table).

These results indicate that more than half of the nonimmune 18-month-old infants did not respond to PRP with protective levels of antibody. Therefore, for infants vaccinated at this time, revaccination at 24 months of age or older, which has been shown to be protective, is appropriate.

Antipolyribosyl Ribitol Phosphate Antibody Concentrations 4–6 Weeks After Vaccination in 17- to 22-Month-Old Infants Who Were Not Immune Before Vaccination*

Age (mo)	Polyribosyl Ribitol Phosphate			Polyribosyl Ribitol Phosphate-Diphtheria Toxoid		
	No. Tested	No. (%) of Vaccinees With Antibody Concentration (µg/mL)		No. Tested	No. (%) of Vaccinees With Antibody Concentration (µg/mL)	
		≥0.15	≥1.0		≥0.15	≥1.0
17	5	2 (40)	2 (40)	7	4 (57)	3 (43)
18	11	4 (36)	0	9	8 (89)	6 (67)
19	11	4 (36)	2 (18)	14	11 (79)	10 (71)
20	4	3 (75)	2 (50)	7	6 (86)	3 (43)
21	4	2 (50)	1 (25)	3	3 (100)	3 (100)
22	0			2	2 (100)	1 (50)

*Not immune = < .15 µg/mL of antibody in prevaccine serum.
(Courtesy of Hendley JO, Wenzel JG, Ashe KM, et al: Pediatrics 80:351–354, September 1987.)

Efficacy of *Haemophilus influenzae* Type b Polysaccharide-Diphtheria Toxoid Conjugate Vaccine in Infancy

Eskola J, Peltola H, Takala AK, Käyhty H, Hakulinen M, Karanko V, Kela E, Rekola P, Rönnberg P-R, Samuelson JS, Gordon LK, Mäkelä PH (Natl Public Health Inst, Helsinki; Connaught Labs, Swiftwater, Pa; Connaught Research Inst, Willowdale, Ont)
N Engl J Med 317:717–722, Sept 17, 1987

1–33

Recent research has shown that *Hemophilus influenzae* type b capsular polysaccharide-diphtheria toxoid conjugate vaccine can induce antibodies to *H. influenzae* in infants. A study was done to assess the clinical efficacy of the vaccine.

Sixty thousand children in Finland were enrolled in an open trial. Children born on odd-numbered days between October 1, 1985, and September 30, 1986, were given the vaccine at 3, 4, 6, and 14 months. Children born on even-numbered days comprised the comparison group. All reactions occurring within 48 hours of vaccination were followed in detail in a cohort of 99 infants.

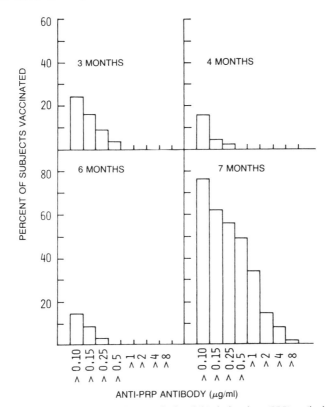

Fig 1–9.—Percentage of infants with anti-polyribosylribitol phosphate (PRP) antibody concentrations of 0.1 to 8 µg/ml in a cohort of 99 infants vaccinated with PRP-D at 3, 4, and 6 months of age. (Courtesy of Eskola J, Peltola H, Takala AK, et al: *N Engl J Med* 317:717–722, Sept 17, 1987.)

Invasive H. influenzae Type B Disease In 14 Children in Evaluation of PRP-D Vaccine

Subject No.	Sex	Age at Entry	Diagnosis	Confirmation of Diagnosis*		Vaccines Given†			Anti-PRP Antibody	
				BLOOD CULTURE	CSF CULTURE	PRP-DT	DPT	IPV	ACUTE PHASE‡	CONVALESCENT PHASE§
		mo				no. of doses			µg/ml	
Children born on odd days (PRP-DT vaccine group)										
1	M	9	Meningitis	+	+	3	3	1	0.20	1.70
2	M	11	Meningitis	+	+	3	3	1	0.318	12.85
Children born on even days (control group)										
3	M	7	Meningitis	+	+	0	3	1	ND	ND
4	M	7	Pneumonia	+	ND	0	3	1	<0.03	0.03
5	F	8	Arthritis	+	ND	0	3	1	ND	ND
6	M	8	Meningitis	+	+	0	3	1	0.118	1.585
7	F	9	Meningitis	+	+	0	3	1	0.207	0.328
8	M	10	Meningitis	+	+	0	3	1	0.069	0.026
9	M	10	Meningitis	+	+	0	3	1	<0.03	0.031
10	M	10	Meningitis	+	+	0	3	1	0.081	0.497
11	M	11	Cellulitis	+	−	0	3	1	0.39	<0.03
12	M	13	Meningitis	+	+	0	3	1	<0.03	0.31
13	M	14	Pneumonia	+	ND	0	3	2	ND	ND
14	M	15	Meningitis	+	+	0	3	2	ND	ND

*CSF, cerebrospinal fluid; ND, not determined.
†DPT, diphtheria-pertussis vaccine; IPV, inactivated poliomyelitis vaccine; MMR, measles-mumps-rubella vaccine; PRP-D, H. influenzae type b capsular polysaccharide (polyriboslyribitol phosphate)-diphtheria toxoid conjugate vaccine. All children received 3 doses of DPT and 1 dose of IPV; those given PRP-D received 3 doses of the vaccine.
‡Antibody level in blood obtained within 11 days (median, 2) after hospitalization.
§Antibody level in blood obtained 16–45 days (median, 26) after acute phase sample.
(Courtesy of Eskola J, Peltola H, Takala AK, et al: N Engl J Med 317:717–722, Sept 17, 1987.)

In this cohort, the geometric mean antibody titer rose from a prevaccination level of 0.08 µg/ml at 3 months of age to 0.42 µg/ml at 7 months. Antibody concentrations of more than 0.15 or 1 µg/ml were present in 62% and 34% of the samples obtained at age 7 months, 1 month after the third dose (Fig 1–9). Adverse reactions were minor, e.g., increased irritability, fever higher than 38.5C, and local soreness. By February 1987 invasive H. influenzae had occurred in 2 children receiving 3 doses of vaccine and in 12 children who were not vaccinated (table). Thus, at an average follow-up of 5 months, the rate of protection provided by this conjugate vaccine in infancy was 83%.

In this study, 83% of the children vaccinated with H. influenzae type b capsular polysaccharide covalently coupled to diphtheria toxoid, 0.5 mL, were protected from invasive H. influenzae. This response rate was better than was anticipated on the basis of previous experience with antibody responses to unconjugated capsular polysaccharide vaccine.

Prevention of *Haemophilus influenzae* Type b Infections in High-Risk Infants Treated With Bacterial Polysaccharide Immune Globulin

Santosham M, Reid R, Ambrosino DM, Wolff MC, Almeido-Hill J, Priehs C, As-

pery KM, Garrett S, Croll L, Foster S, Burge G, Page P, Zacher B, Moxon R, Siber GR (Johns Hopkins Univ; Francis Scott Key Med Ctr, Baltimore; Dana-Farber Cancer Inst, Boston; Harvard Med School; Massachusetts Dept of Public Health, Jamaica Plain, Mass; et al)
N Engl J Med 317:923–929, Oct 8, 1987   1–34

Apache Indian infants have been reported to have a high incidence of *Haemophilus influenzae* type b (Hib) and pneumococcal infections. Forty percent of Hib infections in this population occur before the age of 6 months, when active immunization may not protect them. To assess the efficacy of passive immunization with a human hyperimmune globulin—bacterial polysaccharide immunoglobulin (BPIG)—which was prepared from the plasma of immunized adult donors, the authors conducted a double-blind test of 703 infants who were randomly assigned to receive BPIG, 0.5 ml/kg, or 0.5 ml of saline intramuscularly at ages 2, 6, and 10 months.

The treatment group consisted of 353 babies; the control group included 350. Levels of Hib antibody were significantly higher in recipients of BPIG than in recipients of placebo at 4, 6, and 10 months (Fig 1–10). In the first 90 days after injection of BPIG or placebo no Hib or pneumococcal infections were noted in the BPIG group, whereas 7 Hib infections and 4 pneumococcal infections developed in the placebo group (Tables 1 and 2)., During the fourth month 1 case of Hib meningitis and 2 cases of

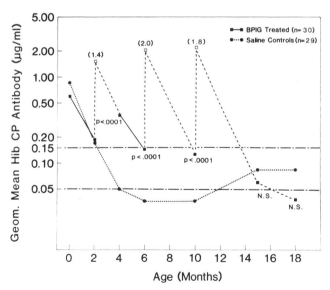

Fig 1–10.—Mean concentration of Hib capsular polysaccharide (Hib CP) antibody in BPIG and placebo recipients. *Interrupted horizontal lines* represent estimates of minimum protective concentration of IgG class Hib antibody. In BPIG recipients peak antibody concentrations *(open squares)* were extrapolated from observed values *(solid squares)*, assuming a half-life of 30 days for antibody. Extrapolated points are connected to observed values by interrupted lines. P values represent significance of differences between means according to *t* statistic. (Courtesy of Santosham M, Reid R, Ambrosino DM, et al: N Engl J Med 317:923–929, Oct 8, 1987.)

TABLE 1.—Comparison of Bacterial Polysaccharide Immunoglobulin (BPIG) and Pneumococcal Bacteremia and Meningitis

	BPIG GROUP	PLACEBO GROUP	P VALUE*
No. of patients at risk	353	350	
No. of doses	858	838	
Cases of invasive Hib disease			
Before treatment period	0	1	
1–90 days after immunization	0	7	0.007
91–120 days after immunization	1	0	
1–120 days after immunization	1	7	0.04
After treatment period†	2	4	
Cases of invasive pneumococcal infections			
Before treatment period	1	0	
1–90 days after immunization	0	4	0.06
91–120 days after immunization	2	0	
1–120 days after immunization	2	4	
After treatment period†	6	6	
Combined no. of cases of invasive Hib and pneumococcal infections			
Before treatment period	1	1	
1–90 days after immunization	0	11	<0.001
91–120 days after immunization	3	0	
1–120 days after immunization	3	11	0.03
After treatment period†	8	10	
Total number of cases	12	22	

*By 2-sided Fisher's exact test. P value is given only if $P < .1$.
†At 121 days to 2 years after third dose.
(Courtesy of Santosham M, Reid R, Ambrosino DM, et al: N Engl J Med 317:923–929, Oct 8, 1987.)

pneumococcal bacteremia occurred in the BPIG group, compared with none in the placebo group.

When BPIG is given at 4-month intervals, it can provide significant protection against serious Hib disease for 3 months. In infants at high risk it may be used alone at 3-month intervals or in conjunction with active immunization.

▶ The need to immunize susceptible young infants to Haemophilus influenzae type b at an age when their response to polysaccharide antigens is poor is a dilemma affecting the efficacy of Hib vaccines. The first study (Abstract 1–32) shows that a protein conjugate polyribosyl phosphate (PRP) vaccine is better than the plain PRP vaccine in the 17- to 22-month-old group and that it may be given with DTP booster without additional side effects. On the other hand, less than half of the PRP vaccinees had an acceptable antibody titer, showing once again that the response is unreliable in the infants younger than 2 years. The wisdom of the American Academy of Pediatrics recommendation that a second dose be given at age 24 months to children receiving PRP at an earlier age is therefore reinforced by this study. Plain PRP is likely to go the way of killed measles vaccine: to be replaced by a more effective product.

TABLE 2.—Comparison of Bacterial Polysaccharide Immunoglobulin (BPIG) and Placebo in Prevention of Various Outcomes*

	BPIG GROUP	PLACEBO GROUP	P VALUE†
No. of children at risk	353	350	
No. of episodes of pneumonia	29	35	
No. of children with ≥3 episodes of pneumonia	0	7	0.007‡
No. of children with consolidative pneumonia	3	9	0.09‡
No. of episodes of gastroenteritis	620	581	
No. of episodes of impetigo	24	30	
No. of children hospitalized with any illness	154	164	
No. of children hospitalized with temperature ≥39°C	100	123	0.05§

*At 1–120 days after treatment.
†P value is given only if P < .1.
‡By 2-sided Fisher's exact test.
§By chi-square test.
(Courtesy of Santosham M, Reid R, Ambrosino DM, et al: *N Engl J Med* 317:923–929, Oct 8, 1987.)

The second study (Abstract 1–33) is a large-scale field trial among some 60,000 Finnish babies, half of whom received a PRP-diphtheria toxoid conjugate vaccine beginning at 3 months of age, the controls receiving the same vaccine at 24 months. After 2 doses only 12% of subjects responded, but by the third dose, there was a good antibody response in most infants (82%). Protection efficiency from invasive *H. influenzae* disease was 87% during a 9-month follow-up after 3 doses of vaccine, in comparison to the control group who had not yet received PRP-DT. These results are impressive.

The third study (Abstract 1–34) shows that passive immunization with bacterial polysaccharide immunoglobulin (BPIG) appears to work in high-risk infants. However, the protection wanes and was not demonstrable 90 days after the last administration of BPIG. This product will clearly not replace Hib vaccine but may be useful to protect high-risk groups very early in life until active immunization can be given.—G.T. Keusch, M.D.

Large-Scale Field Trial of Ty21a Live Oral Typhoid Vaccine in Enteric-Coated Capsule Formulation
Levine MM, Ferreccio C, Black RE, Germanier R, Chilean Typhoid Committee (Univ of Maryland School of Medicine; Ministry of Health, Santiago, Chile; Swiss Serum and Vaccine Inst, Berne, Switzerland)
Lancet 1:1049–1052, May 9, 1987   1–35

Typhoid fever remains an important disease in many parts of the world. An important advance was the development of Ty21a, an attenu-

TABLE 1.—Results of 36 Months of Surveillance

	Enteric-coated capsules		Gelatin capsules with NaHCO$_3$		
—	Long interval	Short interval	Long interval	Short interval	Placebo
No of children	21 598	22 170	21 541	22 379	21 906
No of classes	861	863	864	862	862
Cases	34	23	46	56	68
Incidence/10^5	157·4[a]	103·7[b]	213·5[c]	250·3[d]	310·4[e]
Efficacy	49% (24–66%)	67% (47–79%)	31% (0–52%)	19% (0–43%)	—
Classes with typhoid	34	23	46	54	64
Classes with typhoid/ 100 classes	3·95[f]	2·67[g]	5·32[h]	6·26[i]	7·42[j]
Efficacy	47%	64%	28%	16%	—

*Long interval = 3 doses, 21 days between; short interval = 3 doses, 1–2 days between. Values in parentheses are 95% confidence intervals of vaccine efficacy.

†a vs. e, $P = .0006$; b vs. e, $P < .00001$; c vs. e, $P = .023$; d vs. e, $P = .21$; a vs. c, $P = .23$; b vs. d, $P = .00052$; a + b vs. c + d, $P = .001$; f vs j, $P = .00135$; g vs. j, $P = .0000031$; h vs. j, $P = .07$, i vs. j, $P = .35$; g vs. i, $P = .00032$; f + g vs. h + i, $P = .00024$ (all statistical comparisons by chi square test).

(Courtesy of Levine MM, Ferreccio C, Black RE, et al: Lancet 1:1049–1052, May 9, 1987.)

ated strain of *Salmonella typhi*, that can be used in an orally administered vaccine. A randomized, placebo-controlled field study of the efficacy of this vaccine was conducted with 109,000 schoolchildren in Santiago, Chile.

Group 1 received 3 doses of vaccine in gelatin capsules with sodium bicarbonate, with 2 days between doses. Group 2 received the 3 doses in enteric-coated capsules. Group 3 received 3 doses in enteric-coated capsules with 21 days between the doses. Group 4 received 3 doses of vaccine in the gelatin/bicarbonate formulation with 21 days between doses. Group 5 received placebo with 2 days between the doses.

In group 2, the vaccine had a 67% efficacy over at least 3 years (Table 1). Increasing the time between dosages to 21 days did not enhance protection (group 3). There was significantly less protection with the gelatin/bicarbonate formulation (groups 1 and 4).

The Ty21a protects against typhoid as well as the heat/phenol-inactivated whole-cell parenteral vaccine but is not associated with adverse reactions (Table 2). The Ty21a can now be regarded as an effective alternative vaccine.

Prevention of Typhoid Fever in Nepal With the Vi Capsular Polysaccharide of *Salmonella typhi*: A Preliminary Report

Acharya, IL, Lowe CU, Thapa R, Gurubacharya VL, Shrestha MB, Cadoz M, Schulz D, Armand J, Bryla DA, Trollfors B, Cramton T, Schneerson R, Robbins JB (Infectious Disease Hosp and Central Health Lab, Teku, Nepal; Natl Insts of

TABLE 2.—Comparison of Results of World Health Organization-Sponsored Controlled Field Trials of Heat/Phenol-Inactivated Parenteral Killed Whole Cell Typhoid Vaccine (L) and Attenuated *Salmonella typhi* Ty21A Live Oral Vaccine

Field site, dates	Age groups	Vaccine (no of doses)	No vaccinated	Duration of surveillance	Incidence of typhoid per 10^5	Vaccine efficacy	Ref
Yugoslavia 1960-63	2-50 yr; mostly schoolchildren	L (2)	5028	$2\frac{1}{2}$ yr	727[a]	51%	10
		Control (2)	5039	$2\frac{1}{2}$ yr	1488[b]	–	
Guyana, 1960-67	5-15 yr (schoolchildren)	L (2)	24 241	7 yr	198[c]	67%	11
		Control (2)	27 756	7 yr	605[d]	–	
USSR, 1962-65	Schoolchildren and young adults (92% age 7-15 yr)	L (2)	36 112	$2\frac{1}{2}$ yr	55[e]	66%	13
		Control (2)	36 999	$2\frac{1}{2}$ yr	162[f]	–	
Egypt, 1978-81	Schoolchildren 6-7 yr	Ty21a (3)*	16 486	3 yr	6[a]	96% (77-99%)‡	17
		Control (3)	15 902	3 yr	138[b]		
Chile, 1983-86	Schoolchildren 6-21 yr	Ty21a (3)†	22 170	3 yr	104[i]	67% (47-79%)‡	
		Control (3)	21 906	3 yr	310[j]		

*Liquid formulation, 3 doses given within 1 week;
†Enteric-coated capsule formulation, 3 doses given within 1 week. Values in parentheses are 95% confidence interval of vaccine efficacy.
‡a vs. b, $P < .0004$; c vs. d, $P < .000005$; e vs. f, $P = .000021$; i vs. j, $P < .00001$ (comparisons by chi square test).
(Courtesy of Levine MM, Ferreccio C, Black RE, et al: *Lancet* 1:1049–1052, May 9, 1987.)

Typhoid fever has not been controlled by vaccinations, because of limitations of the 2 existing vaccines. The role of the capsular polysaccharide

Occurrence of Typhoid Fever Within 17 Months After Immunization*

Typhoid Fever	Vaccine		P Value†	Efficacy
	Vi	Pneumo		
				%
Culture-positive	9	32	0.004	72
Clinically suspected	5	25	0.0003	80
Combined	14	57	0.00001	75

*A total of 6,907 individuals received with Vi capsular polysaccharide of *Pneumococcus* polysaccharide (pneumo) vaccine (control).
†P values for differences in the attack rate of typhoid fever between the Vi group and the control group, calculated by Fisher's exact test.
(Courtesy of Acharya IL, Lowe CU, Thapa R, et al: N Engl J Med 317:1101–1104, Oct 29, 1987.)

of *Salmonella typhi* (Vi antigen) in immunity to typhoid fever was evaluated in a pilot study involving 274 Nepalese and a double-blind, randomized clinical trial involving Nepalese residents, aged 5 to 44 years, of 5 villages west of Kathmandu.

In the pilot study, Vi was given intramuscularly at doses of 25 μg or 50 μg, dissolved in 0.5 ml saline. There were no significant side effects of Vi vaccine, and about 75% responded with a fourfold or greater increase in serum antibodies. In the clinical trial, 6,907 participants were vaccinated with either Vi (n = 3,457) or pneumococcus vaccine (control) (n = 3,450). Persons with temperatures of 37.8C or higher for 3 consecutive days were examined and asked to give blood for culture. Within 17 months after immunization, 71 patients met the criteria for typhoid fever defined as either having blood culture-positive (n = 41) or being clinically suspected on the basis of bradycardia, splenomegaly, and fever with negative blood culture (n = 30) (table). The attack rate of typhoid fever was significantly higher among controls (16.2 per 1,000) than among those immunized with Vi (4.1 per 1,000). The protective efficacy of Vi was 72% in the culture positive group, 80% in the clinically suspected group, and 75% in the two groups combined.

Serum antibodies to the Vi antigen confer immunity to typhoid fever. Despite an efficacy of only 75%, Vi offers some advantages over the cellular and attenuated strain Ty-21a vaccines, such as rare adverse reactions, use of only 1 dose, reliable standardization by physicochemical methods verified for other capsular polysaccharide vaccines, and stability at ambient temperatures simplifying its use in the field. Surveillance still continues regarding the duration of Vi-induced immunity.

Protective Activity of Vi Capsular Polysaccharide Vaccine Against Typhoid Fever

Klugman KP, Gilbertson IT, Koornhof HJ, Robbins JB, Schneerson R, Schulz D, Cadoz M, Armand J, Vaccination Advisory Committee (Univ of the Witwatersrand; Natl Inst for Tropical Diseases; Medical Univ of Southern Africa; Letaba Hosp; Univ of Pretoria; et al)

The key to the elimination of typhoid fever lies in the provision of adequate sewage disposal and protected water supplies. However, the provision of a safe water supply to everyone is unlikely, at least in the next decade. An effective, safe vaccine, especially in children, could lessen the incidence of typhoid fever in endemic areas. The efficacy of a single intramuscular injection of the Vi capsular polysaccharide (CPS), 25 μg, was evaluated in a randomized, double-blind, controlled trial. A total of 23,075 children, aged 5–16 years, was enrolled in the 36 participating schools. Of these, 11,834 were vaccinated. The children were followed up for 21 months. Forty-seven blood-culture-proved cases of typhoid occurred in children who received meningococcal A + C CPS vaccine, compared with 19 cases among those vaccinated with Vi CPS (Table 1). Calculated from the day of vaccination, protective efficacy was 60%. Calculated from 6 weeks after vaccination, it was 64%. Of the 11,691 children not vaccinated, 173 cases of typhoid occurred. Compared with the unvaccinated group, protective efficacy was 77.4% and 81% after 21 months, calculated immediately and 6 weeks after vaccination, respectively. Vaccinations were associated with minimal local side effects (Table 2). Also, an increase in anti-Vi antibodies occurred, as measured by radioimmunoassay and enzyme-linked immunosorbent assay. Antibody levels continued to be significantly increased at 6 and 12 months after vaccination.

The duration of immunity with 25 μg of Vi CPS vaccine beyond 21 months is yet to be determined. However, these initial favorable results indicate safety and efficacy of single-dose preparation in the prevention of typhoid fever.

▶ The protection afforded by the enteric-coated live typhoid vaccine given 3 times a week to a group of children in Santiago, Chile, was good (67% vaccine efficacy) but not as good as the 96% achieved in an earlier trial in Alexandria,

TABLE 1.—Typhoid Fever Cases Among School Children 21 Months after Immunization

	Vaccine			
—	Vi	Meningococcal	Efficacy	P value*
Culture-positive total	19	47	60% (31%–76%)†	<0.001
Cases >6 wk after vaccination	16	44	64% (36%–79%)†	<0.001

*Chi-squared test with Yates modification.
†95% confidence intervals.
(Courtesy of Klugman KP, Gilbertson IT, Koornhof HJ, et al: *Lancet* 2:1165–1169, Nov 21, 1987.)

TABLE 2.—Side Effects of Meningococcal A + C Versus Typhoid Vl Vaccination

Vaccine*	Vaccination site			
	Pain	Erythema	Induration	Fever
Meningococcal A + C 50 μg (n = 129)	89 (*69%*)	23 (*18%*)	21 (*16%*)	2 (*2%*)
Typhoid Vi 25 μg (n = 127)	78 (*61%*)	10 (*8%*)	2 (*2%*)	1 (*1%*)
Typhoid Vi 50 μg (n = 126)	86 (*68%*)	9 (*7%*)	9 (*7%*)	0

*These vaccines were identified as vaccines A, C, and B, respectively, in the pilot study.
(Courtesy of Klugman KP, Gilbertson IT, Koornhof HJ, et al: *Lancet* 2:1165–1169, Nov 21, 1987.)

Egypt. One reason may be the difference in formulation of vaccine: enteric-coated vs. reconstituted lyophilate given with bicarbonate. Another, perhaps more important, reason is the 3-fold greater incidence of typhoid in Santiago, which constitutes a significantly increased challenge for the vaccine to work against. So, not bad for Ty21a, and nice study, Dr. Levine and colleagues (Abstract 1–35).

The second paper (Abstract 1–36) reports a different strategy for a typhoid vaccine using the Vi antigen. This capsular polysaccharide has always been suspect as a target for protective immunity, and the trial suggests that it offers something of value. Over a 17-month period, a vaccine efficacy of 72% was found, evaluating only culture-positive cases.

The third paper (Abstract 1–37) is icing on the cake. Nearly 12,000 children were immunized with the same Vi vaccine; controls received a meningococcal A and C polysaccharide vaccine. Efficacy approached 80% over 21 months of observation. One can only wonder what a combined oral vaccine plus Vi immunization could achieve. I'm certain we will see trials of other oral vaccines being developed and more Vi trials before such a combined approach will be tested. Anyway, after well over half a century of the same old killed parenteral vaccine, there is clearly progress being made in the attack on typhoid.— G.T. Keusch, M.D.

Antimicrobial Therapy

Univariate and Multivariate Analyses of Risk Factors Predisposing to Auditory Toxicity in Patients Receiving Aminoglycosides
Gatell JM, Ferran F, Araujo V, Bonet M, Soriano E, Transerra J, SanMiguel JG (Hosp Clinic, Faculty of Medicine, Barcelona, Spain)
Antimicrob Agents Chemother 31:1383–1387, September 1987   1–38

Aminoglycosides still are important antimicrobial drugs, but renal dysfunction and ototoxicity are possible side effects. Risk factors for audi-

Relationship Between Development of Auditory Toxicity and Type of Aminoglycoside Administered

Aminoglycoside	No. in study population	No. (%) with auditory toxicity:	
		≥15 dB*	≥20 dB †
Netilmicin	68	3 (4.4)	0 (0)
Tobramycin	102	11 (10.8)	8 (7.8)
Amikacin	17	4 (23.5)	2 (11.8)
Total	187	18 (9.6)	10 (5.3)

*Chi-square = 6.5; P = .04. Chi-square for linear trend = 6.2; P = .01.
†Chi-square = 6.1; P = .05. Chi-square for linear trend = 5.6; P = .02.
(Courtesy of Gatell JM, Ferran F, Araujo V, et al: *Antimicrob Agents Chemother* 31:1383–1387, September 1987.)

tory toxicity were studied in a series of 187 patients enrolled in 3 prospective trials comparing netilmicin, tobramycin, and amikacin for 3 days or longer. At least 2 serial audiograms were available in all cases.

Slight or mild hearing loss of 15–20 dB occurred in 9.6% of patients, and loss of 20 dB or greater occurred in 5.3%. Auditory toxicity was least frequent with netilmicin and most frequent with amikacin therapy (table). Univariate analysis showed that patients with auditory toxicity were older than the others and more often had trough levels of netilmicin or tobramycin above 2 mg/L or amikacin levels above 5 mg/L.

A final logistic regression analysis showed that only age independently influenced the occurrence of auditory toxicity. Factors without significance included the serum aminoglycoside level, total drug dose, duration of treatment, previous otic pathology, and the development of renal toxicity. Age appears to the chief factor disposing to auditory toxicity in patients given aminoglycosides, at least in certain patient populations.

▶ Nephrotoxicity caused by aminoglycosides is much more easily detected and measured than is ototoxicity; however, ototoxicity may be a more significant event because it is so often irreversible. This group of investigators has carried out a well-designed series of investigations of the ototoxicity of major aminoglycosides. The only variable that independently could be shown to influence the rate of auditory ototoxicity was age. As shown in the accompanying figure, the incidence of ototoxicity increased steadily with age but rose most steeply after 60 years of age. If one were to select arbitrarily a 5% risk of ototoxicity as a maximum acceptable threshold, one would have to avoid giving aminoglycosides to patients older than 30 years of age.—M.J. Barza, M.D.

What Is the Cost of Nephrotoxicity Associated with Aminoglycosides?

Eisenberg JM, Koffer H, Glick HA, Connell ML, Loss LE, Talbot GH, Shusterman NH, Strom BL (Univ of Pennsylvania, Philadelphia Assoc for Clinical Trials)
Ann Intern Med 107:900–909, December 1987

The monobactam antibiotics, with a solely gram-negative spectrum of activity, may influence medical costs through eliminating nephrotoxicity associated with aminoglycosides. Costs of aminoglycoside use were examined in 111 patients with nephrotoxicity and 149 others who received aminoglycoside antibiotics without developing nephrotoxicity. Gentamicin, tobramycin, or amikacin was given for 72 hours or longer to study patients, who were aged 18 years or older.

Patients with nephrotoxicity were older than the others and received larger doses of aminoglycoside for a longer time. The length of stay was nearly twice as long for patients with nephrotoxicity. Costs were significantly greater for these patients. The added cost of hospital ancillary services per case of nephrotoxicity was $446, and the added cost of hospital stay was $825 for routine days and $1,152 for intensive care days. The mean total additional cost of aminoglycoside-associated nephrotoxicity was $2,501, and the average added cost per treated patient was $183. Estimated costs of aminoglycoside-associated nephrotoxicity depend on its prevalence.

Aminoglycoside use imposes a significant economic burden on the health care system because of the associated nephrotoxicity. Other complications such as vestibular and auditory toxicity may add significantly to the costs of this treatment.

▶ Because of the low acquisition cost of aminoglycosides, especially gentamicin, there is a tendency to recommend these drugs over the new broad-spectrum beta-lactam antibiotics on a cost basis. This study provides documentation of the cost of nephrotoxicity associated with the use of the aminoglycosides. In addition to the cost of nephrotoxicity, there are added expenses of monitoring of the serum concentration of creatinine and of the aminoglycoside. Accordingly, the true cost differential between the aminoglycosides and the new beta-lactam drugs such as third-generation cephalosporins, aztreonam, imipenem, or combinations of penicillins with beta-lactamase inhibitors may be slight.—M.J. Barza, M.D.

Clinical Response to Aminoglycoside Therapy: Importance of the Ratio of Peak Concentration to Minimal Inhibitory Concentration
Moore RD, Lietman PS, Smith CR (Johns Hopkins Univ School of Medicine)
J Infect Dis 155:93–99, January 1987

Aminoglycosides still are important in the treatment of aerobic gram-negative infections. The peak drug level may interact with the minimal inhibitory concentration (MIC), a strong determinant of clinical response. The value of the trough or geometric mean aminoglycoside level as a determinant of response was studied in 236 patients with gram-negative bacterial infections who participated in clinical trials of gentamicin, tobramycin, and amikacin. Urinary tract infection was most prevalent. More than one third of the patients were bacteremic.

Eighty percent of patients had clinical responses to aminoglycoside

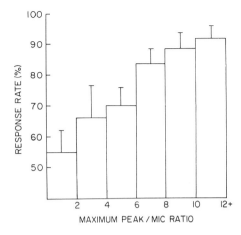

Fig 1-11.—Relationship between the maximal peak level/MIC ratio and rate of clinical response. *Vertical bars* represent SE values. (Courtesy of Moore RD, Lietman PS, Smith CR: *J Infect Dis* 155:93–99, January 1987.)

therapy. Elevated maximum and mean peak aminoglycoside concentration/MIC ratios were closely associated with clinical response. A graded dose-response relation was evident between an increasing maximal peak concentration/MIC ratio and the clinical response (Fig 1–11). This relationship persisted after adjustment for the severity of illness and other response-related factors.

Previous studies have associated higher minimal and peak aminoglycoside levels with clinical efficacy. In the present study, the rate of clinical response increased in a graded manner with increasing peak concentration/MIC ratios. A relatively low MIC is required to keep maximal peak drug levels at nonnephrotoxic concentrations while achieving an adequate response rate. If gentamicin or tobramycin is used alone, a MIC of 2 μg/ml or lower in patients with serious infection or a poor underlying prognosis may be needed in order to keep the maximal serum concentration lower than 10 μg/ml while maintaining an 80% response rate.

▶ Of the various factors predictive of a response to treatment, the most potent was the underlying prognosis (rapidly fatal, ultimately fatal, or nonfatal underlying illness) followed by the maximal peak/MIC ratio. Negative prognostic factors were *Pseudomonas* infection and cutaneous or wound infection.—M.J. Barza, M.D.

Decrease of Caffeine Elimination in Man During Co-Administration of 4-Quinolones
Stille W, Harder S, Mieke S, Beer C, Shah PM, Frech K, Staib AH (Univ of Frankfurt, West Germany)
J Antimicrob Chemother 20:729–734, November 1987   1–41

The pharmacokinetics of theophylline can be altered by simultaneous administration of enoxacin or ciprofloxacin but not ofloxacin. To investigate further, the single-dose pharmacokinetics of caffeine (similar to those of theophylline) were evaluated in a crossover fashion in 12 healthy male volunteers before and during 5-day treatment with ofloxacin (200 mg); ciprofloxacin (250 mg); and enoxacin (400 mg), all given twice a day.

Co-administration of enoxacin caused on average a 2.6-fold prolongation of the elimination half-life of caffeine, while ciprofloxacin caused on average a 15% prolongation. In contrast, ofloxacin had little or no effect on the kinetics of caffeine.

Treatment with ciprofloxacin and enoxacin may have a significant inhibitory effect on caffeine elimination. The therapeutic use of 4-quinolones in patients with liver disease, cardiac arrhythmias, or latent epilepsy may result in unexpected effects following caffeine intake as a result of elevated plasma concentration. Available data suggest that the 4-oxo metabolite of quinolones, rather than the parent drug, inhibits theophylline clearance.

▶ It seems possible that many of the reports of anxiety, tremulousness, and insomnia attributed to the use of enoxacin and ciprofloxacin may be related to caffeine intoxication because of the effect of these drugs on the pharmacokinetics of caffeine. Physicians should remind patients given ciprofloxacin or enoxacin of this possible side effect and of the many beverages including coffee, tea, and cola drinks that contain caffeine.—M.J. Barza, M.D.

Prospective Randomized Controlled Study of Ciprofloxacin Versus Imipenem-Cilastatin in Severe Clinical Infections

Lode H, Wiley R, Höffken G, Wagner J, Borner K (Freie Universität Berlin, West Germany)
Antimicrob Agents Chemother 31:1491–1496, October 1987   1–42

Infection remains a major problem in immunocompromised patients and those with serious underlying disease. The authors evaluated 2 antibiotics covering a broad spectrum of significant pathogens, imipenem and ciprofloxacin, in a prospective study of 66 adult patients with bacterial infection of the respiratory tract, skin, urinary tract, bones or joints, or abdomen. These patients received 500–1,000 mg of imipenem by infusion at 6- or 8-hour intervals. Ciprofloxacin was given in an infusion dose of 100 mg every 8–12 hours, or orally in a usual dose of 1,000 mg daily.

Two thirds of causative organisms were eradicated by ciprofloxacin therapy, and 79%, by imipenem. Two patients failed to respond to ciprofloxacin, and 6 did not respond to imipenem treatment. All the unresponsive patients had fatal underlying disease. Side effects occurred in 25% of imipenem-treated patients and 18% of those given ciprofloxacin. Gastrointestinal and CNS effects predominated in both treatment groups.

Both ciprofloxacin and imipenem give good to excellent clinical results in patients with severe bacterial infections. Both drugs cover most of the causes of complicated respiratory tract infection and septicemia in patients with serious underlying illness. Patterns of resistance must be followed carefully in patients treated with these antimicrobials.

▶ This study showed that intravenously administered ciprofloxacin was about as effective as imipenem in the treatment of severe clinical infections. However, the number of patients studied was small, and important differences in the efficacy and toxicity rates between the two drugs may have been missed. One patient treated with imipenem developed seizures.—M.J. Barza, M.D.

Emergence of Vancomycin Resistance in Coagulase-Negative Staphylococci
Schwalbe RS, Stapleton JT, Gilligan PH (North Carolina Mem Hosp, Chapel Hill; School of Medicine, Univ of North Carolina)
N Engl J Med 316:927–932, April 9, 1987   1–43

Coagulase-negative staphylococci are the cause of many hospital infections, and most isolates are resistant to penicillins. Vancomycin has become the antibiotic of choice for these infections. A case of peritonitis caused by vancomycin-resistant coagulase-negative staphylococci is described.

Man, 37, with diabetes and end-stage renal disease presented with nausea, pain, and cloudy peritoneal fluid from which coagulase-negative staphylococci were isolated. He was treated with cefazolin and tobramycin, but the peritonitis worsened. The isolate was noted to be methicillin-resistant, and vancomycin therapy was initiated. Peritonitis continued, and vancomycin therapy was increased. However, 8 coagulase-negative staphylococcal isolates displayed a stepwise increase in vancomycin resistance from a minimal inhibitory concentration (MIC) of 2 μg/ml to 8 μg/ml in an 88-day period. Treatment with rifampin was initiated, and the peritoneal fluid became clear. Nevertheless, as soon as the rifampin was withdrawn, the patient relapsed. Tobramycin was added, and the symptoms disappeared.

All peritoneal fluid isolates were identified as *Staphylococcus haemolyticus*. An MIC of 8 μg/ml is interpreted as being in the intermediate (relatively resistant) range; thus the clinical isolates were not truly resistant in vivo. However, all of the peritoneal fluid isolates contained stable subpopulations capable of growth on BHI-agar plates containing 8 μg of vancomycin per milliliter. In vitro, a subpopulation was recovered for which the MIC was 128 μg/ml with a starting inoculum of 10^6 colony-forming units. These findings strongly suggest that coagulase-negative staphylococci have the ability to acquire vancomycin resistance. Whether this will become a serious problem is impossible to predict, and current therapeutic alternatives to vancomycin are limited. It would seem wise to identify alternative antibiotics for these infections and to use vancomycin sparingly in prophylaxis.

▶ This is only the third report of the development of resistance of coagulase-negative staphylococci to vancomycin in vivo, which suggests that such an occurrence is remarkably rare. It should be noted that the stresses upon this poor isolate of *Staphylococcus haemolyticus* were impressive: resistance emerged slowly over 88 days of vancomycin treatment. The total bacterial inoculum in the peritoneal fluid was probably also very large, which might facilitate the selection of a resistant subpopulation.—M.J. Barza, M.D.

Adverse and Beneficial Effects of Immediate Treatment of Group A Beta-Hemolytic Streptococcal Pharyngitis With Penicillin
Pichichero ME, Disney FA, Talpey WB, Green JL, Francis AB, Roghmann KJ, Hoekelman RA (Elmwood Pediatric Group, Rochester, NY; Univ of Rochester)
Pediatr Infect Dis J 6:635–643, July 1987

The availability of the "quick strep test" for diagnosis of group A beta-hemolytic streptococcal (GABHS) pharyngitis has created pressure for immediate treatment that would allow patients more prompt relief from the symptoms. A prospective, randomized, double-blind study was conducted to evaluate the effects of immediate penicillin treatment on symptomatic response and recurrent infection in 142 children with GABHS pharyngitis.

Specimens for throat culture, white blood cell count, and acute streptococcal antibody serology were obtained at the initial visit from children with a clinical picture indicating GABHS pharyngitis. A 48-hour supply of penicillin V or placebo was dispensed, and parents were instructed to administer aspirin or acetaminophen as needed for fever and discomfort as well as to keep a diary of temperature, use of analgesic, and clinical symptoms. On day 3, penicillin-treated patients received an additional 8-day supply of penicillin, while children treated with placebo were given a 10-day supply of antibiotic. At a follow-up visit 3 weeks after enrollment, throat culture was repeated; total follow-up for recurrence was extended for 4 months.

Positive cultures for GABHS infection were obtained in 114 children. Immediate treatment was associated with a *higher* incidence of recurrent infections in these children. Early recurrences developed in 14 patients treated with penicillin immediately versus 8 children treated with penicillin after 48 hours, a difference not considered statistically significant ($P = .115$, table). Significantly more late recurrences occurred in the immediately treated group (8 cases) compared to the delayed treatment group (1 case) (see table). There was no significant difference between groups with regard to intrafamilial spread.

Penicillin treatment had a beneficial effect on symptomatic improvement. On day 2, fever was significantly reduced in the group that was treated immediately. Sore throat, dysphagia, lethargy, headache, abdominal pain, and anorexia were also significantly better in children receiving immediate treatment. These patients also used significantly less aspirin or acetaminophen on day 2 than did placebo-treated patients. No statistical difference between treatment groups was found in culture-negative patients. This study demonstrated that immediate treatment of GABHS

Adverse Effects of Immediate Treatment of GABHS
Pharyngitis With Penicillin

Variable	Treatment Group		P*
	Penicillin (n = 59)	Placebo (n = 55)	
Relapse	10 (17)†	8 (15)	0.382
Early recurrence	14 (24)	8 (15)	0.115
Late recurrence	8 (14)	1 (2)	0.035‡
Early and late recurrence	22 (37)	9 (16)	0.025‡

*Treatment groups compared by chi square or Fisher's exact test as appropriate, 1-tailed probability.
†Numbers in parentheses, percent.
‡Significant difference observed.
(Courtesy of Pichichero ME, Disney FA, Talpey WB, et al: *Pediatr Infect Dis J* 6:635–643, July 1987.)

pharyngitis produces both beneficial and adverse effects that should be considered by physicians when managing patients with these infections.

▶ The possible reasons for the finding of a higher rate of recurrence in the patients given immediate as opposed to delayed treatment are worthy of inquiry. There was a suggestion of a lower and less consistent rise in the Streptozyme titer for the group given immediate treatment, but the difference between the groups was not statistically significant. These authors previously showed that penicillin treatment seemed to prevent the development of type-specific immunity to GABHS. Nevertheless, as they point out, other data indicate that type-specific serum bactericidal antibody is not protective against pharyngeal colonization by homologous GABHS. Thus, the authors speculate that the most important effect of early penicillin treatment may be to suppress the formation of secretory IgA in the pharynx; however, this point was not examined specifically. Given that early treatment has now been well shown to ameliorate the symptoms of streptococcal pharyngitis but may also predispose to recurrences, the physician is faced with a therapeutic dilemma.—M.J. Barza, M.D.

Plasmid-Mediated Resistance to Nalidixic Acid in Shigella Dysenteriae Type 1
Munshi MH, Sack DA, Haider K, Ahmed ZU, Rahaman MM, Morshed MG (Internatl Ctr for Diarrhoeal Disease Research, Dhaka, Bangladesh; Johns Hopkins Univ School of Public Health)
Lancet 2:419–421, Aug 22, 1987

Shigellosis is a major diarrheal disease in developing countries. *Shigella dysenteriae* type 1 strains isolated from a Bangladeshi epidemic proved to be resistant to nalidixic acid. These strains, isolated from 161 patients, were also resistant to tetracycline, ampicillin, streptomycin, co-trimoxazole, and chloramphenicol, but were sensitive to mecillinam. All 19 of the resistant strains analyzed contained a 20-megadalton (Mdal) plasmid that was not found in sensitive strains. During conjugation experiments, transfer of this plasmid to *Escherichia coli* strains was associated with resistance to nalidixic acid. The resistance to nalidixic acid, apparently mediated by a 20-Mdal conjugative plasmid, is especially problematic because nalidixic acid is the drug that has been used in the past to treat resistant strains of *S. dysenteriae*.

▶ If these data are true and confirmed, it will be of importance for treatment of invasive diarrhea in the Third World, where nalidixic acid has become a mainstay for drug-resistant shigellosis. If there is plasmid transmissible resistance, nalidixic acid resistance will spread rapidly, and unless the new quinolones can be shown to be safe for children (they are certainly effective) and cheap enough to be readily available, I am afraid many will die of untreatable infections.—G.T. Keusch, M.D.

Second Episodes of *Haemophilus influenzae* Type b Disease Following Rifampin Prophylaxis of the Index Patients
Cates KL, Krause PJ, Murphy TV, Stutman HR, Granoff DM (Univ of Connecticut School of Medicine; Univ of Texas Southwestern Med School; Univ of California, Irvine; Washington Univ School of Medicine)
Pediatr Infect Dis J 6:512–515, June 1987   1–46

Patients treated with ampicillin or chloramphenicol for *Hemophilus influenzae* type b disease are at increased risk of recurrence, as those patients often remain nasopharyngeal carriers of the organism and fail to develop protective levels of antibodies against the organism. Rifampin prophylaxis in the index patient may prevent such recurrence by eliminating *H. influenzae* type b carriage. The authors report their experience in 9 children who had recurrent invasive *H. influenzae* type b disease despite prophylactic treatment with rifampin.

Six boys and 3 girls, aged 5–17 months, with *H. influenzae* type b disease, were treated for 10 days or longer with drug regimens that included rifampin for prophylactic purposes. All 9 patients developed a second episode of *H. influenzae* type b disease after periods ranging from 9 to 138 days following discharge from hospitalization for the first episode (table).

Analysis of biotypes and outer membrane protein polyacrylamide gel electrophoresis patterns of paired isolates obtained from 8 children revealed that the second episodes in 2 children were caused by a new type of *H. influenzae* type b strain. In the other 6 children, the second episodes were caused by isolates that were indistinguishable from those obtained during the first episodes of disease. Rifampin prophylaxis of the index patient may prevent some episodes of recurrent disease, but in some patients, second episodes may be caused by organisms acquired from contacts who did not receive rifampicin prophylaxis or from acquisition of new *H. influenzae* type b strains.

Patients With Recurrent Invasive *Hemophilus influenzae* Type B Disease*

Patient	Age (mos) First Infection	Site of First Infection †	Duration (Days) of Antimicrobial Therapy (Including Rifampin)	Interval (Days) between End of Rifampin and Start of Second Infection	Site of Second Infection	Outer Membrane Protein Subtype (Biotype)	
						First infection	Second infection
1	6½	Meningitis	10	9	Suppurative arthritis	2 H (I)	2 H (I)
2	5½	Meningitis	10	11	Meningitis	1 H (I)	1 H (I)
3	17	Meningitis	13	13	Epiglottitis	2 L (I)	2 L (I)
4	5½	Meningitis	14	80	Meningitis	1 H (I)	1 H (I)
5	5	Meningitis	14	107	Meningitis	1 H (I)	1 H (I)
6	9	Meningitis	14	138	Septic arthritis	1 H (I)	1 H (I)
7	11	Pneumonia	10	70	Pneumonia	3.1 L (IV)	1 H (I)
8	10½	Meningitis	14	91	Pneumonia	3‒‡(II)	3 L (I)
9	5½	Left buccal cellulitis	14	13	Right buccal cellulitis, meningitis	ND	ND

*ND = not done.
†All episodes of infection were accompanied by *Hemophilus influenzae* type b bacteremia except for the first episode in patient 3, which was documented by a positive cerebrospinal fluid culture for *H. influenzae* type b.
‡The H/L protein was absent from this *H. influenzae* type b isolate.
(Courtesy of Cates KL, Krause PJ, Murphy TV, et al: *Pediatr Infect Dis J* 6:512–515, June 1987.)

Malignant External Otitis: Comparison of Monotherapy Vs Combination Therapy
Meyers BR, Mendelson MH, Parisier SC, Hirschman SZ (Mount Sinai School of Medicine, New York)
Arch Otolaryngol Head Neck Surg 113:974–978, September 1987   1–47

Pseudomonas aeruginosa is the major cause of malignant external otitis (MEO) in diabetic patients. Cases of MEO are treated primarily with an antipseudomonal penicillin and an aminoglycoside for a minimum of 6 weeks. For this study, 20 patients with MEO were given either standard therapy or an antipseudomonal cephalosporin (cefsulodin sodium) monotherapy and were retrospectively compared.

The clinical features and patient course are summarized in the table. Among the patients who received standard therapy, 64% were cured. Among the patients who received monotherapy, 70% were cured. Follow-up ranged from 5 to 57 months. Less extensive infection was correlated with a more favorable outcome in both groups. Monotherapy with cefsulodin compared favorably with conventional therapy in MEO patients.

▶ There have been progressive refinements in our recognition and treatment of patients with malignant external otitis. Early reports emphasize the need for extensive surgical débridement, which was often not successful. The advent of antipseudomonal penicillins and aminoglycosides led to a more conservative approach that included a long course of these antibiotics coupled to local débridement only.

In this report, patients were treated with an antipseudomonal cephalosporin that was found to be as effective as the combination of an antipseudomonal penicillin and aminoglycoside. It is noteworthy, however, that the patients in the historical control group who received combination therapy may have had more extensive disease, at least as judged by the incidence of cranial nerve palsies or paresis. Only 33% of the patients in the cephalosporin group had cranial nerve abnormality, whereas 64% in the historical controls presented with

Clinical Features and Course of Patients

Age	Sex		Total
	Male	Female	
1 month to 18 years	144	129	273
19 to 65 years	885	623	1,508
65 years or older	472	286	758
Unknown	1	1	2
Total	1,501	1,038	2,539
Mean (years)	50.1	47.3	49.0
Range (years)	9–94	0–99	0–99

(Courtesy of Meyers BR, Mendelson MH, Parisier SC, et al: Arch Otolaryngol Head Neck Surg 113:974–978, September 1987.)

this problem. Therefore, the equality of the outcome may not reflect an equality of therapeutic efficacy for patients whose disease is recognized late in its course.—M.S. Klempner, M.D.

Platelet-Mediated Bleeding Caused by Broad-Spectrum Penicillins
Fass RJ, Copelan EA, Brandt JT, Moeschberger ML, Ashton JJ (Ohio State Univ)
J Infect Dis 155:1242–1248, June 1987   1–48

The β-lactam antibiotics have been implicated in clinically significant bleeding, possibly through producing platelet dysfunction. Hospitalized patients who received ticarcillin, piperacillin, or mezlocillin were followed prospectively, along with others given cefotaxime, a β-lactam antibiotic not known to cause platelet dysfunction. The study included 156 adults given intravenous antibiotic therapy.

An increased bleeding time was most frequently associated with ticarcillin therapy. Both the total incidence of bleeding and the incidence of serious bleeding also were more frequent with ticarcillin, followed by piperacillin. Bleeding was associated with an increase in bleeding time of 5 minutes or more from baseline, a prolonged pretreatment bleeding time, and a maximal bleeding time of 16 minutes or more during treatment. Choice of antibiotic was not a significant factor when adjusted for an increased bleeding time or the peak observed bleeding time, indicating that the mechanism of bleeding was platelet dysfunction.

Penicillin-induced platelet dysfunction is an important risk factor for bleeding and is additive to other risk factors such as thrombocytopenia, hypoprothrombinemia, and azotemia. Monitoring treated patients for platelet dysfunction by measuring the bleeding time will identify those at increased risk for developing clinical bleeding.

Antibiotic Penetration Into Rabbit Nucleus Pulposus
Eismont FJ, Wiesel SW, Brighton CT, Rothman RH (Univ of Miami; George Washington Univ; Univ of Pennsylvania)
Spine 12:254–256, April 1987   1–49

Disk space infection in adults is a serious illness with high morbidity, but the lack of a vascular supply in the human adult intervertebral disk means that metabolites must diffuse passively into the disk space. Penetration of various antibiotics was examined in a model using rabbit nucleus pulposus. Oxacillin, cephalothin, clindamycin, and tobramycin were administered by serial intramuscular injection on varying schedules.

Penetration of clindamycin into nucleus pulposus averaged 62% of serum levels; the average serum level was 9.3 μg/ml. Tobramycin levels in serum averaged 8.7 μg/ml, and penetration averaged 58% of the serum level. Cephalothin concentrations in the disk averaged less than 4% of serum levels. Oxacillin penetrated to only 22% of the serum level.

Both clindamycin and tobramycin diffuse readily into the rabbit intervertebral disk. Equivocal results can be obtained with cephalothin; the situation with oxacillin is uncertain. The findings are probably applicable to antibiotic penetration into human nucleus pulposus, for the rabbit and human disks are anatomically and biochemically similar. Less limited penetration of antibiotics is expected in children, in whom a vascular supply to the disk space is present.

▶ We do not, as a rule, select animal studies for YEAR BOOK, unless the data are unique. This is the case in this study of antibiotic penetration into rabbit nucleus pulposus, a study just not possible in humans. Four drugs with antistaphylococcal activity were studied including a n-lactam (oxacillin), a first-generation cephalosporin (cephalothin), an aminoglycoside (tobramycin), and clindamycin. Unfortunately, the drugs were given by intramuscular injection, a now less common (and inhumane) way to give prolonged antimicrobial treatment. The results show that clindamycin and tobramycin achieved the best levels in the nucleus pulposus, approaching 60% of serum levels, and exceeding by many times the minimal inhibitory concentration for *Staphylococcus aureus*.

While penetration of cephalothin and oxacillin were poor under the conditions of the study, this is not tantamount to saying neither drug would work in disk space infection. Rather the message is that you may get more for your money from antibiotics penetrating the disk well. Clinical studies are always the bottom line, and patients certainly respond to oxacillin. Whether or not there is an important advantage to clindamycin could only be shown by a comparative clinical trial.—G.T. Keusch, M.D.

Miscellaneous Topics

Outbreak of Fever Caused by *Streptobacillus moniliformis*
McEvoy MB, Noah ND, Pilsworth R (Public Health Lab Service Communicable Disease Surveillance Ctr, London)
Lancet 2:1361–1363, Dec 12, 1987   1–50

Forty-three percent of the 700 students and staff members at a boarding school in Britain became ill with streptobacillary fever in 1983. This outbreak was the first of its kind in the United Kingdom. The fever is caused by *Streptobacillus moniliformis,* an organism usually found in rats. Such an epidemic, occurring without direct contact with rats, is rare. An outbreak in Haverhill, Massachusetts, in 1926 was apparently caused by raw milk, and the 1983 epidemic described here was likely a result of infected water.

The cases appeared over a 10-day period in February. Symptoms included a rash concentrated on the extremities, fever, and severe pain in the joints. Boarding students had a significantly higher incidence of the disease than day students because of their greater exposure to contaminated water. Although raw milk served at the school was first suspected, investigation showed that spring water probably carried the organism.

Many of the students remained in bed for weeks and relapses were common, but no deaths occurred and no complications developed among the young victims. After the organism was isolated, erythromycin was administered.

Although streptobacillary fever is rare, the possibility of an outbreak exists when a water supply is open to contamination. Public health officials recommend monitoring of water not supplied by mains and control of the rat population as effective preventive measures.

▶ A nice epidemiologic study of a large number of cases of Haverhill fever.—S.M. Wolff, M.D.

Seasonal Variation of Transmission Risk of Lyme Disease and Human Babesiosis
Piesman J, Mather TN, Dammin GJ, Telford SR III, Lastavica CC, Spielman A (Univ of Alabama in Birmingham; Harvard Univ; Tufts Univ)
Am J Epidemiol 126:1187–1189, December 1987   1–51

In the Midwestern and Northeastern United States, Lyme disease and babesiosis are transmitted by nymphal *Ixodes dammini*. The authors sought to determine when the maximal risk of contact with an infected tick occurs.

Host-seeking ticks were collected, and the number of ticks collected per person-hour was determined during at least 3 hours on 2 days of each month between April and September inclusively (table, p. 60). Nymphs were examined for *Babesia* sporozoites and Lyme disease spirochetes.

The proportion of ticks infected with *Babesia* did not differ from that of ticks infected with Lyme disease. There was a significant seasonal variation in the transmission risk for both diseases. The number of host-seeking infected ticks was largest in May and June but fell sharply in July.

Because of seasonal tourism, the number of persons exposed to infection by *I. dammini*-borne pathogens is increased. Visitors to sites endemic for tick-borne zoonotic diseases are at greatest risk if they begin their vacations during May and June.

▶ This paper reminds us that the peak incidence of ticks infected with *Babesia* and *Borrelia* occurs in the spring and early summer and decreases in July, August, and September in Nantucket. What is even more striking is the coincidence of infection of ticks by both *Babesia* and *Borrelia*. In patients who are diagnosed with one or the other of these illnesses, failure to respond to therapy should prompt a search for the other pathogen.—M.S. Klempner, M.D.

The Clinical Evolution of Lyme Arthritis
Steere AC, Schoen RT, Taylor E (Yale Univ School of Medicine)
Ann Intern Med 107:725–731, November 1987   1–52

Seasonal Variation of Transmission Risk for Lyme Disease (Borrelia burgdorferi) and Babesiosis (Babesia microti) on Nantucket Island, 1985

Month	No. of nymphs per person-hour	% nymphs infected		No. of infected nymphs per person-hour	
		Babesia	Borrelia	Babesia	Borrelia
April	11.0	20.0	50.0	2.2	5.5
May	37.3	46.5	43.5	17.3	16.2
June	35.4	43.3	45.0	15.2	15.9
July	6.6	23.1	44.4	1.5	2.9
August	4.6	36.4	30.0	1.7	1.4
September	2.0	20.0	28.6	0.4	0.6

(Courtesy of Piesman J, Mather TN, Dammin GJ, et al: *Am J Epidemiol* 126:1187–1189, December 1987.)

Lyme disease, a complex infection caused by the tick-borne spirochete *Borrelia burgdorferi,* was first described in 1975 in a group of children in Lyme, Connecticut. Joint involvement in these children was characterized by brief, recurrent attacks of asymmetric swelling and pain in some large joints, particularly the knees. A previous annular skin lesion, erythema chronicum migrans, was then recognized as the first illness manifestation. In the late 1970s, before the role of antibiotic therapy in treating patients with Lyme disease was known, patients were enrolled in a prospective study to determine the natural history of Lyme arthritis.

Through a surveillance system of community-based physicians, an attempt was made to find all patients with erythema chronicum migrans in the Lyme area. The 55 patients who did not receive antibiotic therapy for this condition were followed longitudinally for a mean of 6 years. The frequency, duration, and spectrum of joint involvement were studied. Eleven patients, or 20%, had no subsequent manifestations of Lyme disease beyond the erythema chronicum migrans. One day to 8 weeks after disease onset, 10 patients, or 18%, began to suffer brief episodes of joint, periarticular, or musculoskeletal pain for up to 6 years but never developed objective joint abnormalities.

Four days to 2 years after disease onset, 28 patients, or 51%, had 1 episode of or began to have intermittent attacks of frank arthritis, especially in large joints. A few patients had polyarticular movement. The number of patients who continued to have recurrences decreased by 10%–20% each year (Fig 1–12). The remaining 6 patients, or 11%, developed chronic synovitis later in the illness. Of these, 2 had erosions, and 1 had permanent joint disability.

This study was begun soon after Lyme arthritis was first recognized with the goal of determining the disorder's natural history. The spectrum

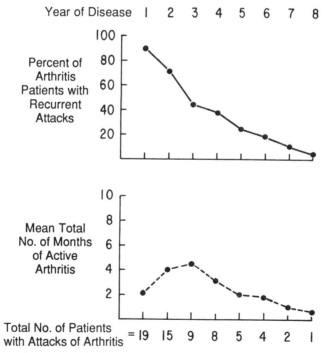

Fig 1–12.—The percentage of arthritis patients with recurrent attacks *(top)* and the mean total number of months of active arthritis by year of disease *(bottom)*. Nineteen of the 21 patients had attacks of arthritis during the first year of illness, and the number of patients who continued to have recurrences decreased by 10% to 20% each year. The mean total number of months of active arthritis was 4 months and 5 months during the second and third years of illness and decreased to 2 months or less by the fifth year. (Courtesy of Steere AC, Schoen RT, Taylor E: *Ann Intern Med* 107:725–731, November 1987.)

of Lyme arthritis was found to range from subjective joint pain to intermittent attacks of arthritis to chronic erosive disease.

▶ We now know that the arthritis of Lyme disease is due to the presence of *B. burgdorferi* (see the 1988 YEAR BOOK OF INFECTIOUS DISEASES, pp 59–61) and is treatable with penicillin or ceftriaxone (see the 1987 YEAR BOOK OF INFECTIOUS DISEASES, pp 57–59; Dattwyler RJ et al: *J Infect Dis* 155:1322–1325, 1987). This study provides an overview of the natural history of untreated Lyme arthritis.—D.R. Snydman, M.D.

Lyme Disease: Cause of a Treatable Peripheral Neuropathy
Halperin JJ, Little BW, Coyle PK, Dattwyler RJ (State Univ of New York, Stony Brook)
Neurology 37:1700–1706, November 1987
1–53

Lyme disease, caused by the spirochete *Borrelia burgdorferi*, is a multisystem infection with neurologic involvement. Mild peripheral neuropathy was present in 14 patients with proven Lyme disease. The average age was 43 years (Table 1), and the average duration of Lyme disease was 35 months.

Neurologic symptoms ranged from severe meningoencephalitis to mild intermittent paresthesias of the fingers (Table 2). Sensory conduction was

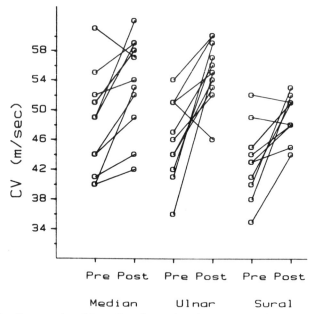

Fig 1–13.—Representation of the median, ulnar, and sural sensory potential conduction velocity (m/sec) before (pre) and several months after (post) antibiotic treatment. (Courtesy of Halperin JJ, Little BW, Coyle PK, et al: *Neurology* 37:1700–1706, November 1987.)

TABLE 1.—Patient Characteristics

	Age	Sex	Tick bite	ECM	Anti-Lyme Ab	Arthritis	Duration	Prior Rx	Definitive Rx
Symptomatic patients:									
1	51	M	+	+	*	+	4 mos	TCN, PCN	CFTX
2	55	M	?	+	+	+	?6 yrs	PCN	PCN
3	40	F	?	+	+	−	?5 yrs	PCN	CFTX
4	30	M	+	+	*	−	1 mo	—	CFTX
5	39	M	?	−	+	+	1 yr	TCN, PCN	CFTX
6	69	F	?	?	+	+	3 mos	PCN, TCN	PCN
7	48	F	?	+	+	−	3 yrs	PCN	CFTX
8	33	M	+	+	+	−	4 mos	PCN	CHLOR
9	37	F	?	+	+	−	9 mos	—	PCN PO
10	59	M	+	+	+	+	5 yrs	—	PCN PO
11	47	M	+	+	+	+	?10 yrs	PCN, proben	AMOX PO
12	48	M	?	+	+	+	6 yrs	PCN	PCN
13	29	F	?	−	+	+	6 mos	PCN, proben	PCN PO
14	17	M	+	+	+	+	2 yrs	—	CFTX
Asymptomatic patients:									
15	32	M	+	+	+	+	2 yrs	—	
16	26	M	+	−	+	+	2.5 yrs	PCN; PCN & proben	
17	35	M	?	+	+	+	1 yr	TCN; PCN & proben	

*Negative Lyme serology but positive assay of cell-mediated immune response to Lyme spirochete.
ECM, erythema chronicum migrans.
Prior Rx: PCN, penicillin orally; TCN, tetracycline orally; proben, probenecid.
Definitive Rx: CFTX, ceftriaxone, 2 gm twice daily for 14 days; PCN, 24 million units intravenously daily for 10 days; PCN PO, penicillin VK, 4 gm orally, and probenecid, 2 gm daily for 30 days; CHLOR, chloramphenicol, 4 gm intravenously daily for 10 days; AMOX PO, amoxicillin, 2 gm orally, and probenecid, 2 gm daily for 30 days.
(Courtesy of Halperin JJ, Little BW, Coyle PK, et al: *Neurology* 37:1700–1706, November 1987.)

64 / Infectious Diseases

TABLE 2.—Neurologic Findings

	History		Mental status change	Radic pain	Exam			
	Pares-thesias	Bell's palsy			Sensory	Motor	DTRs	Misc
1	+	−	−	−	NL	NL	NL	Mild L V, VII
2	+	+	−	−	Mild SG	NL	NL	
3	+	−	+	−	NL	NL	NL	Headache, tinnitus
4	+	−	−	−	Mild SG	NL	NL	
5	+	−	+	+	Mild SG + Ulnar dig	NL	NL	
6	+	+	−	−	Mod SG	Mod	Decr	Dysarthria, confusion, dizzy, headache
7	+	−	+	+	NL	NL	NL	
8	+	−	+	−	NL	NL	NL	
9	+	−	−	+	NL	NL	NL	+Tinel's
10	+	−	−	−	NL	NL	NL	Low back pain
11	+	−	−	−	NL	NL	NL	"sciatica"
12	−	−	−	−	NL	NL	NL	
13	+	−	−	−	NL	NL	NL	Facial m. twitching
14	+	−	−	−	NL	NL	NL	
15	−	−	−	−	NL	NL	NL	
16	−	−	−	−	NL	NL	NL	
17	+	−	−	+	NL	NL	NL	"Sciatica," left cts

NL, normal; Decr, decreased; Mod, moderate; SG, stocking-glove neuropathy; V, VII, mild dysfunction of cranial nerves V and VII.
(Courtesy of Halperin JJ, Little BW, Coyle PK, et al: *Neurology* 37:1700–1706, November 1987.)

abnormal in 13 patients, and motor terminal latencies were prolonged in 10. After antibiotic treatment, all patients had significant clinical improvement, especially in sensory conduction velocity (Fig 1–13), amplitude, and motor terminal latency.

▶ A large number of neurologic complications of Lyme disease have been reported, including Bell's palsy, aseptic meningitis, brachial neuritis, painful polyradiculoneuritis, mononeuritis multiplex, a Guillain-Barré-like syndrome, and encephalopathy. While the authors have seen a considerable number of patients with Lyme disease, the incidence of these complications has been rare indeed, and the most common neurologic complaint has been intermittent paresthesias. Extensive peripheral nerve testing was performed on 36 patients with late Lyme disease and revealed peripheral nerve dysfunction in 13 of the 14 patients with prominent limb paresthesias. Almost all of the patients had received previous antibiotic therapy (penicillin or tetracycline), but further therapy with ceftriaxone, penicillin, amoxicillin, or chloramphenicol in 1 patient each led to a marked improvement in symptoms in 11 of the 12 patients. Similar improvement was documented by the nerve conduction studies.

Since paresthesias are such an easily dismissible symptom and are often associated with a normal neurologic exam, this paper should certainly heighten the awareness of practitioners in Lyme endemic areas to this treatable manifestation of the disease. The pathogenesis of this syndrome remains unclear.—M.S. Klempner, M.D.

Brazilian Purpuric Fever: Epidemic Purpura Fulminans Associated With Antecedent Purulent Conjunctivitis
Brazilian Purpuric Fever Study Group (Instituto Adolfo Lutz, São Paulo, Brazil; São Paulo Ministry of Health; Promissao Gen Hosp, São Paulo; Parana Ministry of Health, Londrina, Brazil; Hosp Emilio Ribas; et al)
Lancet 2:757–761, Oct 3, 1987   1–54

In 1984, 10 children in Promissao, Brazil developed high fever, vomiting, and abdominal pain. Within 12–48 hours, purpura, vascular collapse, and peripheral necrosis developed. All 10 children died.

Cerebrospinal fluid examinations did not indicate meningitis (table). Other examinations did not identify the cause. Another cluster of cases was uncovered in another town, as well as sporadic cases in 5 other cities. Two case-control studies found that those children who became ill were significantly more likely to have had conjunctivitis during the month preceding illness. The conjunctivitis was purulent and resolved before the onset of fever. *Hemophilus aegyptius* was the most common pathogen isolated from conjunctival cultures during this time.

This report summarizes the characteristics of the purpuric illness that occurred in Brazil in 1984. This illness, called Brazilian purpuric fever, affected young children and was fulminant and often fatal. The data suggest that Brazilian purpuric fever is a previously unknown illness, possibly associated with *H. aegyptius*.

Summary of Clinical Laboratory Evaluations of Children
With Brazilian Purpuric Fever: 1984–1985

Laboratory test	No of cases tested	Mean (median; range)
CSF:		
White blood cells (/μl)	22	26 (19; 1–57)
Polymorphs (%)	18	6 (5; 0–19)
Lymphocytes (%)	18	18 (19; 2–38)
Glucose (mg/dl)	21	54 (56; 21–108)
Protein (mg/dl)	22	28 (28; 12–61)
Blood:		
Haemoglobin (g/dl)	7	11·1 (11·4; 9·1–12·7)
Haemotocrit (%)	17	35·9 (35·8; 29·0–48·0)
White blood cells (1000/μl)	19	13·2 (12·0; 3·5–34·0)
Bands (%)	14	14 (13; 2–32)
Polymorphs (%)	16	56 (55; 21–90)
Lymphocytes (%)	12	29 (31; 1–57)
Platelets (1000/μl)	14	77 (50; 12–247)
Fibrinogen (mg/dl)	10	312 (310; 30–573)
PT (s)	11	36 (27; 16–98)
Serum protein (g/dl)	9	5·6 (6·4; 2·2–7·3)

(Courtesy of Brazilian Purpuric Fever Study Group: Lancet 2:757–761, Oct 3, 1987.)

Haemophilus aegyptius Bacteraemia in Brazilian Purpuric Fever

Brazilian Purpuric Fever Study Group (Instituto Adolfo Lutz, São Paulo, Brazil; São Paulo Ministry of Health; Univ of São Paulo; Hosp das Clinicas; Ctrs for Disease Control, Atlanta)
Lancet 2:761–763, Oct 3, 1987

1–55

Brazilian purpuric fever (BPF) was first observed in the town of Promissao, Brazil, in 1984. It was associated with a preceding purulent conjunctivitis. In 1986, another cluster of BPF cases occurred in Serrana, Brazil. The study group reports on the isolation of *Hemophilus aegyptius* from these BPF patients.

Nine patients had positive blood cultures, 1 patient had a positive cerebrospinal fluid culture (contaminated with blood), and 1 patient had a positive conjunctival culture. Each case was compared to 2 age-matched controls. The patients were aged 1–6 years. Five of the 11 patients died. Ten of the patients had a recent history of conjunctivitis, whereas only 6 of 20 controls had a recent history of conjunctivitis. Brazilian purpuric fever patients who received systemic antibiotics prior to the onset of petechiae or purpura had a better chance of survival.

The isolation of *H. aegyptius* from patients with BPF suggests that this organism plays a role in the pathogenesis of this disease. Blood cultures appear to be a sensitive method for BPF diagnosis. Early antibiotic therapy is associated with improved survival. Further study is necessary to determine optimal therapeutic approaches.

▶ A very unusual disease presenting as a "culture-negative meningococcemia"-like illness associated with a resolving conjunctivitis apparently due to *H. aegyptius* (*H. influenzae* biotype III) and high plasma levels of endotoxin probably from *H. aegyptius* bacteremia. These two papers (Abstracts 1–54 and 1–55) describe results from 2 outbreaks of BPF in 1984 and 1986. Only in *Lancet* could you separate the 2 papers, but we will provide just 1 comment.

The Brazilian purpuric fever group deserves credit for the initial observations suggesting the connection between BPF and *H. aegyptius* from the 1984 outbreak and for being ready to jump on the next outbreak and to culture the organism from blood from a significant number of subjects. The data suggest that the strains may have plasmid virulence markers, that topical treatment of the conjunctivitis does not prevent BPF, and that a parenteral antibiotic be given to patients with high fever following conjunctivitis in the endemic zone for BPF. I can't argue.—G.T. Keusch, M.D.

Placebo-Controlled Trial of Intravenous Penicillin for Severe and Late Leptospirosis
Watt G, Padre LP, Tuazon ML, Calubaquib C, Santiago E, Ranoa CP, Laughlin LW (US Naval Med Research Unit 2, San Lazaro Hosp, Manila, Philippines)
Lancet 1:433–435, Feb 27, 1988   1–56

Antibiotics may be effective against leptospirosis only if given early in the course of disease. Parenteral penicillin is standard treatment for late or severe leptospirosis, or Weil's syndrome, in the Philippines and other developing countries. A double-blind placebo-controlled trial was undertaken in 42 patients with severe, advanced leptospirosis in Manila. Penicillin was given intravenously in a daily dose of 6 million units for 1 week.

No patient died, and none required dialysis. Penicillin shortened the time of fever and the time of elevated creatinine. The hospital stay also was shortened significantly by penicillin therapy. Positive cultures for leptospires were more frequent among placebo patients than among those given penicillin. After the start of treatment, leptospires were isolated from 58% of placebo recipients and only 13% of penicillin-treated patients.

Intravenously administered penicillin is effective in patients with severe leptospirosis, even if given late in the course of illness. Good results are obtained in the patients for whom optimal treatment is most important, those with potentially fatal disease. The beneficial effect of penicillin on the affected kidney is particularly salutary. By eradicating leptospires, penicillin shortens the time of renal dysfunction, and thereby the period of susceptibility to renal failure and death.

▶ Previous studies have suggested that the usual treatments of leptospirosis, i.e., penicillin G or one of the tetracyclines, are of uncertain benefit or at most are beneficial only if given in the first few days of symptomatic disease. This study showed a significant clinical benefit from the administration of penicillin G even when treatment was started a mean of at least 9 days after the onset of illness. Among the differences between this and previous studies was that the penicillin G was given in high dosage and intravenously in this study, though not in previous ones.—M.J. Barza, M.D.

The Relationship of Tampon Characteristics to Menstrual Toxic Shock Syndrome
Berkley SF, Hightower AW, Broome CV, Reingold AL (Ctrs for Disease Control, Atlanta)
JAMA 258:917–920, Aug 21, 1987

Early studies of toxic shock syndrome (TSS) showed the use of tampons to be a risk factor. Furthermore, some brands increased this risk, though the reasons for the danger in using certain tampons was not adequately explained. A study of the relationship between tampons and TSS could provide a safer product and a better understanding of the disease.

The authors used data from their records as well as information from a national survey taken in 1983 and 1984. Women who used only a single brand of tampon were included in the study. Various brands were categorized according to their composition and degree of absorbency. The number of cases of TSS among users of different brands was determined, and these statistics were compared to the incidence of cases among non-tampon users.

Of the 399 cases of menstrual-related TSS reported to the Centers for Disease Control in 1983 and 1984, 392 involved women using tampons. All of the brands proved to offer a higher risk for TSS than nonuse of tampons. A tampon's absorbency was found to be significant in its degree of risk: for each 1-gm increase in absorbency, the likelihood of TSS increased 37%. Tampons made of polyacrylate fiber were associated with higher risk, but when their greater absorbency was taken into account, the risk factor might actually be lower than that of cotton/rayon tampons.

Since a tampon's safety seems linked to its absorbency, manufacturers should consider lowering absorbency and adopting a standardized classification for tampons. Although TSS is a rare disease, even the small degree of risk that now exists with tampons could be eliminated.

▶ In 1982, I was the chairman of the Institute of Medicine's Committee on the Toxic Shock Syndrome. In our report (*Toxic Shock Syndrome: Assessment of Current Information and Future Research Needs.* National Academy Press, 1982), we advised the use of low-absorbency tampons (if tampons were used) to lower the risk of toxic shock syndrome. The paper by Berkley et al. provides further epidemiologic support for such a recommendation.—S.M. Wolff, M.D.

Impact of Intensive Care Management on the Prognosis of Tetanus: Analysis of 641 Cases
Trujillo MH, Castillo A, España J, Manzo A, Zerpa R (Univ Hosp of Caracas, Venezuela)
Chest 92:63–65, July 1987

TABLE 1.—Causes of Death in ICU-Treated Patients

Cause	No. of Patients	% of Total
Cardiovascular		
Cardiac arrest	18	39.13
Myocardial infarction	5	10.87
Pulmonary embolism	2	4.34
Hemorrhage from erosion of innominate artery	2	4.34
Respiratory		
Aspiration pneumonitis	3	6.52
Barotrauma	2	4.34
Massive hemoptysis	1	2.17
Displaced tracheostomy tube	1	2.17
Infection		
Puerperal sepsis	4	8.69
Nonpuerperal sepsis	4	8.69
Other		
Upper GI bleeding	4	8.69
Total	46	100.00

(Courtesy of Trujillo MH, Castillo A, Espaā J, et al: Chest 92:63–65, July 1987.)

TABLE 2.—Stages of Tetanus According to Clinical Course and Management

Phase	Clinical Course	Management
1	Severe tetanospasms Autonomic overactivity	Ventilatory support Tracheostomy Curarization, sedation β-blockers, penicillin Wound excision, immunization Total enteral nutrition
2	Opportunistic infections	Add appropriate antibiotic therapy
3	Tonic muscle spasms Residual coma due to sedation	Add active physical therapy Wean curarization, sedation, and ventilatory support
4	Tonic muscle spasms, inadequate deglution, and management of secretions	Airway protection, continue physical therapy, early mobilization, and wean tube feeding

(Courtesy of Trujillo MH, Castillo A, Espaā J, et al: Chest 92:63–65, July 1987.)

Tetanus remains an important health problem in the third world. The authors describe the impact of intensive care management on 306 tetanus patients, compared to 335 patients treated prior to the creation of the intensive care unit (ICU).

Tetanus was the most common cause of admission to the ICU, composing 9.63% of admissions. The mortality in the ICU-treated tetanus group was 15.03%. In the group of tetanus patients treated prior to the creation of the ICU, mortality was 43.58%. The leading cause of death among the ICU patients was cardiac arrest, whereas among the non-ICU patients, it was respiratory failure (Table 1). All patients in the ICU-treated group were maintained for 23 ± 12 days, allowing observation of the natural history of tetanus (Table 2).

Use of the ICU in the treatment of tetanus results in an almost fourfold reduction in mortality. The most common cause of death among these patients was cardiac failure, which has been attributed to overactivity of the autonomic nervous system. It is clear that treatment of tetanus must take place in an ICU.

▶ Let us not forget this is an entirely vaccine-preventable disease. Nearly 10,000 ICU days were used in the care of 306 patients. That's a lot of resources for a preventable disease. The cost of care and the cost of prevention are probably not that different, with a considerable savings in human life and suffering.—G.T. Keusch, M.D.

Expression of *Campylobacter jejuni* Invasiveness in Cell Cultures Coinfected With Other Bacteria
Bukholm G, Kapperud G (Univ of Oslo; Norwegian College of Veterinary Medicine, Oslo)
Infect Immun 55:2816–2821, November 1987   1–59

Campylobacter jejuni frequently is found in mixed infections with other bacterial enteropathogens. The authors attempted to learn whether coinfection with other pathogens influences the interaction of *C. jejuni* with cultured cells and found that coinfectants enhance the ability of *C. jejuni* to localize in epithelial cells. Six strains of *C. jejuni* and 2 of *C. coli* isolated from human clinical specimens were used in the study, which employed monolayers of the human epithelial cell lines HEp-2 and A-549.

Pure cultures of either *Campylobacter* failed to invade the cell monolayers. Four of the 8 strains, however, localized intracellularly when cells were challenged with a mixture of campylobacters and enteroinvasive *Salmonella typhimurium, Shigella flexneri, Shigella boydii, Shigella sonnei*, or *Escherichia coli* strains. Invasiveness also was induced by a nonenteroinvasive *E. coli* strain. *Salmonella typhimurium* was most effective in inducing internalization of campylobacters. None of the *Campylobacter* strains was pathogenic in the guinea pig eye, even if coinfectants were present.

It appears that *C. jejuni* metabolism is essential for its invasiveness, but the mechanisms involved are uncertain. A microaerobic atmosphere is necessary for intracellular localization of the organism.

► This in vitro study was interesting to me because it suggests that interactions between microorganisms in mixed infections can influence the expression of putative virulence traits such as cell invasiveness. Invasion is generally thought to be an intrinsic property of a pathogen, although it may be specific for cells possessing certain surface characteristics. This study suggests that *Campylobacter jejuni* can become invasive in the presence of other microorganisms, but it does not tell us whether the influence of coinfection is on the *C. jejuni* itself (? altered metabolism) or on the host cell to alter permissiveness. Moreover, the importance of this for the real world of infection has yet to be demonstrated. We'll keep you posted on this one.— G.T. Keusch, M.D.

Microbial Endophthalmitis Resulting From Ocular Trauma
Affeldt JC, Flynn HW Jr, Forster RK, Mandelbaum S, Clarkson JG, Jarus GD
(Univ of Miami School of Medicine)
Ophthalmology 94:407–413, April 1987   1–60

The authors reviewed 27 cases of culture-positive endophthalmitis developing after ocular trauma. The intraocular antibiotics used were gentamicin and, until 1980, cephaloridine. Cefazolin was used thereafter. Amphotericin B was given intraocularly when fungal endophthalmitis was suspected.

Gram-positive organisms were isolated in 59% of cases, and fungi, in 19%. The most frequent specific isolates were *Bacillus* species and *Staphylococcus epidermidis*. Only six eyes (22%) achieved vision of 20/400 or better. Four of five eyes with fungal infection achieved this degree of vision. None of three eyes with mixed flora achieved 20/400 or better vision. Nineteen eyes had phthisis bulbi, pre-phthisis, or pain with blindness; 8 of these patients had enucleation or evisceration. All 7 patients who had retinal detachment or retinal breaks from the impact of a foreign body became phthisical or had enucleation after initial management.

The microbiology of traumatic endophthalmitis differs from that of other forms of exogenous endophthalmitis. Antibiotics effective against *Bacillus* sp. should be used because of the frequency and fulminant course of this infection. Vancomycin offers excellent coverage of the full range of gram-positive organisms causing traumatic endophthalmitis. Its intraocular use, along with gentamicin, may be the best approach. Prophylactic intravitreal antibiotics probably are not warranted except when a large amount of intraocular foreign material is present or there is a strong clinical suspicion of early infection. If an eye is severely injured, topical gentamicin should be used preoperatively.

► The authors do not recommend prophylactic intravitreal antibiotics in penetrating trauma "except in eyes with large amounts of intraocular foreign material or a strong clinical suspicion of early infection." They mention a previous study in which only 4 of 122 patients with corneal scleral lacerations developed endophthalmitis after repair of the initial injury. They also cite the risk of retinal toxicity from an excessive dose of intraocular antibiotics. However, they recommend the use of topical gentamicin sulfate at regular intervals before reparative surgery, as well as periocular antibiotics (gentamicin and vancomycin) at the time of primary repair.—M.J. Barza, M.D.

2 Viral Infections

Hepatitis Viruses

Outbreak of Severe Hepatitis Due to Delta and Hepatitis B Viruses in Parenteral Drug Abusers and Their Contacts
Lettau LA, McCarthy JG, Smith MH, Hadler SC, Morse LJ, Ukena T, Bessette R, Gurwitz A, Irvine WG, Fields HA, Grady GF, Maynard JE (Ctrs for Disease Control, Atlanta; Worcester Dept of Public Health, Mass; Hahnemann Hosp, Worcester, Mass; St Vincent Hosp, Worcester, Mass; Massachusetts Dept of Public Health, Boston)
N Engl J Med 317:1256–1262, Nov 12, 1987   2–1

Several outbreaks of hepatitis B infection with excessive mortality have been reported among parenteral drug abusers in the United States. Clusters of such infection may be explained by an unusually virulent strain of hepatitis B virus, the concomitant action of hepatotoxic chemicals, or simultaneous infection with a second hepatotropic virus, such as non-A, non-B virus or delta virus. However, such a factor has rarely been actually implicated. An unusually large, severe outbreak of hepatitis B involving parenteral drug abusers and their sexual contacts over 21 months was investigated.

The outbreak occurred in Worcester, Massachusetts from 1983 to 1985. Of the 135 patients with drug-related acute hepatitis B, 80% were parenteral drug abusers, and 19% had had sexual contact with drug abusers. There were 13 fulminant cases, resulting in 11 deaths. Among all the patients with hepatitis B, evidence of delta virus infection was observed in 54% of drug abusers, in 33% of their sexual contacts, and in 9% of other patients with acute hepatitis B (Table 1). Eighty-six percent

TABLE 1.—Results of Testing for Delta Virus According to Risk Group

Risk Group*	Total Identified	No. Tested	Delta-Positive	Type of Delta Infection	
				Coinfection	Superinfection
			no. (%)		
PDAs	110	83	45 (54)	39	6
PDA contacts	25	24	8 (33)	7	1
Other patients with acute hepatitis B	55	34	3 (9)	2	1

*PDA, parenteral drug abuser.
(Courtesy of Lettau LA, McCarthy JG, Smith MH, et al: *N Engl J Med* 317:1256–1262, Nov 12, 1987.)

TABLE 2.—Delta Infection as a Risk Factor Affecting Disease Severity in Drug-Related Cases

Hepatitis	Total Identified	No. Tested	Delta-Positive
			no. (%)
Fulminant	13	11	10 (91)*
Nonfulminant			
Patients hospitalized	27	21	12 (57)
Patients not hospitalized	94	74	31 (42)
Total†	122	96	43 (45)*

*$P = .0037$, Fisher's exact test.
†The totals for nonfulminant disease include a delta-negative patient whose hospitalization status was unknown.
(Courtesy of Lettau LA, McCarthy JG, Smith MH, et al: N Engl J Med 317:1256–1262, Nov 12, 1987.)

of the delta infections were coinfections with hepatitis B virus. The remainder were superinfections. Delta infection appeared strongly associated with fulminant hepatitis: 91% of the patients with a fulminant outcome had delta infection, whereas 45% of the less severely ill drug abusers and their sexual contacts did (Table 2). Alcohol, other drugs, and other hepatitis viruses were not hepatotoxic cofactors in fulminant disease.

This outbreak of hepatitis B apparently resulted from the concurrent spread of hepatitis B and delta viruses among new drug users. Physicians were given guidelines on prophylaxis in contacts of patients with hepatitis B, health education for drug abusers, and a hepatitis B vaccination program. Despite these efforts to control the outbreak, it continued unabated until the number of new cases began to slowly decline late in 1986.

▶ This outbreak illustrates the importance of delta-virus coinfection with hepatitis B in association with fulminant hepatitis B. Many of the cases in this epidemic had a biphasic course of illness. The association with parenteral drug abuse is well known and consistent with other outbreaks (see the 1986 YEAR BOOK OF INFECTIOUS DISEASES, pp 85–88). In addition to the association of hepatitis delta virus (HDV) and fulminant hepatitis, evidence that HDV is more frequently associated with chronic liver disease is accumulating (see Abstract 2–2).—D.R. Snydman, M.D.

Influence of Hepatitis Delta Virus Infection on Progression to Cirrhosis in Chronic Hepatitis Type B
Fattovich G, Boscaro S, Noventa F, Pornaro E, Stenico D, Alberti A, Ruol A, Realdi G (Univ of Padua, Italy)
J Infect Dis 155:931–935, May 1987

2–2

The hepatitis delta virus (HDV) is very pathogenic, and HDV infection may be associated with severe liver disease in chronic carriers of hepatitis

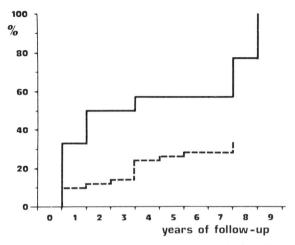

Fig 2–1.—Product life-table analysis of evolution from chronic active hepatitis to cirrhosis in patients with hepatitis delta virus (HDV) infection *(solid line)* and in patients without HDV infection *(broken line)*. The 2 curves are significantly different ($P < .001$). (Courtesy of Fattovich G, Boscaro S, Noventa F, et al: *J Infect Dis* 155:931–935, May 1987.)

B virus. Serologic markers of HDV infection were sought in 146 consecutive patients with chronic hepatitis B. The histologic state of the liver was followed for 1 to 15 years, the mean time being 4.7 years. Forty-three patients received steroids in conventional doses for 6 to 45 months.

Anti-HDV was detected in initial serum samples in 12% of the patients and persisted in high titer in all instances. No patient seroconverted during follow-up. Previous overt acute hepatitis was significantly more frequent in the anti-HDV-positive patients. The HDV infection was present in 15% of patients with chronic active hepatitis and in the same proportion of those with cirrhosis, but not in any of 24 patients with chronic persistent hepatitis. The risk of cirrhosis developing in patients presenting with chronic active hepatitis was significantly greater for those who were anti-HDV-positive (Fig 2–1).

The HDV infection was relatively infrequent in chronic carriers of hepatitis B surface antigen in this study. Young men who are anti-HBe-positive are chiefly affected. The presence of HDV infection is associated with a more rapid progression to cirrhosis.

Adenine Arabinoside Monophosphate (Vidarabine Phosphate) in Combination With Human Leukocyte Interferon in the Treatment of Chronic Hepatitis B: A Randomized, Double-Blinded, Placebo-Controlled Trial
Garcia G, Smith Cl, Weissberg Jl, Eisenberg M, Bissett J, Nair PV, Mastre B, Rosno S, Roskamp D, Waterman K, Pollard RB, Tong MJ, Brown BW Jr, Robinson WS, Gregory PB, Merigan TC (Stanford Univ School of Medicine; Univ of Texas, Galveston; Huntington Mem Hosp, Pasadena, Calif)
Ann Intern Med 107:278–285, September 1987

There is no effective and safe treatment for the liver disease associated with chronic hepatitis B infection. To determine the usefulness of adenine arabinoside monophosphate (Ara-AMP) alone or in combination with human leukocyte interferon in the treatment of hepatitis B surface antigen carriers, a randomized, double-blind, placebo-controlled trial was carried out in 25 patients with chronic active hepatitis and 39 patients with chronic persistent hepatitis.

Thirteen patients were treated with 2.5 mg/kg Ara-AMP intramuscularly twice daily, alternated monthly with 5 million units of subcutaneous human leukocyte interferon twice daily, for 6 months. Twenty-four patients received Ara-AMP alternated with placebo. Twenty-seven patients received placebo alone.

There was a much higher dropout rate in the group receiving Ara-AMP. This was mainly due to painful paresthesia of the legs. The placebo group was the least symptomatic at 12 months. All groups were equally symptomatic at 24 months. Loss of markers of infection was the same in all 3 groups. At 12 months, there was less erosion of the limiting plate in the Ara-AMP group, but this difference disappeared by 24 months of follow-up. Neither Ara-AMP alone nor Ara-AMP combined with human leukocyte interferon was useful in the treatment of chronic hepatitis B.

A Serologic Follow-Up of the 1942 Epidemic of Post-Vaccination Hepatitis in the United States Army
Seeff LB, Beebe GW, Hoofnagle JH, Norman JE, Buskell-Bales Z, Waggoner JG, Kaplowitz N, Koff RS, Petrini JL Jr, Schiff ER, Shorey J, Stanley MM (VA Med Ctrs in Washington DC, Los Angeles, Boston, Miami, Dallas, Hines, Ill; et al)
N Engl J Med 316:965–970, April 16, 1987

2-4

In 1942, a dramatic outbreak of hepatitis occurred that affected approximately 50,000 U.S. Army servicemen. This epidemic was thought to have resulted from receipt of yellow-fever vaccine stabilized with pooled human serum. A study was conducted to identify the responsible virus and the consequences of the epidemic.

Five hundred ninety-seven veterans who had been in the army in 1942 were interviewed and serologically screened. These subjects were selected from 3 groups. Group I was made up of patients who had received the implicated vaccine and had jaundice; group II was made up of patients who had received the implicated vaccine and had remained well; and group III was made up of patients who had received a new, serum-free vaccine, with no subsequent jaundice. Ninety-seven percent of group I, 76% of group II, and 13% of group III registered positive for antibodies to hepatitis B virus (HBV). Only 1 patient exhibited hepatitis B surface antigen, and this yielded a carrier rate of 0.26% among recipients of the implicated vaccine. The prevalence of hepatitis A antibody was similar in all 3 groups, and no subject had antibody to hepatitis delta virus.

It is likely that hepatitis B caused the outbreak, that about 330,000 persons may have been infected, that the HBV carrier state was a rare consequence, and that the outbreak induced hepatitis B antibodies that persist for life.

▶ The rate for carriers of hepatitis B surface antigen in this study was much lower than the 5% to 10% that one might have expected based on previous studies. Reasons for these discrepancies are not clear and could include virus or host factors not yet defined. An additional point to note is that in symptomatic individuals, anti-hepatitis B core as a single serologic marker was more common than anti-HBs. This contrasts with findings in exposed populations such as hospital employees where anti-HBs may frequently be present as a single marker. That 98% of infected symptomatic individuals retain at least one marker for HBV infection for 40 years attests to the lifelong immunity associated with HBV infection.—D.R. Snydman, M.D.

Should All Pregnant Women Be Screened for Hepatitis B?
Kumar ML, Dawson NV, McCullough AJ, Radivoyevitch M, King KC, Hertz R, Kiefer H, Hampson M, Cassidy R, Tavill AS (Cleveland Metropolitan Gen Hosp, Case Western Reserve Univ School of Medicine)
Ann Intern Med 107:273–277, September 1987   2–5

The U.S. Public Health Service currently recommends hepatitis B surface antigen (HBsAg) screening for pregnant women at high risk for hepatitis B infection. To assess the sensitivity of historical risk factors for identification for HBsAg-positive parturients, 4,399 consecutive pregnant women were screened for HBsAg. Information regarding risk for hepatitis B infection was obtained from each HBsAg-positive parturient.

Twenty-three HBsAg-positive subjects were identified (5.2/1,000 deliveries). The HBsAg carrier rate was significantly higher in women of black, Asian, or Hispanic origin (18/2,231, or 8.1/1,000 deliveries) than in the remaining ethnic groups (non-Hispanic white women plus all others, 5/2,168 or 2.3/1,000 deliveries). Only 1 of 23 HBsAg-positive parturients was identified antepartum. Routine screening showed an additional 22 asymptomatic carriers, of which only 10 had defined risk factors for hepatitis B infection on detailed historical evaluation.

The sensitivity of multiple historical risk factors for detection of asymptomatic HBsAg-positive parturients is disappointingly low (table). In addition, much of the information required to assess these risk factors involves detailed questioning and is unlikely to be obtained in the context of conventional obstetrical care. Moreover, the cost of preventing a single case of posttransfusion hepatitis B infection is comparable with that of preventing a single case of perinatally acquired infection. Hence, routine maternal HBsAg screening programs may be necessary to prevent transmission of hepatitis B from mothers to infants.

▶ This study and several others (Jonas MM et al: *Ann Intern Med* 107:335–

Sensitivity and Specificity of Ethnic Group Status as a Risk Factor for Detection of Positivity for Hepatitis B Surface Antigen (HBsAg)

Criteria	HBsAg-Positive*	Sensitivity	95% CI†	Specificity	95% CI‡
	n/n	%			
Clinical hepatitis B§	1/23	4.3	0.1 to 22.0	100	99.9 to 100
Asian	2/23	8.7	1.1 to 28.0	99.4	99.1 to 99.6
Asian plus Hispanic	5/23	21.7	7.5 to 43.7	93.8	93.0 to 94.5
Asian, Hispanic, black	18/23	78.3	56.3 to 92.5	49.4	47.9 to 50.9
All deliveries	23/23	100	85.2 to 100	0	0.0 to 0.1

*Cumulative prevalence, includes 13 asymptomatic blacks (1 with clinical hepatitis B also was black).
†"Exact" 95% confidence interval (CI).
‡Approximate 95% CIs.
§Assumes that current prevalence is too low to warrant routine testing—only symptomatic patients would be tested (1 in the present study).
(Courtesy of Kumar ML, Dawson NV, McCullough AJ, et al: *Ann Intern Med* 107:273–277, September 1987.)

337, 1987; McQuillan GM et al: *Am J Epidemiol* 126:484–491, 1987; Summers PR et al: *Obstet Gynecol* 69:701–704, 1987) illustrate the problem inherent in screening only those mothers thought to be at risk for HbsAg carriage. All 3 studies demonstrate that the use of "high risk" demographic characteristics for screening criteria will miss more than 50% of HbsAg-positive individuals.

As illustrated below (Abstract 2–6) the most cost-effective approach is to screen everyone for HbsAg and immunize those infants born to HbsAg carrier mothers. The Advisory Committee for Immunization Practices has recently changed its recommendations to screen all pregnant women for HbsAg and immunize those infants born to HbsAg-positive mothers (*MMWR CDC Surveill Summ* 37:341–351, 1988).—D.R. Snydman, M.D.

Cost-Effectiveness of Prenatal Screening and Immunization for Hepatitis B Virus
Arevalo JA, Washington AE (Univ of California at Davis, Sacramento; Univ of California School of Medicine, San Francisco; Stanford Univ School of Medicine)
JAMA 259:365–369, Jan 15, 1988   2–6

The Centers for Disease Control recommend that all prenatal patients from designated high-risk groups be screened for the presence of hepatitis B surface antigens (HbsAg) and that neonates of mothers who are HbsAg-positive should receive hepatitis B vaccine and hepatitis B immune serum globulin (HBIg) at birth and repeated hepatitis B vaccine at ages 1 and 6 months.

To evaluate the cost-effectiveness of such a screening and immunization program, a decision analysis model was formulated from data obtained from published reports, chart reviews, and a Delphi survey to determine the outcome probabilities and costs. Prevalence of HbsAg in the various groups that were studied ranged from 0.1% to 15%.

It was calculated that a routine screening program could prevent 2 to 140 cases of acute neonatal hepatitis and 18 to 1,400 cases of chronic liver disease per year for every 100,000 pregnant women who were screened. The calculated cost of the screening and immunization program would total between $2.5 and $4 million for populations with prevalences between 0.2% and 15%, respectively. With an annual national rate of 3.5 million births, a national policy of routine screening of all pregnant women would result in an annual net savings of more than $105 million to as much as $765 million at a prevalence of 15%.

When direct and indirect costs are considered, the screening and immunization program would be cost-effective at a prevalence of 0.06% and higher, a prevalence much lower than the national prevalence of 0.2%. This analysis demonstrates the cost-effectiveness of such programs and supports the practice of screening all pregnant women in the United States for hepatitis B virus infection.

Yeast-Recombinant Hepatitis B Vaccine: Efficacy With Hepatitis B Immune Globulin in Prevention of Perinatal Hepatitis B Virus Transmission
Stevens CE, Taylor PE, Tong MJ, Toy PT, Vyas GN, Nair PV, Weissman JV, Krugman S (New York Blood Ctr; New York Univ; Univ of California, San Francisco; Huntington Mem Hosp, Pasadena, Calif)
JAMA 257:2612–2616, May 15, 1987

A yeast-recombinant hepatitis vaccine was compared with a plasma vaccine in 122 high-risk Asian-American newborns. These infants were also given hepatitis B immune globulin. They were followed for a minimum of 9 months.

The infants were born to mothers positive for both hepatitis B surface antigen and the e antigen. If such infants would not receive immunoprophylaxis, 70%–90% would become infected and develop the chronic carrier state. Among those who received the recombinant vaccine and hepatitis immune globulin, only 4.8% became chronic carriers. Among those who received the plasma-derived vaccine 10.2% became carriers.

Among high-risk newborns the yeast-recombinant hepatitis B vaccine is as effective as the plasma-derived vaccine in preventing infection with hepatitis B virus and the establishment of the carrier state. For those afraid to use a plasma-derived product, this provides a viable alternative.

▶ Although this study is not comparative and relies on historic information in the neonatal group, significant evidence of protection by the recombinant yeast-derived hepatitis B vaccine is provided. In my experience the recombinant product is clearly the choice of most individuals who need prophylaxis even though the safety record of the plasma-derived vaccine is outstanding (see the 1988 YEAR BOOK OF INFECTIOUS DISEASES, p 84).—D.R. Snydman, M.D.

Herpes Viruses

Detection of Antibodies to Herpes Simplex Virus in the Cerebrospinal Fluid of Patients With Herpes Simplex Encephalitis
Kahlon J, Chatterjee S, Lakeman FD, Lee F, Nahmias AJ, Whitley RJ (Univ of Alabama at Birmingham; Emory Univ)
J Infect Dis 155:38–44, January 1987

Early therapy for herpes simplex encephalitis (HSE) improves the outcome. However, the only certain method of diagnosis is the isolation of the virus from the brain by biopsy. Intrathecal synthesis of antibody to the virus has been reported in HSE patients and would provide another assay. Therefore, specimens of cerebrospinal fluid and serum from 35 patients with biopsy-proven HSE were compared to 22 specimens from biopsy-negative patients.

Using immunoblotting, it was shown that antibodies to the herpes simplex virus were present in serum from biopsy-positive individuals. When purified glycoprotein B was used as the antigen, this assay had a 97% sensitivity and a 73% specificity. If this assay was controlled for cross-reactivity to adenovirus, the specificity was 100%. Therefore, immunologic assays are useful in the retrospective analysis of cerebrospinal fluid obtained from patients who are believed to have HSE.

Magnetic Resonance Imaging of the Brain in Childhood Herpesvirus Infections
Bale JF Jr, Anderson RD, Grose C (Univ of Iowa)
Pediatr Infect Dis J 6:644–647, July 1987

Magnetic resonance (MR) imaging is helpful in evaluating the CNS in children, particularly the white matter. Study therefore was made of 9 children having CNS herpesvirus infections. Both spin-echo and inversion-recovery techniques were used. Infants and uncooperative young children were sedated with chloral hydrate. Computed tomography (CT) studies of the head also were obtained.

All but 1 of the 9 patients had abnormal MR findings (table). The abnormalities included cystic encephalomalacia, ventricular dilatation, cerebral atrophy, and lesions of white matter. The MR findings were comparable to the CT findings in patients with severe congenital or perinatal infections caused by herpesvirus, varicella-zoster virus, and cytomegalovirus. Magnetic resonance imaging showed parenchymal abnormalities in a child with Epstein-Barr virus (EBV) encephalitis who had a normal CT study. In 2 neonates, parenchymal abnormalities were defined more clearly by MR imaging than by CT. Magnetic resonance imaging also was more informative in an infant having congenital varicella infection and nearly complete destruction of cerebral and cerebellar tissues.

Magnetic resonance imaging is of considerable value in assessing children with neurologic disorder secondary to herpesvirus infection. It defines the extent of parenchymal lesions more sensitively than CT and also is better in identifying abnormalities of the cerebral white matter. Sagittal MR images display multiple levels of the neuroaxis, including the spinal cord, simultaneously.

▶ While I am not sure that this small study of 9 children with evidence of CNS herpesvirus infections supports the authors' suggestion that MR imaging may be the preferred neuroimaging technique in children with these infections, anyone who has seen MR images of the brain must be awed by their incredible clarity. For many things, CT scan in comparison to MR imaging looks like a fuzzy brain scan. In neonates with herpesvirus infections, there was no difference in sensitivity between MR imaging and CT scans and both were consistent in their ability to pick up significant lesions. The only normal CT scan with an abnormal MR image occurred in a 10-year-old girl who had major neurologic symptoms (coma, seizures, left hemiparesis, and aphasia) after an apparent EBV virus infection. The MR imaging was done several days later and revealed

Clinical and Virologic Findings

Case	Age	Virus	Neurologic Features	CT	MRI
1	22 days	HSV	Lethargy	ND	Normal
2	16 days	HSV	Coma, seizures	Cystic encephalomalacia	Cystic encephalomalacia
3	10 days	HSV	Chorioretinitis	Left thalamic hypodensity	Left hemisphere atrophy, abnormal signal periventricular white matter, abnormal signal left thalamus
4	3 days	CMV	Full fontanel, split sutures, hypotonia	Hydrocephalus, subependymal cysts	Ventriculitis, hemorrhage, abnormal signals in parenchyma bilaterally
5	13 days	CMV	Hypotonia, weak Moro response	Subependymal cysts, hemorrhage	Subependymal cysts, hemorrhage, abnormal signals in parenchyma bilaterally
6	5 days	CMV	Microcephaly	Normal	Focal white matter lesion
7	1 day	VZV	Macrocephaly, hypotonia, absent respirations	Hydrocephalus, brainstem and basal ganglia calcifications	Hydrocephalus, cerebellar aplasia, hypervascularity of deep nuclei
8	5 years	VZV	Coma, long tract signs	ND	Abnormal signals in midbrain and middle cerebellar peduncle
9	10 years	EBV	Coma, seizures, left hemiparesis, aphasia	Normal	Bilateral areas of abnormal signal

*ND = not done.
(Courtesy of Bale JF Jr, Andersen RD, Grose C: Pediatr Infect Dis J 6:644–647, July 1987.)

"bilateral areas of abnormal signal" at a time when the patient was fully alert with paucity of speech. It is not apparent that the MR imaging altered the course of diagnosis or therapy in any of these patients.

We need to continue to systematically evaluate these various imaging methods so that we can define those CNS infections that are better detected by 1 or the other of the 3 major imaging methods. As it stands, we are often in the dilemma of obtaining 2 or 3 of these, and they are repeated several times as we follow the patient. This is becoming especially critical for both children and adults with acquired immunodeficiency syndrome who have multiple different kinds of CNS lesions that need therapy and sequential follow-up. It has generally been our practice here that in this subset of patients, when an abnormality is seen on the CT scan, this is used as the modality for subsequent follow-up.—M.S. Klempner, M.D.

Young Children as a Probable Source of Maternal and Congenital Cytomegalovirus Infection
Pass RF, Little EA, Stagno S, Britt WJ, Alford CA (Univ of Alabama in Birmingham)
N Engl J Med 316:1366–1370, May 28, 1987   2–10

Recent population-based studies have shown that from 1.6% to 3.7% of women acquire cytomegalovirus (CMV) infections for the first time during pregnancy and that the virus is transmitted to the fetus in 30% to 40% of these primary maternal infections. Although most newborns with congenital CMV infection develop normally, 10% to 20% of the infected

Virologic Features of Five Families Containing Newborns With Congenital or Perinatal Cytomegalovirus Infection

FEATURE	FAMILY 1	FAMILY 2	FAMILY 3	FAMILY 4	FAMILY 5
Newborn's infection	Perinatal	Congenital	Congenital	Congenital	Congenital (symptomatic)
Maternal seroconversion during gestation	17–23 wk	12–40 wk	12–40 wk	23–40 wk	Time unknown
Paternal serologic status	Unknown	Negative	Negative	Negative	Positive
Sibling's age at birth of newborn	24 mo	25 mo	10 mo*	19 mo	23 mo
Sibling attending day care	Yes	Yes	Occasionally	Yes	Yes
First isolate of cytomegalovirus					
Newborn	2-12-86† Saliva	12-8-85 Urine	12-13-85 Urine	3-26-86 Urine	8-6-85 Urine
Sibling	2-12-86 Urine	12-20-85 Urine	2-27-86 Urine	4-23-86 Urine	8-6-85 Urine
Mother	2-12-86 Milk	12-20-85 Urine	None	None	None

*Cousin of newborn.
†Negative at 1–14–86.
(Courtesy of Pass RF, Little EA, Stagno S, et al: N Engl J Med 316:1366–1370, May 28, 1987.)

infants have some degree of impaired hearing, mental ability, neuromuscular function, or vision. Seven families with a recent congenital or maternal CMV infection were studied in an effort to identify possible sources of viral transmission.

The study comprised 5 families with either confirmed maternal seroconversion during pregnancy or a recent birth of a newborn with congenital CMV infection and 2 nonpregnant mothers with recently acquired CMV infection, who each had a child known to be shedding CMV (table). Serum samples were collected, and restriction-endonuclease techniques were used to compare the DNA of viral isolates collected from all family members in the immediate households.

In each of the first 5 families, a young child was attending a day-care center at least part-time and CMV strains from family members were identical. It is most likely that the toddler attending a day-care center was the source of CMV infection for both the mother and the fetus or newborn infant. In the other 2 families, both mothers also seroconverted after their children had been infected with CMV in a day-care center. These findings confirm that maternal CMV infection can be acquired from a young child, then transmitted to the fetus when the mother becomes pregnant again.

Effects on Infants of a First Episode of Genital Herpes During Pregnancy
Brown ZA, Vontver LA, Benedetti J, Critchlow CW, Sells CJ, Berry S, Corey L
(Univ of Washington; Children's Hosp and Med Ctr, Seattle)
N Engl J Med 317:1246–1251, Nov 12, 1987   2–11

Genital herpesvirus infection during pregnancy is associated with neonatal and maternal complications. To evaluate the perinatal effects of infection, 29 women who acquired genital herpes during pregnancy were prospectively followed.

A primary first episode of herpes simplex virus type 2 (HSV-2) occurred in 15 of these women, and a nonprimary first episode occurred in 14. Six of the 15 with primary genital herpes had serious perinatal morbidity without disseminated disease. None of the infants in the nonprimary group had serious perinatal morbidity. Four of the 5 infants with mothers who acquired primary HSV-2 in the third trimester were premature and exhibited growth retardation and neonatal HSV-2 infection. This was also true for 1 of 5 infants whose mothers acquired primary HSV-2 in the first trimester and in 1 of 5 whose mothers acquired it in the second trimester. Asymptomatic HSV-2 shedding was detected 10.6% of the time after a primary first episode and 0.5% of the time after a nonprimary first episode.

Infants born to women who acquire primary genital herpes during pregnancy are at high risk for exposure to HSV-2. There is a 40% incidence of serious perinatal morbidity in such cases. Studies are needed to determine what preventive measures can be taken.

▶ It is important to note that the patients referred to this group were clinically symptomatic. Clearly the rate of perinatal complications after symptomatic primary disease was high. The rate of perinatal complications following asymptomatic primary genital HSV-2 infection would require a very large cohort (see the 1988 YEAR BOOK OF INFECTIOUS DISEASES, pp 86–87). The most significant practical point from this analysis is that the clinical manifestations of primary genital herpes were of prognostic importance for pregnancy outcome. In this very high-risk group use of prophylactic acyclovir may need to be explored.— D.R. Snydman, M.D.

Use of Cytomegalovirus Immune Globulin to Prevent Cytomegalovirus Disease in Renal-Transplant Recipients

Snydman DR, Werner BG, Heinze-Lacey B, Berardi VP, Tilney NL, Kirkman RL, Milford EL, Cho SI, Bush HL Jr, Levey AS, Strom TB, Carpenter CB, Levey RH, Harmon WE, Zimmerman CE II, Shapiro ME, Steinman T, LoGerfo F, Idelson B, Schröter GPJ, Levin MJ, McIver J, Leszczynski J, Grady GF (New England Med Ctr, Brigham and Women's Hosp, Children's Hosp, Beth Israel Hosp, Univ Hosp, Boston; et al)
N Engl J Med 317:1049–1054, Oct 22, 1987   2–12

Cytomegalovirus (CMV) is the main viral pathogen in renal-transplant recipients. Cytomegalovirus-seronegative recipients of transplants from CMV-seropositive donors are at high risk for serious CMV disease. A multi-institutional, randomized, controlled trial was done to investigate the use of a CMV hyperimmune globulin modified for intravenous (IV) administration to prevent primary CMV disease.

Fifty-nine CMV-seronegative recipients of kidneys from donors with antibodies against CMV were assigned to receive IV CMV immune globulin or no treatment. The immune globulin was given in doses of 150 mg/

TABLE 1.—Outcomes in 24 Patients Receiving CMV Immune Globulin and 35 Control Patients

OUTCOME	GLOBULIN	CONTROLS
	no. (%)	
Clinical		
Virologically confirmed CMV syndrome	5 (21)	21 (60)*
Fungal or parasitic opportunistic infection	0	7 (20)†
Death	1 (4)	5 (14)
Graft loss	4 (17)	10 (29)
Virologic		
CMV viremia	6 (25)	15 (43)
Viral isolation (any site)	13 (54)	20 (57)
Seroconversion	17 (71)	27 (77)

*Chi-square = 8.86; $P < .01$.
†Fisher's exact test, $P = .05$.
(Courtesy of Snydman DR, Werner GG, Heinze-Lacey B, et al: N Engl J Med 317:1049–1054, Oct 22, 1987.)

TABLE 2.—Effects of Therapy for Rejection and of CMV Immune Globulin on Serious CMV Disease*

Rejection Therapy	Study Group		P Value
	GLOBULIN	CONTROLS	
	disease total		
Any	2/13 (15%)	14/26 (54%)	0.04
None	1/11 (9%)	2/9 (22%)	NS
Total	3/24 (13%)	16/35 (46%)	<0.01

*Rejection therapies included antithymocyte globulin, methylprednisolone sodium succinate pulse, monoclonal antibody, and plasmapheresis. Serious CMV disease is that occurring in association with at least 1 of the following: leukopenia < 3,000 white cells (WBC); CMV pneumonia; fungal or parasitic superinfections; retinitis; or CNS involvement. NS, not signficant.

(Courtesy of Snydman DR, Werner BG, Heinze-Lacey B, et al: 317:1049–1054, Oct 22, 1987.)

kg body weight within 72 hours of transplantation, then 100 mg/kg 2 and 4 weeks after transplantation, followed by 50 mg/kg at 6, 8, 12, and 16 weeks after surgery.

The incidence of virologically confirmed CMV-associated syndromes was 60% in control subjects and 21% in immune globulin recipients (Table 1). Fungal or parasitic superinfections occurred in 20% of control subjects and in none of the immune globulin recipients. Rates of graft loss and mortality did not significantly differ between the two groups. One globulin recipient died from CMV pneumonia complicated by pseudomonas sepsis. Immune globulin was found to have no effect on overall rates of viral isolation or of seroconversion. In patients who received therapy for graft rejection, immune globulin reduced the attack rate of serious CMV disease from 54% to 15% (Table 2). Of the 205 immune globulin infusions, 6% were associated with possible side effects. Therapy did not need to be stopped for any of the reactions noted.

Prophylactic use of CMV immune globulin provides substantial protection for the renal-transplant recipient at risk for primary CMV disease. All CMV-seronegative candidates receiving kidneys from CMV-seropositive donors should be considered for globulin prophylaxis.

▶ The results reported above (Abstract 2–12) are the best controlled data to demonstrate a reduction of CMV disease by the prophylactic administration of CMV hyperimmune globulin. The results are biologically consistent with several studies in bone marrow transplantation (see the 1988 Year Book of Infectious Diseases, pp 91–93). Unanswered questions remain concerning use of nonselected intravenous immune globulin, usage in other transplant settings, or usage of immune globulin combined with antiviral therapy.

Another approach is antiviral prophylaxis. Until now there have been a number of trials of antiviral agents that have demonstrated only a limited antiviral effect. The study cited below by Meyers and others is intriguing (Abstract 2–13). The authors used a currently available antiviral agent, acyclovir, which has some in vitro activity against CMV in a prophylactic manner. It should be noted that the acyclovir was being given to prevent reactivation of herpes simplex virus and CMV disease.

The results showed a dramatic reduction in oropharyngeal and urine excretion of CMV, a reduction in CMV pneumonia occurring at less than 100 days, and a reduction in mortality among acyclovir recipients. The results are curious in that the probability of CMV pneumonia and the survival curves only begin to diverge at 60 days posttransplant (30 days after stopping acyclovir). Also, the authors chose to ignore those events after 100 days posttransplant. Furthermore, we know that acyclovir had no impact on CMV viremia, which has been a marker for more serious CMV disease in some transplant settings.

One variable the authors do not state in the methods is blood product usage. Although this trial is of considerable interest, I do not think that acyclovir prophylaxis for CMV disease can be justified on the basis of these data. There are clearly too many potential confounding variables. Furthermore, the results should not be translated to those transplant populations at risk for primary CMV disease, since only reactivation CMV disease was studied. A controlled, prospective, randomized trial of CMV prophylaxis is clearly warranted.— D.R. Snydman, M.D.

Acyclovir for Prevention of Cytomegalovirus Infection and Disease After Allogeneic Marrow Transplantation
Meyers JD, Reed EC, Shepp DH, Thornquist M, Dandliker PS, Vicary CA, Flournoy N, Kirk LE, Kersey JH, Thomas ED, Balfour HH Jr (Fred Hutchinson Cancer Research Ctr, Seattle; Univ of Washington; Univ of Minnesota, Minneapolis; Burroughs Wellcome Co, Research Triangle Park, NC)
N Engl J Med 318:70–75, Jan 14, 1988
2–13

Cytomegalovirus infection remains a significant obstacle to the success of allogeneic marrow transplantation. A study was undertaken to determine the efficacy of intravenously given acyclovir for the prevention of cytomegalovirus infection and disease after allogeneic bone marrow transplantation. Acyclovir was administered intravenously from 5 days before and 30 days after allogeneic marrow transplantation in 86 patients seropositive for both cytomegalovirus and herpes simplex virus, and 65 patients seropositive only for cytomegalovirus served as control. This format was chosen because acyclovir was the standard prophylactic agent against herpes simplex virus.

Active cytomegalovirus infection developed in 51 of 86 acyclovir recipients (59%) during the first 100 days after transplantation, compared with 49 of 65 control patients (75%). The probability that cytomegalovirus infection would develop was 0.70 among acyclovir recipients and 0.87 among control patients at medians of 62 and 40 days after transplantation, respectively ($P = .0001$). Significantly fewer acyclovir recipients developed invasive cytomegalovirus disease (22%), i.e., cytomegalovirus pneumonia and gastrointestinal disease, compared with control patients (38%) (Fig 2–2). Significantly fewer acyclovir recipients died

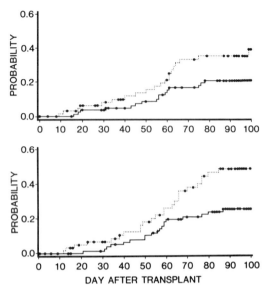

Fig 2–2.—Probability of pneumonia *(upper panel)* or any invasive disease *(lower panel)* caused by cytomegalovirus during the 100 days after transplantation. Acyclovir recipients *(solid line)* and control patients *(broken line)*. The probability of pneumonia is different at $P = .04$, and the probability of invasive disease at $P = .008$ (log-rank test). (Courtesy of Meyers JD, Reed EC, Shepp DH, et al: *N Engl J Med* 318:70–75, Jan 14, 1988.)

during the first 100 days after transplantation (29%) compared with control patients (54%) (table). The probability of survival within the first 100 days after transplantation was significantly better among acyclovir recipients. Proportional-hazards regression analysis showed that acyclovir prophylaxis was associated with a relative risk of 0.5 or less for the development of cytomegalovirus infection or disease or death within the first 100 days after the transplantation.

Prophylaxis with high-dose intravenously administered acyclovir significantly reduces the risk of both cytomegalovirus infection and disease for seropositive patients after allogeneic bone marrow transplantation. More important, acyclovir prophylaxis improves survival in these patients.

Ganciclovir for the Treatment and Suppression of Serious Infections Caused by Cytomegalovirus

Laskin OL, Cederberg DM, Mills J, Eron LJ, Mildvan D, Spector SA, Ganciclovir Study Group (Cornell Univ Med College; Wellcome Research Lab, Research Triangle Park, NC; San Francisco Gen Hosp; Fairfax Hosp, Falls Church, Va; Beth Israel Med Ctr, New York; Univ of California, San Diego)
Am J Med 83:201–207, August 1987   2–14

Cytomegalovirus is a major cause of morbidity and mortality among patients with acquired immunodeficiency syndrome (AIDS). Ganciclovir

Pneumonia, Graft-Versus-Host Disease, Relapse, and Death
Before and After Day 100 After Transplantation

	ACYCLOVIR GROUP	CONTROL GROUP
	no. of patients (percent)	
Cytomegalovirus pneumonia		
≤100 days	16 (19)*	20 (31)
>100 days	3	1
Other interstitial pneumonia		
≤100 days	7† (8)‡	10§ (15)
>100 days	3	1
Acute graft-versus-host disease¶	27 (31)	25 (38)
Leukemic relapse	7 (8)	3 (5)
Death	25 (29)‖	35 (54)

*Significantly different from control ($P = .04$ by log-rank test).
†One patient with herpes simplex virus pneumonia, and 6 with confirmed or suspected idiopathic interstitial pneumonia.
‡Not significantly different from control ($P = .11$ by log-rank test).
§One patient with herpes simplex virus pneumonia, 1 with varicella-zoster virus pneumonia, and 8 with confirmed or suspected idiopathic interstitial pneumonia.
‖Significantly different from control $\chi^2 = 8.5$, $P < .01$).
¶Clinical grade of 2 or more.
(Courtesy of Meyers JD, Reed EC, Shepp DH, et al: N Engl J Med 318:70–75, Jan 14, 1988.)

is an analogue of acyclovir with activity against herpesviruses, such as cytomegalovirus. In this open trial, 97 AIDS patients with a serious cytomegalovirus infection received 3.0–15 mg/kg per day of ganciclovir. The mean duration of therapy was 14 days.

In 88% of these patients, viremia cleared during ganciclovir therapy. Viral shedding was not detectable in the throat in 68% and in the urine in 78% of the patients. Among those patients with retinitis, 87% had improvement or stabilization. When the drug was discontinued, the retinitis always recurred or progressed. Long-term ganciclovir therapy, 5.0 mk/kg

Effect of Long-Term Suppressive Ganclicovir Therapy on
Recurrence Rate of Cytomegalovirus Retinitis in Patients
With AIDS

Suppressive Therapy after Treatment for Cytomegalovirus Retinitis	Number of Patients with Recurrent Disease
No suppressive therapy (n = 21)	21 (100%)*†
2.5 mg/kg 3 or 5 times weekly (n = 15)	11 (73%)*‡
5.0 mg/kg 5 to 7 times weekly (n = 8)	0 (0%)†‡

*Statistically significant ($P = .02$, Fisher exact test, 2-tailed).
†$P < 10^{-6}$, Fisher exact test, 2-tailed.
‡$P = .001$, Fisher exact test, 2-tailed.
(Courtesy of Laskin OL, Cederberg DM, Mills J, et al: Am J Med 83:201–207, August 1987.)

5 to 7 times per week, prevented the recurrence of cytomegalovirus retinitis (table). The drug was eliminated by renal excretion with a mean half-life of 4.2 hours in patients without renal impairment. Adverse effects included significant neutropenia in 55% and significant leukopenia in 32% of the patients.

Ganciclovir is the first antiviral drug with a therapeutic effect on cytomegalovirus in patients with AIDS. However, as this study was conducted without a placebo control, the results should be interpreted conservatively. It is clear that long-term ganciclovir therapy suppresses cytomegalovirus retinitis in a dose-dependent manner. However, since neutropenia is associated with the use of ganciclovir, long-term trials are necessary to determine how useful this therapy will be. It appears from this open trial of ganciclovir in AIDS patients that this drug induces improvement of cytomegalovirus infection and suppresses recurrence for several months during long-term therapy.

▶ The data indicate that ganciclovir is useful therapy for serious cytomegalovirus disease, especially retinitis in AIDS patients (see the 1987 YEAR BOOK OF INFECTIOUS DISEASES, pp 97–99). This study is the first to demonstrate a dose-dependent maintenance regimen necessary to prevent CMV retinitis relapse.—D.R. Snydman, M.D.

Other Viruses

Temporal Relations Between Maternal Rubella and Congenital Defects
Munro ND, Sheppard S, Smithells RW, Holzel H, Jones G (Gen Infirmary at Leeds, England; Hosp for Sick Children, London)
Lancet 2:201–204, July 25, 1987   2–15

The risk of damage to a fetus following maternal rubella in early pregnancy is well recognized, but the risk after the 16th week of pregnancy appears small. To elucidate further on the relation between congenital defects and maternal rubella at known gestational ages, the records of

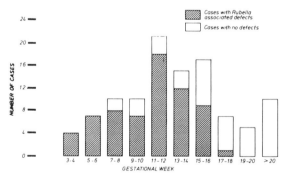

Fig 2–3.—Confirmed congenital rubella with proven maternal infection (group A cases) by time of infection (n = 106). (Courtesy of Munro ND, Sheppard S, Smithells RW, et al: *Lancet* 2:201–204, July 25, 1987.)

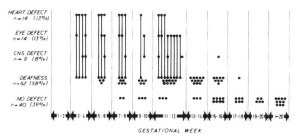

Fig 2-4.—Combinations of defects developing after proven maternal rubella by time of infection (n = 106). (Courtesy of Munro ND, Sheppard S, Smithells RW, et al: *Lancet* 2:201-204, July 25, 1987.)

422 children with confirmed congenital rubella registered in the National Congenital Rubella Surveillance Programme were reviewed. Two groups of cases were studied: group A consisted of 106 infants in whom maternal rubella infection was confidently assessed with laboratory procedures, and group B consisted of 316 infants in whom maternal rubella infection was deduced from a history of rubella-like illness or contact with rubella.

Of the 106 infants born after proved maternal infection, 62% had defects: 67% were exposed between the 3rd and 12th weeks of pregnancy, and 33% were exposed between the 13th and 17th weeks. No defects were recorded among the 20 children exposed after the 17th week (Fig 2-3). Defects of the heart, eye, and CNS followed in children exposed between 3 and 12 weeks of pregnancy, while multiple defects were not recorded in children exposed after 12 weeks (Fig 2-4). Deafness was the most common defect. Patent ductus arteriosus was the most common heart defect reported. In group B cases, 84% had rubella-associated defects following maternal infection between 2 and 33 weeks of gestation. In contrast to group A, 48% of infants exposed after the 16th week of pregnancy had defects. The striking difference between the two groups underlines the importance of serologic investigation of pregnant women who present with rashes or histories of contact with rubella. A total of 148 children were followed up to school age; 27% attended normal schools, with some needing special help, and three quarters attended special schools. It appears that if exposure to rubella occurs later than the 16th week of pregnancy, the danger of fetal damage will be very small.

▶ This study seems to lay to rest the issue of late second trimester rubella causing congenital defects. There were 106 cases of laboratory confirmed rubella at a known point in pregnancy. The percentage with defects dropped sharply from those infected at the end of the first trimester to the middle of the second trimester. After this, as I count the cases from Figure 2-3, there were 15 pregnancies with rubella after week 18 of gestation, with no defects noted. The authors, who no doubt know better, state there were 0 defects found in 20 pregnancies with infection after week 18. Either way, the data are clear.

The other set of data included in the paper includes 316 children with confirmed congenital rubella for whom timing of maternal infection was inferred by history of compatible illness or rubella contact. Twelve of the 31 mothers assumed to have had rubella after week 18 of gestation gave birth to infants with defects, a result totally different from the well-defined, timed 106 cases, Appropriate counseling is thus very dependent on accurate timing of diagnosis in the mother.—G.T. Keusch, M.D.

Human Papillomavirus Infections in Women With and Without Abnormal Cervical Cytology
de Villiers E-M, Wagner D, Schneider A, Wesch H, Miklaw H, Wahrendorf J, Papendick U, zur Hausen H (Deutsches Krebsforschungszentrum, Heidelberg; Evangelisches Diakoniekrankenhaus, Freiberg; Universitäts-Frauenklinik, Ulm; Salem Krankenhaus, Heidelberg; Dr K Thomas Pharmaceuticals, Biberach, West Germany)
Lancet 2:703–706, Sept 26, 1987   2–16

There is evidence to suggest that human papillomavirus (HPV) infection influences the development of human genital cancer. Gynecologic smears obtained from 9,295 women were examined for HPV infection by filter in situ hybridization. The distribution of HPV infection by age and its correlation with cervical neoplasia were determined.

Normal smears comprised 94% of the total; koilocytotic HPV infection was noted in 2%, mild to moderate dysplasia in 2%, carcinoma in situ in 1%, and invasive carcinoma in 1% of the smears. Of HPV-positive patients who were reexamined after 3–6 months, only 30% were still positive. Of the 8,755 patients with normal smears, 9% were HPV DNA positive. The peak of HPV positivity occurred between 15 and 50 years. Beyond age 55 years only 2% to 5% of the patients were HPV-positive. Cervical intraepithelial neoplasia was most common among women aged 20–30 years. Invasive carcinoma was most common among those aged 55–80 years. Among women with cervical intraepithelial neoplasia and carcinoma, between 35% and 40% were positive for HPV. The high prevalence of HPV infection and the fact that the age prevalences for HPV infection and neoplasia are not the same indicate that HPV infection is not the only factor responsible for cervical malignancy.

A Case-Control Study of the Clinical Diagnosis and Course of Lassa Fever
McCormick JB, King IJ, Webb PA, Johnson KM, O'Sullivan R, Smith ES, Trippel S, Tong TC (Ctrs for Disease Control, Atlanta; Nixon Mem Hosp, Segbwema; Panguma Hosp, Panguma; and the Peace Corps, Sierra Leone)
J Infect Dis 155:445–455, March 1987   2–17

Lassa fever is an acute febrile disease occurring in West Africa. A prospective case-control study was undertaken in rural Sierra Leone to determine the frequency and case-fatality ratio of the disease among febrile hospital patients and to define the clinical course. A total of 441 cases were confirmed among 1,087 adult medical admissions with fever. Cases predominated during the dry season months of February to May.

Lassa fever begins gradually after an incubation period of 7–18 days. Fever peaked at 39C to 41C in the early morning and early evening. Many patients also had aching in the large joints, lower back pain, and a dry cough. Many patients appeared severely ill and anxious when admitted. About 20% of patients had fine, dry, diffuse rales. Neurologic manifestations were infrequent. Bleeding and edema were closely associated with a diagnosis of Lassa fever. The most predictive cluster of clinical variables included pharyngitis, retrosternal pain, and proteinuria. Complications included mucosal bleeding, eighth-nerve deafness, and pleural and pericardial effusions.

Lassa fever is a more common cause of hospitalization and death than previously recognized. It is important to include it in the differential diagnosis of febrile illness in West Africa.

▶ This is a landmark study on the clinical aspects of Lassa fever. The disease presents in a very nonspecific fashion, and even in an endemic region, it is difficult to diagnose. The presence of the predictors of Lassa described in the paper is reason to isolate the patient. Management is supportive, with delicate problems in fluid balance and bleeding to contend with.—G.T. Keusch, M.D.

Human Monkeypox: Clinical Features of 282 Patients
Ježek Z, Szczeniowski M, Paluku KM, Mutombo M (WHO, Geneva; Monkeypox Surveillance Team, Kinshasa, Zaire)
J Infect Dis 156:293–298, August 1987   2–18

This report describes the clinical course of 282 patients, aged 1 month to 69 years, with monkeypox. More than 90% of those infected with monkeypox were younger than age 15 years. The clinical appearance of monkeypox was similar to smallpox. In most patients, the illness started with fever. Another common symptom was headache. This was generally followed by skin rash, which usually first appeared on the face. Temporary enlargement of the lymph nodes was more common in those patients who had not been vaccinated for smallpox. The illness generally lasted 2 to 4 weeks. Serious complications occurred in 43% of unvaccinated and 9% of vaccinated subjects. The most common sequela was scarring.

The prognosis of patients with monkeypox depended on the occurrence of severe complications. The occurrence of these complications depended on initial health, concurrent illness, and vaccination status. Those who had been vaccinated for smallpox had a significantly better prognosis than those who had not. No deaths occurred among vaccinated patients, but there were 27 deaths among 250 unvaccinated patients. There was a much higher death rate among young children.

▶ Monkeypox is a smallpox-like illness occurring in Central and West Africa. It has been clinically confused as smallpox in countries already certified as smallpox-free. This paper describes the clinical features of 282 patients with monkeypox. Clinical severity was increased among the young (< 10 years) and was decreased among those immunized with vaccinia: these effects may be directly related as immunization to smallpox disappears.

The infection begins with fever, and rash develops later, usually on the face at first. It then spreads, with crops appearing as in smallpox. In some, the rash is primarily on the trunk, spares the face, palms, and soles, and is reminiscent of chickenpox. Lymphadenopathy is the only feature more characteristic of monkeypox than of the other two infections. Complications occur primarily in the unvaccinated, and include secondary skin infections, pneumonia, diarrhea with severe dehydration, and corneal ulcers.

The authors consider monkeypox "the most important orthopox virus infection presently occurring in humans." While the disease in individuals is or can be severe, it is still overshadowed globally by morbidity and (in the Third World) mortality associated with varicella.—G.T. Keusch, M.D.

Vaccine-Associated Paralytic Poliomyelitis: United States: 1973 Through 1984
Nkowane BM, Wassilak SGF, Orenstein WA, Bart KJ, Schonberger LB, Hinman AR, Kew OM (Ctrs for Disease Control, Atlanta)
JAMA 257:1335–1340, March 13, 1987   2–19

Since the introduction of inactivated poliomyelitis vaccine and oral poliomyelitis vaccine (OPV), the incidence of poliomyelitis in the United States has decreased dramatically. Whereas before 1955 the average annual incidence of paralytic poliomyelitis was about 16,000 cases, the average annual incidence during the early 1980s was only about 10 cases.

Of 138 cases of paralytic poliomyelitis reported between 1973 and 1984, 85 cases (62%) were vaccine-associated, occurring in individuals with no known immune deficiencies. Of these 85 cases, 35 (41%) had

Ratios of Vaccine-Associated Paralytic Poliomyelitis to Doses of OPV Distributed*

Epidemiologic Classification	Overall		First Dose		Subsequent Doses	
	No. of Cases	Cases:10^6 Doses	No. of Cases	Cases:10^6 Doses	No. of Cases	Cases:10^6 Doses
Recipients	35	1:7.8	33	1:1.2	2	1:116.5
Contacts	50	1:5.5	41	1:1.0	9	1:25.9
Subtotal	85	1:3.2	74	1:0.55	11	1:21.2
Immune deficient‡	14	1:19.6	5	1:8.2	8	1:29.1
Other VA§	6	1:45.7	...	...	...	...
Total	105	1:2.6	79	1:0.52	19	1:12.3

*OPV, oral poliomyelitis vaccine, distributed overall and by dose associated: United States, 1973 through 1984.

†One of these patients was a contact of a first-dose vaccine recipient; 1 was a contact of an indeterminate-dose vaccine recipient, herein considered a subsequent dose; another had no history of recent vaccine exposure, and vaccine-like virus was isolated from a stool specimen.

‡VA, other vaccine associated; no history of recent vaccine exposure and vaccine-like viruses were isolated from patient specimens.

(Courtesy of Nkowane BM, Wassilak SGF, Orenstein WA, et al: JAMA 257:1335–1340, March 13, 1987.)

recently received OPV, while 50 (59%) were contacts of OPV recipients. Fourteen more cases occurred in immune-deficient patients, including 11 vaccine recipients, 2 contacts, and 1 patient with no history of recent OPV exposure (table). Of the 35 OPV recipients who contracted paralytic poliomyelitis, 89% were infants younger than 1 year.

The overall frequency of vaccine-associated poliomyelitis was 1 case per 2.6 million doses of vaccine distributed. The incidence of poliomyelitis associated with the first OPV dose was 1 case per 520,000 first doses of OPV vaccine distributed, while the incidence associated with subsequent OPV doses was only 1 case per 12.3 million subsequent doses of OPV vaccine distributed. Thus, it is apparent that the greatest risk of paralytic poliomyelitis occurs with the first dose of OPV. Nevertheless, the overall risk of vaccine-associated paralytic poliomyelitis is extremely low.

Prevention and Control of Type A Influenza Infections in Nursing Homes: Benefits and Costs of Four Approaches Using Vaccination and Amantadine
Patriarca PA, Arden NH, Koplan JP, Goodman RA (Ctrs for Disease Control, Atlanta)
Ann Intern Med 107:732–740, November 1987   2–20

Type A influenza virus infection is a common cause of acute, life-threatening respiratory illness in nursing homes and other chronic-care facilities for the elderly. A model was developed to project morbidity, mortality, and costs attributable to type A influenza virus infections in such facilities and to assess the relative benefits and costs of programs for prevention and control.

A decision tree was created to outline the components of influenza outbreaks and control programs in an average-sized nursing home. Outcomes and costs associated with each alternative were then quantitated. Experiences with the H3N2 subtype were used as the basis for the model, since most type A influenza outbreaks in nursing homes have been caused by this subtype.

Influenza vaccination was most cost-effective in various simulated situations in the model. However, vaccination usually allowed for higher rates of morbidity and mortality compared with other alternatives. The combined use of previous vaccination and chemoprophylaxis during outbreaks in the nursing home was associated with significantly fewer cases compared with vaccination alone and with only modest increases in net program costs. The use of chemoprophylaxis through influenza season without vaccination resulted in the fewest number of illnesses, hospitalizations, and deaths. However, this approach would cost 650% more than the alternatives involving vaccination.

The findings in this study support earlier contentions that influenza control programs in nursing homes are highly beneficial and cost-effective and should be considered a part of standard care in every facility for the elderly in the United States.

Infection With Human T-Cell Leukemia Virus Type I in Patients With Leukemia
Minamoto GY, Gold JWM, Scheinberg DA, Hardy WD, Chein N, Zuckerman E, Reich L, Dietz K, Gee T, Hoffer J, Mayer K, Gabrilove J, Clarkson B, Armstrong D (Mem Sloan-Kettering Cancer Ctr, New York)
N Engl J Med 318:219–222, Jan 28, 1988   2–21

Human T-cell leukemia virus type 1 (HTLV-1) has been associated primarily with adult T-cell leukemia, possibly because of the large quantities of blood products transfused as part of therapy. Because evidence of such infection may be a sensitive indicator of the prevalence of HTLV-1 in the blood-donor population, the presence of HTLV-1 antibody was assessed in 211 adults with leukemia who received multiple transfusions.

Six patients were seropositive for HTLV-1. None of these patients had T-cell leukemia, other illnesses attributable to HTLV-1 infection, or risk factors for HTLV-1 infection other than transfusion. None was positive for human immunodeficiency virus. These patients received a mean 14 ± 12 units of red cells and 78 ± 88 units of platelets prior to collection of positive serum specimens. Serum conversion was documented in 3 patients.

Patients with leukemia who receive large quantities of red-cell and platelet transfusions are at risk for HTLV-1 infection acquired by transfusion. Until the natural history of HTLV-1 infection, its prevalence in donor populations, and the risk of illness from transfusion-associated HTLV-1 infection are defined, strong considerations should be given to routine testing for HTLV-1 donors in areas where screening programs show a marked prevalence. In addition, patients with leukemia, other patients receiving multiple transfusions, and their sexual contacts should be tested for HTLV-1.

▶ The authors estimate that the rate of HTLV-1 positivity was 2.3 per 10,000 units of blood products transfused. This is virtually identical to a recent study they cite in the proof in which 2.5 units per 10,000 were infected (Williams AE et al, unpublished). This rate is about one third the rate of HIV positivity for human immunodeficiency virus in transfused units in the New York City area. The implications for HTLV-1 seropositivity in this patient population are not clear but raise the issues of transfusion screening and potential sexual transmission.—D.R. Snydman, M.D.

Kinins Are Generated During Experimental Rhinovirus Colds
Naclerio RM, Proud D, Lichtenstein LM, Kagey-Sobotka A, Hendley JO, Sorrentino J, Gwaltney JM (Johns Hopkins Univ; Univ of Virginia; Richardson-Vicks Inc, Shelton, Conn)
J Infect Dis 157:133–142, January 1988   2–22

To study the pathophysiology of rhinovirus colds, 40 healthy volunteers with an average age of 20 years, were challenged with rhinovirus type 39, type HH, or placebo. Prior to inoculation and every 4 hours for 5 days postinoculation, nasal lavages were done. The levels of histamine, kinins, [^{3}H]-N-α-p-tosyl-L-arginine methyl ester (TAME)-esterase activity, and albumin were measured in the lavage fluid. The number of neutrophils in the lavage fluid was assessed.

Symptomatic rhinovirus-infected subjects had significant increases in kinins, TAME-esterase activity, albumin, and neutrophil numbers. The total number of symptoms was significantly correlated with increases in the concentrations of kinins, albumin, TAME-esterase activity, and neutrophil numbers. The levels of histamine did not change.

During symptomatic rhinovirus infection, kinins are synthesized, vascular permeability increases, and neutrophils enter nasal secretions. Basophils and mast cells do not appear to participate in the generation of a rhinovirus cold. These results may assist in the treatment of rhinovirus colds.

▶ Rhinovirus colds are an excellent example of it being the host response to the infectious agent and not the infectious agent per se that is bad for you. After experimental rhinovirus infection, only 60% of those individuals who become infected develop symptoms, and it is in those people that this report documents an increase in nasal vascular permeability, the generation of kinins, and the influx of neutrophils into nasal secretions. Remarkably, histamine does not increase locally, and this has been a consistent observation in experimental rhinovirus infection.

Kinins, which are potent basoactive peptides that cause vasodilatation and increased vascular permeability, also stimulate pain production and glandular secretion via neuronal reflexes. Their appearance in nasal secretions closely parallels the development of symptoms after experimental rhinovirus colds. While this does not prove that the kinins are pathophysiologically related to the symptoms of a cold, it certainly is suggestive enough to make us desire a trial of an antagonist. Unfortunately, none are available. While histamine did not go up in nasal secretions, it may be hard to convince everyone that antihistamines don't make some patients feel better. Then again, there are those devotees of chicken soup and orange juice, and it is about time to look for the antikinin activity in them.—M.S. Klempner, M.D.

3 Fungal Infections

Serological Tests for Blastomycosis: Assessments During a Large Point-Source Outbreak in Wisconsin

Klein BS, Vergeront JM, Kaufman L, Bradsher RW, Kumar UN, Mathai G, Varkey B, Davis JP (Wisconsin Division of Health; Univ of Wisconsin Clinical Sciences Ctr, Madison; Trinity Mem Hosp, Cudahy, Wis; Med College of Wisconsin, Milwaukee; Ctrs for Disease Control; et al)
J Infect Dis 155:262–268, February 1987   3–1

A point-source epidemic of acute pulmonary blastomycosis, occurring in Wisconsin in 1984, gave an opportunity to evaluate serodiagnostic tests during acute *Blastomyces dermatitidis* infection. The enzyme immunoassay (EIA), immunodiffusion (ID), and complement fixation (CF) tests for antibody to A antigen of *B. dermatitidis* were compared in 47 patients and 89 control subjects having lower respiratory tract illness.

The EIA was used to detect antibody in 77% of patients, compared to 28% for ID and 9% for the CF test (table). The median EIA titer was 1:128. Whenever antibody was detected by ID or CF it was detected by EIA. The peak seroprevalence rate and peak geometric mean EIA titer occurred 50 to 70 days after the onset, but antibody was detected 13 days after the onset of illness. Antifungal therapy was associated with a significant fall in antibody titer about 6 months after the onset. Eight percent of control subjects had antibody. The EIA was 92% specific in detecting antibody, whereas the other tests were 100% specific.

The EIA is useful in serodiagnostic testing for *B. dermatitidis* infection and may be used in an outbreak as an epidemiologic tool. A titer of 1:32 strongly supports the diagnosis of blastomycosis, and a titer of 1:8 is suggestive.

▶ There have been no generally acceptable immunologic tests for the diagnosis of blastomycosis. The complement fixation and immunodiffusion serologic tests and the blastomycin skin test have lacked sensitivity or specificity or both. The EIA test appears to be the first reasonably reliable test for the serodiagnosis of blastomycosis. In a previous study of *chronic* blastomycosis, elevated EIA titers ≥ 1:64 correlated with extrapulmonary infection. By contrast, in the current outbreak of *acute* blastomycosis, 40% of the patients had EIA titers of 1:64, though none developed extrapulmonary disease. Thus, it appears that high EIA titers have a different implication in acute, as opposed to chronic, blastomycosis.—M.J. Barza, M.D.

Clinical and Serologic Features of Blastomycosis

No. of patient	Case status	Antifungal therapy	Outcome	No. of days from illness onset to specimen collection	Serological test result EIA	Serological test result ID	Serological test result CF
1	Definite	Amphotericin B	Cure	70	1:64	Pos	<1:8
				201	<1:8	Neg	ND*
2	Definite	Amphotericin B	Cure	23	1:128	Neg	<1:8
				169	<1:8	Neg	ND
3	Definite	Amphotericin B	Cure	31	1:128	Neg	<1:8
				189	<1:8	Neg	ND
4	Definite	Amphotericin B	Cure	16	1:16	Neg	<1:8
				147	<1:8	Neg	ND
5	Definite	Amphotericin B	Cure	28	1:128	Pos	<1:8
				178	<1:8	Neg	ND
6	Probable	None	Cure	46	1:32	Neg	<1:8
				177	<1:8	Neg	ND
7	Probable	None	Cure	57	1:32	Neg	<1:8
				197	<1:8	Neg	ND
8	Probable	None	Cure	43	1:32	Neg	<1:8
				167	1:8	Neg	ND
9	Probable	None	Cure	53	1:128	Pos	1:8
				183	1:16	Neg	ND
10	Probable	None	Cure	54	1:512	Pos	<1:8
				185	1:16	Neg	ND
11	Probable	None	Cure	0	<1:8	Neg	<1:8
				161	1:16	Neg	ND
12	Probable	None	Cure	41	<1:8	Neg	<1:8
				182	1:32	Neg	ND

*ND = not done.
†Data are from 12 patients with a known date of onset of illness and with a fourfold rise or fall in titer of antibody between paired serum specimens to the A antigen of *B. dermatitidis*.
(Courtesy of Klein BS, Vergeront JM, Kaufman L, et al: *J Infect Dis* 155:262–268, February 1987.)

Serodiagnosis of Invasive Aspergillosis in Patients With Hematologic Malignancy: Validation of the *Aspergillus fumigatus* Antigen Radioimmunoassay

Talbot GH, Weiner MH, Gerson SL, Provencher M, Hurwitz S (Univ of Pennsyl-

vania School of Medicine; Audie L Murphy Mem VA Hosp; Univ of Texas Health Science Ctr, San Antonio)
J Infect Dis 155:12–27, January 1987   3–2

Invasive aspergillosis (IA) is an important cause of morbidity and mortality in patients with acute leukemia or lymphoma and in organ transplant recipients. Its diagnosis, even by invasive methods, may be difficult. Bronchoscopy and even open lung biopsy can be falsely negative. The authors used the *Aspergillus fumigatus* antigen radioimmunoassay to detect aspergillosis in 79 hematology patients at 152 admissions. A total of 616 serum samples was analyzed.

Invasive aspergillosis was discovered in 22 patients at 24 admissions. Maximal antigenic activity was significantly greater among patients with invasive disease than among controls (Fig 3–1). The assay was 74% sensitive and 90% specific and had a positive predictive value of 82% and a negative predictive value of 85%. Antigen was detected before IA was suspected in nearly one third of admissions and before pathologic evidence of disease was obtained in nearly half the cases. The test would have been useful in diagnosis, management, and prognosis in 80% of the 16 fatal cases.

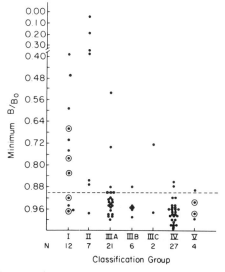

Fig 3–1.—Maximal activity of *Aspergillus* antigen, by patient. The maximal antigenic activity (minimal B/B_0) for each patient in the validation analysis is charted by patient classification group. For patients with 2 or more admissions, a single admission was chosen randomly for analysis. Classification was as follows: group I, definite invasive aspergillosis; group II, probable invasive aspergillosis; group III, indeterminate disease; group IV, probable controls; and group V, controls. Group III patients were further divided as follows: IIIA, a clinically documented infection that did not respond to antibacterial antibiotic therapy during neutrocytopenia; IIIB, fever with no apparent etiology and lasting for 7 or more days during neutrocytopenia; and IIIC, 1 or more cultures positive for *Aspergillus* spp. from sites not clinically infected. The B/B_0 values from previously reported admissions are *circled*. The *dotted line* is drawn at a B/B_0 of 0.90, the cutoff value used in this study. (Courtesy of Talbot GH, Weiner MH, Gerson SL, et al: *J Infect Dis* 155:12–27, January 1987.)

Prospective testing of neutropenic patients for *Aspergillus* antigenemia could facilitate the noninvasive diagnosis of IA and the timely initiation of antifungal treatment. Serologic testing also can help determine the efficacy of therapy.

Diagnosis of Invasive Candidiasis in Patients With and Without Signs of Immune Deficiency: A Comparison of Six Detection Methods in Human Serum

Platenkamp GJ, VanDuin AM, Porsius JC, Schouten HJA, Zondervan PE, Michel MF (Erasmus Univ, Rotterdam, the Netherlands)
J Clin Pathol 40:1162–1167, October 1987
3–3

Invasive candidiasis is a serious and often fatal complication when it occurs in immune-deficient patients. Systemic candidiasis is difficult to diagnose because there is no typical clinical presentation. Confirmation is only by organ biopsy, puncture of a normally sterile body fluid, or at necropsy. The serum concentration of D-arabinitol, a *Candida*-specific metabolite, may help in diagnosis. Three serologic detection methods, two determinations of circulating antigens, and the determination of arabinitol:creatinine ratio were used to distinguish invasive candidiasis from colonization in patients with and without signs of immune deficiency.

Sera and blood samples, where appropriate, were collected and cultured from 56 patients of whom 39 were thought to be immune-deficient. Patients were divided into 2 groups according to whether they had confirmed invasive candidiasis or were colonized without visible lesions. Groups were subdivided into patients with and without evidence of immune deficiency. Whole cell agglutination, hemagglutination, and counterimmunoelectrophoresis were performed to detect antibodies. Hemagglutination inhibition and latex agglutination were used to determine circulating antigens. Arabinitol:creatinine ratios were also determined.

In the suspected immune deficient patients, the best discrimination between visceral candidiasis and colonization was obtained by the combined results of hemagglutination inhibition and arabinitol:creatinine ratio. In the 13 patients in this group who had confirmed candidiasis, the

Percentage of Patients With Positive Results*

Category	No of patients	Percentage WCA	HA	CIE	HAI	LA	A:C
IA	13	15	23	15	54	54	38
IIA	26	19	12	23	12	27	15
IB	10	60	60	80	30	50	40
IIB	7	0	43	14	14	57	0

*Value equal to or greater than the limit value.
(Courtesy of Platenkamp GJ, VanDuin AM, Porsius JC, et al: *Clin Pathol* 40:1162–1167, October 1987.)

tests for antigen and metabolite detection were more often positive than those for the detection of antibodies (table). Counterimmunoelectrophoresis provided the best discrimination for patients without signs of immune deficiency.

A combination of detection methods may be useful in differentiating between invasive candidiasis and colonization in patients with and without signs of immune deficiency. Further research may lead to other approaches: monoclonal antibodies might possibly be used to characterize circulating *Candida* antigens.

▶ Both of these studies (Abstracts 3–2 and 3–3) share the goal of trying to improve our ability to recognize invasive fungal infections by serologic methods. This continues to be an important goal as invasive fungal infections now constitute a major cause of morbidity and mortality in immunocompromised patients, particularly those with hematologic malignancies or those receiving corticosteroid therapy. In the first study, Talbot et al. (Abstract 3–2) have focused on detecting circulating antigen as a predictor of invasive aspergillosis in patients with hematologic malignancies. This is a logical focus since antibody detection methods have been of highly variable success, and antigen detection should have an advantage over antibody detection because antibody production may be attenuated, delayed, or absent in severely immunocompromised patients. Previous studies (e.g., Weiner MH: *Ann Intern Med* 92:793–796, 1980; and Shaffer PJ et al: *Am J Med* 67:627–630, 1979) have shown encouraging results for antigen detection.

This report demonstrates an excellent specificity for the antigen detection method but is limited by a false-negative rate that approaches 25%. If patients who had clinically documented infection that did not respond to antibacterial antibiotic therapy during persistent neutropenia without a documented microbiologic etiology (group 3) are considered in the data analysis, the false-negative rate rises to almost 50%. Nevertheless, application of the results of this test would have affected the management of a substantial portion of their patients.

The second study (Abstract 3–3) compares several different serodiagnostic methods for invasive candidiasis, including a measurement of the serum concentration of D-arabinitol in patients who were either normal hosts or patients immunocompromised by virtue of neoplasms, hemodialysis, total body irradiation, or the use of corticosteroids or other immunosuppressive drugs. It is interesting to note that in the nonimmunocompromised patients, an antibody detection method (CIE) was the best discriminator between colonization and invasive candidiasis, whereas in the immunocompromised group, the antigen detection test (hemagglutination inhibition) combined with an arabinitol:creatinine ratio provided the best results. The sensitivity was still only 62%, whereas the predicted value of the combination was 100%.

It should be emphasized that most of the reagents used in both of these studies are not commercially available and cannot easily be broadly applied to the routine microbiology laboratory. While we are making progress in the serodiagnosis of invasive fungal infection, the sensitivity of these reagents does not allow reliance on a negative result and empiric antifungal therapy in the appropriate situation seems a prudent course. Interested readers are referred to a review on the current trends in immunodiagnosis of candidiasis and aspergillosis (Rev Infect Dis 6:301–312, 1984) by Repetigny, L., and Reese, E.—M.S. Klempner, M.D.

Malassezia furfur Fungemia in Infancy
Alpert G, Bell LM, Campos JM (Univ of Pennsylvania)
Clin Pediatr (Phila) 26:528–531, October 1987   3–4

Malassezia furfur, a lipophilic yeast causing tinea versicolor, rarely causes invasive disease in pediatric patients. Seven infants with M. *furfur* catheter-related fungemia were encountered in 1981–1984. Nearly 6,300 infants were hospitalized in neonatal intensive care units during this period.

Five infants were premature and had serious underlying disease. Five underwent major surgery, which in 3 cases was partial bowel resection. All the infants received 10% or 20% lipid emulsion infusions, usually via a superior caval Broviac catheter. The catheters were in place for a mean of 25 days before fungemia was evident. Two of the infants were asymptomatic, but 5 had signs and symptoms of sepsis, and 1 of them had endocarditis. Only blood obtained through indwelling lines was positive for M. *furfur* in these infants. All 4 catheter tips cultured after removal were sterile. Two patients received antifungal therapy.

It appears that M. *furfur* can colonize indwelling central venous catheters and cause clinically significant infection. A majority of infants may respond to removal of the intravenous catheter. Antifungal therapy should be individualized according to the severity of the clinical findings and whether other explanations for the symptoms are present. The authors presently do not routinely use modified medium to isolate M. *furfur* from the blood.

▶ There has been an upsurge of interest in systemic infection caused by this usually indolent fungus in neonates over the past few years. This organism is part of the normal skin flora in more than 90% of adolescents and adults. Up to 50% of infants in a neonatal intensive care unit may harbor M. *furfur* on the skin. There is a striking association between infection and the administration of intravenous lipid emulsions. Alpert et al. point out that M. *furfur* lacks the ability to synthesize medium- and long-chain fatty acids and therefore requires an exogenous supply of these lipids. The organisms do not grow readily in ordinary blood culture media but grow better in lipid containing media. Indeed, Alpert et al. suggest that in some patients, the presence of lipid emulsion in the venous blood sent for culture may facilitate growth of the yeasts.

The clinical significance of positive "line" cultures for M. *furfur* is not known at this time. Indeed, it is not clear whether symptoms should be attributed to the fungemia or to the other underlying diseases usually present in these ill infants. Based on the very limited number of cases reported so far, it appears that simple removal of the colonized intravenous catheter without administration of antifungal drugs is sufficient to arrest the fungemia.—M.J. Barza, M.D.

Percutaneous Central Venous Catheter Colonization With *Malassezia furfur:* Incidence and Clinical Significance
Aschner JL, Punsalang A Jr, Maniscalco WM, Menegus MA (Univ of Rochester)
Pediatrics 80:535–539, October 1987   3–5

Systemic infections by *Malassezia furfur*, a lipid-dependent yeast, have occurred in neonates with central venous catheters conveying intravenous lipid emulsions. Catheter colonization was studied prospectively in a neonatal intensive care unit, where 25 consecutively removed percutaneous central venous (CV) catheters were evaluated. The catheters were rinsed with saline, and the rinse fluid was plated on Sabouraud dextrose agar overlaid with olive oil. Infants received up to 3.5 gm/kg of lipid emulsion (20% Liposyn) daily.

Of 25 catheters from 19 infants, 8 were positive for *M. furfur*, 5 in large quantity. Ten catheters were colonized by coagulase-negative staphylococci. *Malassezia furfur* was cultured from the skin of two thirds of the infants. Six of 8 infants whose catheters were colonized by *M. furfur* had no objective evidence of systemic infection. Two other infants had systemic infection, and 1 had *M. furfur* cultured from a postmortem lung aspirate.

Although *M. furfur* frequently colonizes the skin and percutaneous CV catheters of neonatal infants in intensive care units, the factors contributing to systemic disease remain to be determined. Several infected infants have had apnea, bradycardia, pulmonary deterioration, and thrombocytopenia. The illness is similar to sepsis with *Staphylococcus epidermidis*, which also frequently colonizes the skin and indwelling catheters.

▶ See Abstract 3–4.—M.J. Barza, M.D.

Treatment of Cryptococcal Meningitis With Combination Amphotericin B and Flucytosine for Four as Compared With Six Weeks
Dismukes WE, Cloud G, Gallis HA, Kerkering TM, Medoff G, Craven PC, Kaplowitz LG, Fisher JF, Gregg CR, Bowles CA, Shadomy S, Stamm AM, Diasio RB, Kaufman L, Soong S-J, Blackwelder WC, Natl Inst of Allergy and Infectious Diseases Mycoses Study Group (Univ of Alabama in Birmingham; Virginia Commonwealth Univ; Ctrs for Disease Control; Natl Insts of Health)
N Engl J Med 317:334–341, Aug 6, 1987   3–6

Cryptococcal meningitis is the most common form of fungal meningitis in the United States and is an important cause of morbidity and mortality in immunocompromised patients. No therapeutic regimen has been uniformly effective or without serious toxicity. In 1979, it was reported that a regimen combining amphotericin B and flucytosine for 6 weeks was as effective as a low-dose regimen of amphotericin B alone for 10 weeks. The duration of this combination was shortened further, from 6 to 4 weeks, to determine whether this would reduce toxicity without compromising efficacy in a multicenter, prospective, randomized clinical trial.

The 194 patients enrolled in the study had cryptococcal meningitis. All patients received intravenous amphotericin B, 0.3 mg/kg/day, for 28 days and oral flucytosine, 150 mg/kg/day, in equal doses every 6 hours, for 28 days. At the end of 4 weeks, patients were randomized to either a 4-week regimen calling for no additional treatment or a 6-week regimen that included 2 more weeks of therapy.

Of the 91 patients who met preestablished criteria for randomization, cure or improvement was seen in 75% of those treated for 4 weeks and in 85% of those treated for 6 weeks. The estimated relapse rate for the group on the 4-week regimen was 27%, compared with 16% of the group on the 6-week regimen. The incidences of toxic effects for the shorter and longer regimens were 44% and 43%, respectively. Among 23 transplant recipients, 4 of 5 treated for 4 weeks relapsed. Thus, the rest were treated for 6 weeks. Only 3 of the 18 treated for 6 weeks relapsed. Of the 80 patients who did not follow the initial protocol and therefore were not randomized, 38 died or relapsed. Three significant predictors of favorable response were identified by multifactorial analysis of treatment factors for all 194 patients: headache as a symptom, normal mental status, and a cerebrospinal fluid white-cell count greater than $20/mm^3$.

These findings are in agreement with other findings that suggest that the 4-week regimen should be reserved for patients with meningitis without neurologic complications, underlying disease, or immunosuppressive therapy: pretreatment cerebrospinal fluid white-cell count greater than $20/mm^3$ and a serum cryptococcal antigen titer below 1:32; and a negative cerebrospinal fluid india ink preparation and serum and cerebrospinal fluid cryptococcal-antigen titers below 1:8 at 4 weeks of therapy.

▶ Another excellent study from the Mycoses Study Group sponsored by the National Institute of Allergy and Infectious Diseases. Such studies would be near impossible for single institutions to carry out, and we should encourage similar endeavors for other similar diseases.— S.M. Wolff, M.D.

Pharmacology and Toxicity of High-Dose Ketoconazole
Sugar AM, Alsip SG, Galgiani JN, Graybill JR, Dismukes WE, Cloud GA, Craven PC, Stevens DA (Stanford Univ Med School; National Inst of Allergy and Infectious Diseases Mycoses Study Group, Bethesda, Md; Univ of Alabama School of Medicine at Birmingham; Univ of Arizona College of Medicine; Univ of Texas Health Sciences Ctr, San Antonio)
Antimicrob Agents Chemother 31:1874–1878, December 1987   3–7

Because of relapse, doses of ketoconazole greater than those currently licensed in the United States have been recommended for the treatment of coccidioidomycosis. The pharmacology of the drug was studied in 160 patients enrolled in 2 multicenter trials, who received 400 to 2,000 mg once a day for meningeal or nonmeningeal disease.

The mean serum drug level exceeded the minimal inhibitory concentration for *Coccidioides immitis* for 24 hours after all doses; trough levels exceeded 1 µg/ml. Mean peak serum levels occurred 4–6 hours after treatment and ranged from 7 to 17 µg/ml. Serum levels tended to increase with prolonged treatment, but not to a significant degree. Very few cerebrospinal fluid samples from patients with meningitis contained more than 1 µg/ml of ketoconazole, and levels could not be related to the dose or the time after dosing. Dosage failed to correlate with toxicity or with the outcome, and serum concentrations also were unrelated to the outcome. Toxic effects were reversible, but doses exceeding 400 mg were significantly more toxic than doses currently licensed. More than half the patients given 1,600 mg of ketoconazole encountered toxic effects.

Higher doses of ketoconazole are more toxic but not demonstrably more effective in patients with coccidioidomycosis. Further studies are needed to show whether high doses are warranted in the treatment of meningitis.

▶ Ketoconazole seems to resemble amphotericin B in that there is some correlation between toxicity and total dosage but no clear correlation between toxicity and serum concentrations of the drug. A disquieting observation was that there was no apparent relation between the daily dosage of ketoconazole and the outcome of treatment of coccidioidomycosis. It will be of interest to see whether similar findings are reported with fluconazole, a related antifungal agent with a number of advantages over ketoconazole.—M.J. Barza, M.D.

Induction of Prostaglandin Synthesis as the Mechanism Responsible for the Chills and Fever Produced by Infusing Amphotericin B
Gigliotti F, Shenep JL, Lott L, Thornton D (St Jude Children's Research Hosp, Memphis, Tenn)
J Infect Dis 156:784–789, November 1987   3–8

Amphotericin B is an effective antifungal agent. However, 50% to 70% of the patients who receive this drug develop chills and fever. The mechanism of this adverse reaction is not known.

To investigate this response, mouse peritoneal macrophages and human mononuclear cells were exposed to 1.0 µg/ml of amphotericin B. Amphotericin B induced the synthesis of prostaglandin E_2, which is involved in the production of fever. Therefore, a double-blind, placebo-controlled clinical trial of 10 mg/kg of ibuprofen, an inhibitor of prostaglandin synthesis, was performed to determine whether preadministration could prevent the adverse effects of amphotericin B in 30 cancer patients. The occurrence of severe chilling reactions was significantly reduced from 69% to 15%.

This suggests that the adverse effects, chilling and fever, caused by the administration of amphotericin B are mediated by the synthesis of prostaglandin E_2. Ibuprofen was useful in this series of patients in ameliorating the side effects of amphotericin B.

▶ Amphotericin B continues to be the most important antifungal agent available to the critically ill patient. This study was undertaken to better understand the mechanism involved in the production of fever and chills after administration of this drug. There are several points worth emphasizing. First, a substantial portion of patients (47%) never experienced an amphotericin B reaction despite no premedication in this and a similar study previously reported (Tynes VS et al: Am Rev Respir Dis 87:264-268, 1963) that when patients received their amphotericin B test dose without premedication and do not get a reaction, it is certainly reasonable not to premedicate them for their subsequent doses unless the complication of fever and chills develops. Second, the in vitro data strongly support the contention that amphotericin B is capable of inducing prostaglandin synthesis in cells that appear to be critical to this overall process (monocyte macrophages), and this concept is further substantiated by the in vivo double-blind study that demonstrated a therapeutic effect of single-dose ibuprofen (10 mg/kg) pretreatment 30 minutes before the amphotericin B administration.

It is important to note that there continues to be a small proportion of patients (15%) who still had severe chilling after this type of premedication, but by and large the therapy was extremely well tolerated and highly efficacious. While many other drugs such as aspirin, diphenhydramine, meperidine, and dantrolene have been used to manage amphotericin B reactions, only hydrocortisone pretreatment has been shown in a controlled study to reduce amphotericin B-associated chills and fever. Based on this and the report of Tynes, the nonsteroidal agents or hydrocortisone are the drugs of choice for treatment of the patients who require this prior to amphotericin B therapy.—M.S. Klempner, M.D.

Amphotericin-B Nephrotoxicity in Humans Decreased by Sodium Supplements with Coadministration of Ticarcillin or Intravenous Saline
Branch RA, Jackson EK, Jacqz E, Stein R, Ray WA, Ohnhaus EE, Meusers P, Heidemann H (Vanderbilt Univ; Medizinische Klinik, Essen, West Germany)
Klin Wochenschr 65:500-506, 1987   3-9

Amphotericin B is widely used to treat systemic mycotic infections, but there is a high incidence of nephrotoxicity with this treatment. Previous studies indicate that salt loading may help to reverse amphotericin B-induced nephrotoxicity. Two groups of patients were studied to determine the role of salt supplementation when amphotericin B is administered.

The first study was a retrospective one at Vanderbilt University. Of 21 patients treated with amphotericin B alone, nephrotoxicity developed in 14, requiring temporary withdrawal of the drug. In contrast, only 2 of 17 patients treated with amphotericin B and ticarcillin, the latter having a high obligatory sodium load, experienced nephrotoxicity. After ticarcillin was withdrawn but amphotericin B was continued in 4 patients, nephrotoxicity developed in all 4 within 1 week.

In the second study, a prospective one at the University of Essen, 20 patients were given 24 courses of amphotericin B with routine daily parenteral salt supplementation: only 2 had nephrotoxicity. Four others with initial evidence of mild renal impairment received amphotericin B and salt supplementation without adverse effects. The results of these 2 studies suggest that nephrotoxicity associated with amphotericin B administration can be substantially reduced by sodium loading.

▶ The authors postulate that nephrotoxicity is mediated via a tubuloglomerular feedback (TGF) mechanism that regulates renal blood flow and glomerular filtration in response to the amount of sodium chloride present in the body. They have previously reported that salt repletion can help to reverse established nephrotoxicity. In the case of aminoglycoside nephrotoxicity, there is evidence that salt loading diminishes the uptake of aminoglycosides by the proximal renal tubule. To my knowledge, such information is not available for amphotericin B.

In this study, some patients received ticarcillin and others received 1 liter per day of 0.9% sodium chloride, that is, 150 ml milliequivalents of sodium chloride; it is not known whether lesser degrees of salt loading would be effective. Further data on this type of interaction would be valuable, but for the moment, it seems reasonable to attempt at least modest salt loading in patients given amphotericin B.—M.J. Barza, M.D.

Short-Course Amphotericin B Therapy for Isolated Candiduria in Children
Kohn DB, Uehling, DT, Peters ME, Fellows KW, Chesney PJ (Univ of Wisconsin, Ctr for the Health Sciences)
J Pediatr 110:310–313, February 1987
3–10

Certain medical and surgical techniques now in use leave children with impaired defenses against fungal infection. This report describes the successful management of candiduria in 6 children receiving short courses of intravenously given amphotericin B.

Initially, regimens thought to be less toxic were tried, including bladder irrigation with amphotericin B, oral administration of ketoconazole and 5-fluorocytosine, and intravenous administration of miconazole. After therapy lasting at least 1 week, these were considered unsuccessful. Treatment with amphotericin B was initiated and increased over a 1- to 4-day period to 1 mg/kg per day intravenously. All patients responded within 1–10 days of therapy. Urine cultures became sterile within 48–96 hours of the initiation of therapy. Candiduria was permanently eradicated in the 5 patients who were followed for 2 months to 5 years.

Low-dose, short-duration amphotericin B therapy is useful in the treatment of candiduria in children, while avoiding most of the toxicity associated with more intensive regimens. Prospective studies are required to compare it to other antifungal therapies and to determine optimal dose and duration.

▶ The results of this study are not surprising in view of the unusual pharmacokinetics of amphotericin B. The drug is readily bound to tissues and epithelial surfaces and is eliminated slowly, producing sustained though low urinary concentrations.—M.J. Barza, M.D.

4 Parasitic Infections

Helminths

Controlled Trial and Dose-Finding Study of Ivermectin for Treatment of Onchocerciasis
White AT, Newland HS, Taylor HR, Erttmann KD, Keyvan-Larijani E, Nara A, Aziz MA, D'Anna SA, Williams PN, Greene BM (Case Western Reserve Univ; Univ Hosps, Cleveland; Johns Hopkins Med Insts; Merck Sharp and Dohme Research Labs, Rahway, NJ; Liberian Agricultural Co, Grand Bassa County, Liberia)
J Infect Dis 156:463–470, September 1987   4–1

Onchocerciasis, caused by the organism *Onchocerca volvulus*, is one of the leading causes of human blindness. Ivermectin has shown promise as a treatment for onchocerciasis. To assess the safety and efficacy of ivermectin, 200 infected Liberians received 100, 150, 200 µg/kg of ivermectin or placebo and were followed for 1 year.

Although therapy was associated with only limited side effects, these adverse effects increased with dosage. All treatment groups had significant reduction in skin parasite counts by day 3. By 3 months, there was a 95% decrease in parasite counts in all groups. However, at 3 months, the proportion of patients with no skin microfilariae was significantly lower in the 100 µg group than in the other 2 groups. After 1 year, the parasite level was reduced by 80%. There was a significant reduction in ocular involvement in all groups.

These results confirm that a single dose of ivermectin is safe and well tolerated. This study suggests that 150 µg/kg of ivermectin may be the optimal therapeutic dose.

▶ A major advance in the struggle against river blindness, one of the leading causes of human blindness. The problem will be in distributing the drug where it is needed while hoping that resistance will not develop.—G.T. Keusch, M.D.

Clinical Study Evaluating Efficacy of Praziquantel in Clonorchiasis
Yangco BG, De Lerma C, Lyman GH, Price DL (Univ of South Florida; James A. Haley VA Hosp, Tampa, Fla; Pinellas County Health Dept, St Petersburg, Fla; Devetec, Inc, Bradenton, Fla)
Antimicrob Agents Chemother 31:135–138, February 1987   4–2

Clonorchiasis, endemic in Southeast Asia, is an infection caused by the liver fluke *Clonorchis sinensis*. The infection is contracted by eating raw or poorly cooked freshwater fish containing encysted larvae. Complications may include cholelithiasis, liver abscesses, portal hypertension, and possibly adenocarcinoma of the liver. The authors evaluated praziquantel, a drug reported to be effective against cestode and trematode infections in animals, in 214 Asian immigrants with diagnoses of clonorchiasis. A double-blind, placebo-controlled trial in 42 patients was followed by an open study in 32 patients. Praziquantel was given in a single-day course of 75 mg/kg.

All treated patients were cured, as were 4 placebo patients (20%). The most frequent adverse drug effects were nausea, vomiting, and vertigo. There were no major changes in laboratory measurements during treatment.

A single-day course of praziquantel was consistently effective in these Asian patients with clonorchiasis. Previous treatment of this disorder has been unsatisfactory. Light infections may resolve without treatment, but the serious complications of infection and the availability of a relatively nontoxic and effective drug warrant its use in treating clonorchiasis.

▶ An important practical question raised by this study is whether all patients with clonorchiasis should be treated or only those with symptomatic infection and a moderate or heavy burden of parasites. Light infestations may resolve without treatment. However, given the fact that treatment is simple and well tolerated, I would tend to treat all patients with clonorchiasis, symptomatic or not and irrespective of the parasite burden.—M.J. Barza, M.D.

Protozoa

Efficacy of Malaria Prophylaxis in American and Swiss Travelers to Kenya
Lobel HO, Roberts JM, Somaini B, Steffen R (Ctrs for Disease Control; Federal Office of Public Health, Bern, Switzerland; Univ of Zurich)
J Infect Dis 155:1205–1209, June 1987   4–3

Malaria infection has increased among American and Swiss travelers to Kenya in recent years, chiefly because of the emergence of chloroquine-resistant strains of *Plasmodium falciparum*. The efficacy of chloroquine alone was compared with that of Fansidar (pyrimethamine/sulfadoxine), alone or combined with chloroquine, in travelers returning from Kenya.

Fifteen of 59 infected travelers from the United States returning from Kenya had not used any prophylaxis. Of all 1,169 travelers returning from Kenya, 7.5% had not used chemoprophylaxis; 44% had regularly used Fansidar with chloroquine, and 3% had used only Fansidar. In Switzerland, 64 cases of *P. falciparum* infection were reported after travel to Kenya. Eleven percent of 2,602 travelers used no chemoprophylaxis. The risk of malaria developing was 9- to 12-fold higher when no prophylaxis was used than when Fansidar was taken, with or without chloroquine. Chloroquine alone was not significantly protective.

Changing patterns of drug susceptibility in Africa make it necessary to continuously evaluate recommended regimens for preventing malaria. No totally effective and safe drug is available for prophylactic use. The use of personal protective measures, such as repellents and mosquito netting, should be emphasized.

▶ This study demonstrates that Fansidar is much more effective than chloroquine in prophylaxis of falciparum malaria where chloroquine-resistant *P. falciparum* (CRPF) is endemic. Nonetheless, the attack rate was reduced by half for the chloroquine users. Fansidar is no longer recommended because of an unacceptable incidence of severe reactions and sudden death. American travelers are recommended to take chloroquine prophylaxis and to seek medical diagnosis and care for febrile illness in areas with CRPF. When such care is not available, the recommendation is to take 3 Fansidar tablets immediately for treatment of otherwise unexplained fevers. All measures to reduce exposure to mosquito bites—netting, screens, protective clothing, and repellent—should be emphasized and employed.—G.T. Keusch, M.D.

Doxycycline Prophylaxis for Falciparum Malaria
Pang LW, Limsomwong N, Boudreau EF, Singharaj P (Armed Forces Research Inst of Med Sciences, Bangkok, Thailand)
Lancet 1:1162–1164, May 23, 1987   4–4

Falciparum malaria has become resistant to many drugs used in the treatment and prophylaxis of malaria in Southeast Asia. Mefloquine has been shown to be effective in the treatment and prophylaxis of malaria, but the WHO has recommended that mefloquine not be used for prophylactic purposes, except under controlled conditions. As a result, there are no approved drugs readily available in Thailand for effective falciparum malaria prophylaxis. Because doxycycline has been shown to be effective in the treatment of falciparum malaria in Thailand, the authors con-

Results
95 subjects received doxycyline and 93 chloroquine. The groups did not differ with respect to age, weight,

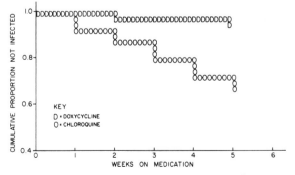

Fig 4–1.—Survival analysis of doxycycline vs. chloroquine. (Courtesy of Pang LW, Linsomwong N, Boudreau EF, et al: *Lancet* 1:1162–1164, May 23, 1987.)

	Drug-Related Side Effects*			
	Doxycycline (n = 95)		Chloroquine (n = 93)	
	Frequency† of complaint	Individuals with complaint	Frequency† of symptoms	Individuals with symptoms
Headache	29 *(0·5)*	16	26 *(0·6)*	15
Fever	27 *(0·5)*	14	11 *(0·2)*	7
Dizziness	65 *(1·1)*	26	64 *(1·4)*	36
Nausea	24 *(0·4)*	19	16 *(0·4)*	3
Vomiting	11 *(0·2)*	7	7 *(0·2)*	1
Abdominal pain	14 *(0·2)*	8	12 *(0·3)*	6
Diarrhoea	9 *(0·2)*	7	10 *(0·2)*	6

*No significant difference in frequency of complaint for any symptom between groups; $P > .05$ chi-square test.

†Entries are number of daily complaints, with percent of total man-days on drugs in parentheses.

(Courtesy of Pang LW, Linsomwong N, Boudreau EF, et al: *Lancet* 1:1162–1164, May 23, 1987.)

ducted a study to determine whether doxycycline would also be effective as a prophylactic agent.

The study was done with 188 schoolchildren, aged 10–15 years, who lived in a malaria-endemic region along the Thai-Burmese border. The children were randomly assigned to treatment with either doxycycline (n = 95) or chloroquine (n = 93) during a 9-week study period of a high rate of *Plasmodium falciparum* transmission. The groups were matched for age, weight, and splenomegaly.

Of 95 children treated with prophylactic doxycycline, 5 developed falciparum malaria, whereas of 93 control children treated with chloroquine, 31 developed falciparum malaria (Fig 4–1). There was no statistically significant difference in incidence or severity of side effects associated with either doxycycline or chloroquine administration (table).

Doxycycline is highly effective in the prophylaxis of falciparum malaria in an area of high multidrug resistance. However, the authors do not advocate its widespread use for long-term prophylaxis but recommend its short-term use only during periods of high-rate malaria transmission.

▶ In Thailand, where chloroquine-resistant *P. falciparum* is prevalent (but not in Bangkok or Chiangmai, so recommend that your traveling patients visit these jewels of Southeast Asia if they possibly can), doxycycline provides significant prophylaxis for malaria. It also protects against traveler's diarrhea, and many patients may be asking for it. A few cautions: the drug (1) is not recommended for children younger than 10 years because of adverse effects on bone and teeth and, (2) because the study was carried out in partially immune children 10–15 years old living in an endemic area, it is not proven effective in malaria virgins.—G.T. Keusch, M.D.

Safety and Immunogenicity in Man of a Synthetic Peptide Malaria Vaccine Against *Plasmodium falciparum* Sporozoites

Herrington DA, Clyde DF, Losonsky G, Cortesia M, Murphy JR, Davis J, Baqar S, Felix AM, Heimer EP, Gillessen D, Nardin E, Nussenzweig RS, Nussenzweig V, Hollingdale MR, Levine MM (Univ of Maryland School of Medicine; Hoffman–La Roche Inc, Nutley, NJ; F Hoffman–La Roche and Co, Ltd, Basel, Switzerland; New York Univ School of Medicine; Biomedical Research Inst, Rockville, Md)
Nature 328:257–259, July 16, 1987   4–5

Plasmodium falciparum malaria is increasing due to the spread of resistant strains of the parasite and its mosquito host. The immunodominant epitope of the circumsporozoite protein was synthesized. This peptide consists of 12 amino acids, $(NANP)_3$. This synthetic epitope was conjugated to tetanus toxoid, with aluminum hydroxide as an adjuvant, and administered intramuscularly in 3 doses at monthly intervals to 35 healthy male volunteers as a malaria vaccine.

Mild soreness at the injection site was common, but no significant adverse reactions were noted. Seroconversion against the synthetic epitope occurred in 53% of those receiving 100 µg and in 71% of those receiving 160 µg. The 3 volunteers with the highest antibody titers and 4 controls who had not been immunized were challenged with infected mosquitos. In all controls, blood stage parasites were detected by day 10. Two of the vaccinees did not manifest infection until day 11 and 1 vaccinee did not have evidence of parasitemia after 29 days of observation (table, p. 116).

This represents the first synthetic peptide parenteral vaccine against a communicable disease that is safe for use in humans and stimulates biologically active antibodies. It is likely that improved formulations and more potent adjuvants can enhance the response to this vaccine.

▶ A synthetic peptide sporozoite malaria vaccine was tested and reported in 1987, a real triumph for science. Even better, 53% to 71% of recipients made antibody, depending on dose. Only 1 of 3 subjects challenged (those with highest counts of antibody) was protected; in the other 2, there was just a slight prolongation in the prepatency period before parasites were detected. From such humble beginnings, however, empires may be built!—G.T. Keusch, M.D.

Construction of Synthetic Immunogen: Use of New T-Helper Epitope on Malaria Circumsporozoite Protein

Good MF, Maloy WL, Lunde MN, Margalit H, Cornette JL, Smith GL, Moss B, Miller LH, Berzofsky JA, (Natl Inst of Health, Bethesda, Md)
Science 235:1059–1062, Feb 27, 1987   4–6

A lot of effort is being devoted to the development of a malarial vaccine. Most of this work has focused on a repeated epitope, $(NANP)_n$, on the circumsporozoite (CS) protein. To determine whether there were

Serologic and Parasitologic Results After *P. falciparum* Sporozoite Inoculation in Vaccinees and Controls

Volunteer	Prevaccination	Reciprocal IgG anti-NANP titres Prechallenge	Day +7	Day +28	Days to patency‡	Peak parasitaemia (parasites mm^{-3})
1	ND†	<25	<25	<25	9	49
2	ND	<25	<25	<25	8	20
3	ND	<25	<25	<25	10	<10
4	ND	<25	<25	<25	7	21
5	<25	400	200	400	11	24
6	<25	400	400	200	§	8
7	<25	200	400	400	11	24

*Volunteers 1–4 were unimmunized controls. Volunteers 5, 6, and 7 were vaccine recipients. Antibody titers were measured by enzyme-linked immunosorbent assay. Parasites mm^{-3} of blood were enumerated microscopically.
†ND = not done. Control volunteers received no vaccine.
‡$P = 0.029$ when prepatent periods between vaccinees and controls are compared using 1-tailed Wilcoxon rank sum test.
§Volunteer 6 did not have parasitaemia during the 29 day post challenge observation period.
(Courtesy of Herrington DA, Clyde DF, Losonsky G, et al: *Nature* 328:257–259, July 16, 1987.)

other sites on the CS protein to which T-cells might respond, congenic strains of mice were immunized with the entire CS protein.

B10.BR and B10.A(4R) mice that do not respond to the $(NANP)_n$ repeat, did respond to the entire CS protein, indicating there are helper T-cell sites other than the repeat unit located on this protein. The computer algorithm, AMPHI, was used to look for such sites by their configuration and their proximity to a B-cell stimulating site. The sequence with the highest amphipathic score was from amino acid 323–349. This peptide was synthesized, injected into mice, and found to be a T-cell site. It was named Th2R.

A synthetic immunogen containing both the repeat unit and this new T-cell site was constructed, Th2R-NP(NANP)$_5$NA. B10.BR and B10.A(4R) mice were immunized with this synthetic immunogen and with another that only contained the repeat unit. Although neither strain responded to the repeat unit, both responded to the conjugate peptide.

Th2R-NP(NANP)$_5$NA represents a synthetic immunogen containing a T-cell site and a B-cell site of parasite origin. The approach described in this paper may be useful in the rational design of recombinant vaccines.

▶ The race is on between logic and the perversity of nature. This is a really lovely study down the logic lane, and it appeals to me. Whether it makes a difference or not remains to be seen.—G.T. Keusch, M.D.

Naturally Acquired Antibodies to Sporozoites Do Not Prevent Malaria: Vaccine Development Implications
Hoffman SL, Oster CN, Plowe CV, Woollett GR, Beier JC, Chulay JD, Wirtz RA, Hollingdale MR, Mugambi M (Naval Med Research Inst, Bethesda, Md; Walter Reed Army Inst of Research, Washington, DC; US Army Med Research Unit–Nairobi, Kenya; Cornell Univ Med College; Biomedical Research Inst, Rockville, Md)
Science 237:639–642, Aug 7, 1987   4–7

Vaccines against malaria have been designed to induce antibodies to the circumsporozoite protein of the parasite. However, it is not known whether naturally acquired antibodies predict resistance to malaria. A prospective study was undertaken to determine whether naturally acquired antibodies to the circumsporozoite protein could predict protection against malaria during a 98-day high-transmission period.

In a malaria-endemic region of Kenya, 83 adults were tested for antibodies to the circumsporozoite protein and then treated for malaria. They were monitored for the development of reinfection for 98 days. Parasitemia developed in 60 of these patients, and in 23, it did not. Antibody levels were indistinguishable between these 2 groups (table). There was no relationship between time of onset and antibody titer. Therefore, unless the antibodies induced by a malarial vaccine are superior to these

Comparison of Sporozoite Antibodies in the Group of 60 Kenyan Adults That Became Infected and the Group of 23 Who Did Not Become Infected During 98 Days

Volunteers	ELISA IgG*	ISI (%)	Samples with >75% ISI (%)	CSP score	IFAT IgG ($-\log_{10}$ titer)
Infected ($N = 60$)	0.53 ± 0.48	67.5 ± 17.6	43	45.2 ± 13.5	2.46 ± 0.42
Not infected ($N = 23$)	0.55 ± 0.37	66.9 ± 17.4	39	36.8 ± 20.1	2.48 ± 0.29

*Serums obtained on study day 0 were tested at a 1:50 serum dilution by ELISA for IgG antibodies to R32LR, by IFAT for IgG antibodies to *P. falciparum* sporozoites for circumsporozoite precipitation (CSP) at a 1:2 serum dilution, and for inhibition of sporozoite invasion of hepatoma cells (ISI) at a 1:20 serum dilution. The results of the assays were similar in the infected and noninfected groups ($P > .05$). Results are expressed as mean ± SD.

(Courtesy of Hoffman SL, Oster CN, Plowe CV, et al: *Science* 237:639–642, Aug 7, 1987.)

naturally acquired antibodies, it is unlikely that these vaccines will prevent infection in malaria-endemic areas.

▶ This paper, appearing in *Science* just 3 weeks after the previous paper was published in *Nature,* comes on somewhat like *The Last Emperor* and reinforces the "don't count your empires before they have been built" caution. In this study, natural antibody to circumsporozoite antigen failed to protect subjects living in an endemic region. The authors conclude that vaccine-induced antibodies are not likely to do better. Want to make a bet?—G.T. Keusch, M.D.

Safety and Efficacy of a Recombinant DNA *Plasmodium falciparum* Sporozoite Vaccine
Ballou WR, Hoffman SL, Sherwood JA, Hollingdale MR, Neva FA, Hockmeyer WT, Gordon DM, Schneider I, Wirtz RA, Young JF, Wasserman GF, Reeve P, Diggs CL, Chulay JD (Walter Reed Army Med Ctr, Washington, DC; US Naval Med Research Inst, Bethesda, Md; National Insts of Health; Biomedical Research Inst, Rockville, Md; Smith, Kline, and French, Swedeland, Pa)
Lancet 1:1277–1281, June 6, 1987   4–8

To date, control of falciparum malaria remains one of the greatest health problems in the world. Widespread drug resistance in the parasite and insecticide resistance in the mosquito vector have seriously hampered the global eradication and control of this disease. Consequently, the direction of malaria research has changed to the prevention of malaria by means of vaccination. A review was made of the results of a human phase I safety and immunogenicity study and of a preliminary efficacy study with a recombinant DNA *Plasmodium falciparum* sporozoite vaccine (FSV-1), produced in *Escherichia coli.*

The study was done with 15 healthy men aged 22–50 years who had no history of malaria. Two agreed to serve as nonimmunized controls in the challenge part of the study. There were no serious side effects. In 12 men (80%), antibody titers of at least 1/50 developed. Maximal antibody responses were sustained for 2–3 weeks but disappeared with a half-life

Immunogenicity and Efficacy of a Fourth Dose of FSV-1

Subject	OD* (1:50)	Dose (µg)	SI†	IFA (1:100)	Prepatent period (days)	Incubation period (days)
C1	0.195	..	ND	–	9	9
C2	0.137	..	ND	–	10	9
11	0.122	300	1.08	–	10	10
7	0.147	100	1.40	–	10	9
10	0.264	300	2.95	–	10	9
8	0.294	100	9.88	–	12	11
13	0.613	800	7.07	2+	13	12
14	1.058	800	4.04	2+	>30	>30

*Enzyme-linked immosorbent assay absorbance.
†Lymphocyte blastogenesis to R32LR; mean SI of four nonimmunized controls was 1.71; ND, not done.
(Courtesy of Ballou WR, Hoffman SL, Sherwood JA, et al.: *Lancet* 1:1277–1281, June 6, 1987.)

of about 28 days. One man who received the maximum dose of vaccine had antibody titers similar to those resulting from lifelong natural exposure to sporozoite-infected mosquitoes (Fig 4–2). After 6 immunized men who had been given a fourth dose of FSV-1 and the 2 nonimmunized controls were challenged by bites of infected mosquitoes, parasitemia did not develop in the man with the highest antibody titer and was delayed in 2 other immunized volunteers (table).

These results indicate that FSV-1 vaccine is safe and well tolerated at the doses studied, but that it did not provide optimal immunity against infection by *P. falciparum*. Higher and more sustained antibody titers are needed before the FSV-1 vaccine can be used for immunization on a wide scale.

▶ We are diligently tracking the malaria vaccine story, represented here by a phase 1 study of a recombinant sporozoite vaccine (it appears to be safe and it induces antibody) and a "we may as well try it" efficacy study (a more positive than negative study which is, in itself, a triumph). So, while there is progress,

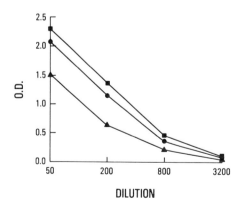

Fig 4–2.—Comparison of antibodies to *P. falciparum* CS protein repeat epitopes after immunization with FSV-1 or natural exposure to infected mosquitoes. Week 10 sera obtained from a volunteer who received 800-gm doses of FSV-1 (▲), and from a hyperendemic region of Indonesia (■) and a holoendemic region of Kenya (●) were assayed by the enzyme-linked immunosorbent method for antibodies against R32LR. (Courtesy of Ballou WR, Hoffman SL, Sherwood JA, et al: *Lancet* 1:1277–1281, June 6, 1987.)

the problem remains, more research is needed, more labs will stay funded (I hope), and some excellent papers will be published. After all, Rome took more than a day to make!—G.T. Keusch, M.D.

Assessment of the Incidence and Prevalence of Clinical Malaria in Semi-Immune Children Exposed to Intense and Perennial Transmission
Trape JF, Zoulani A, Quinet MC (Laboratoire de Parasitologie et d'Entomologie Médicale, Brazzaville, of the Congo Republic)
Am J Epidemiol 126:193–201, August 1987   4-9

The diagnosis of clinical malaria in the semi-immune is difficult in a region of otherwise intense malarial endemicity. A recent study indicates that it is possible to use the parasite:leukocyte ratio to determine whether malaria is responsible for fever in a child living in an area of intense perennial transmission. Using this method and longitudinal temperature surveys, the incidence and prevalence of clinical malaria were defined among 182 children aged 5 to 13 years in Linzolo, Republic of the Congo, a village where malaria is holoendemic. Two surveys were done: a weekly survey over 4 months and a daily survey over 10 days. Axillary temperatures were taken and a thick blood film was taken if temperature was 38C or higher. Only cases of fever with a parasite/leukocyte ratio equal to or more than 2 were considered "confirmed" falciparum malaria cases.

By age group, the prevalence of clinical malaria was between 3.2% and 2.4% at ages 5–6 years; between 2.5% and 1.8% at ages 7–8 years; between 1.6% and 1.1% at ages 9–10 years; and between 0.5% and 0.3% at ages 11–13 years. For these age groups, respectively, the annual incidence of clinical malaria was estimated during the first survey from the data in the table as 3.0, 2.1, 1.8, and 1.2 attacks. There was no difference in the incidence of malarial attacks between children who used bed-nets and those who did not. Although only 53.4% of children with

Incidence of Clinical Malaria in Schoolchildren Over the 4-Month Period of the Weekly Survey, According to Age Group, Linzolo, Republic of the Congo, November 3, 1983–March 1, 1984

Age group (years)	No. of children/ weeks	No. of episodes of clinical malaria		Mean no. of episodes per child during four months of study	
		Minimum*	Maximum†	Minimum	Maximum
5–6	501	22	37	0.75	1.26
7–8	670	20	34	0.51	0.86
9–10	952	19	47	0.34	0.84
11–13	874	8	32	0.16	0.62
Total	2,997	69	150	0.39	0.85

*Confirmed number of clinical malaria infections during the sessions of the weekly survey (schoolchildren present and absent) and those during the intervals between sessions.
†Confirmed and possible clinical malaria infections.
(Courtesy of Trape JF, Zoulani A, Quinet MC: Am J Epidemiol 126:193–201, August 1987.)

episodes of fever or "headache" were examined at the school or medical center, most of those who were not examined received treatment as well, directly from their parents. Persons with fever or "headache" were rapidly treated with antimalarials, and half of these cases were treated by the parents themselves.

The incidence of clinical malaria among semi-immune children exposed to intense and perennial transmission remains high at ages 5–6 years and decreases rapidly until it reaches a very low level in the adolescent and adult. The total consumption of antimalarial drugs by children in Linzolo is high, mainly as a result of the practices of the parents. This explains the fall in mortality from malaria despite a very high level of transmission.

▶ I'm not certain this study measures clinical malaria, since it defines such cases as being in febrile patients who have 2 or more parasites per leukocyte in a malaria smear. This selects those with higher parasitemia, but this is not necessarily the same as a clinical cause and effect. It's surely difficult to get at the latter, however. Using the parasite:leukocyte ratio, the incidence of clinical attacks progressively diminished with age, which is consistent with what is expected. I don't see how this will help in individual cases, and I would personally take antimalarials at the outset of fever in a setting so hyperendemic as this one. The parasite:leukocyte ratio may be a useful index of control measures for malaria, be they vaccine- or vector-directed.—G.T. Keusch, M.D.

Dynamic Alteration in Splenic Function During Acute Falciparum Malaria
Looareesuwan S, Ho M, Wattanagoon Y, White NJ, Warrell DA, Bunnag D, Harinasuta T, Wyler DJ (Mahidol Univ, Bangkok, Thailand; Oxford Univ; New England Med Ctr Hosps, Boston; Tufts Univ School of Medicine)
N Engl J Med 317:675–679, Sept 10, 1987   4–10

Experimental rat studies have shown that erythrocytes infected with plasmodia undergo alteration in rheologic properties and lose their physiologic red blood cell deformability, rendering these cells susceptible to filtration by the spleen. To determine whether splenic filtration is also altered in man, the clearance rates of ^{51}Cr-labeled heated autologous erythrocytes were measured in 25 Thai patients aged 19–49 years being treated for acute *Plasmodium falciparum* malaria and in 10 healthy age-matched Thai volunteers (controls).

Sixteen patients had splenomegaly. In all 16 a markedly accelerated clearance of labeled erythrocytes was noted, whereas in the 9 without splenomegaly the clearance rates were normal (Fig 4–3). After antimalarial chemotherapy was initiated, clearance rates in malaria patients with splenomegaly did not change significantly, but those in malaria patients without splenomegaly accelerated to greater than normal, approaching rates observed in the splenomegalic group (Fig 4–4). Because of these dramatic changes, clearance studies were repeated in 3 of the patients without splenomegaly. Again, markedly increased clearance rates

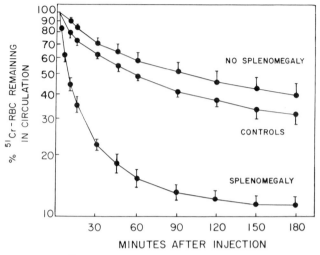

Fig 4–3.—Clearance of ^{51}Cr-labeled heated autologous erythrocytes (RBC) after injection into 10 uninfected controls, 16 malaria patients with splenomegaly, and 9 malaria patients with no detectable splenomegaly. The peak count recorded per minute in the blood samples was assigned a value of 100%; *bars* indicate means ± SD. (Courtesy of Looareesuwan S, Ho M, Wattanagoon Y, et al: *N Engl J Med* 317:675–679, Sept 10, 1987.)

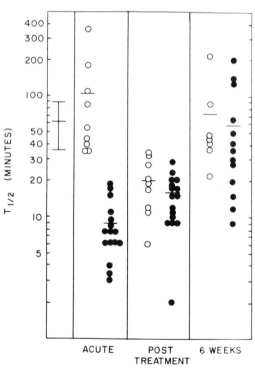

Fig 4–4.—Comparison of clearance half-time (T-1/2) of ^{51}Cr-labeled heated autologous erythrocytes in patients with acute malaria without splenomegaly *(open circles)* and in patients with splenomegaly *(closed circles)*, on admission (acute), 7–10 days after institution of therapy, and 6 weeks after admission. The *bar* on the left represents the mean and 95% confidence interval of the clearance half-time in 10 controls. (Courtesy of Looareesuwan S, Ho M, Wattanagoon Y, et al: *N Engl J Med* 317:675–679, Sept 10, 1987.)

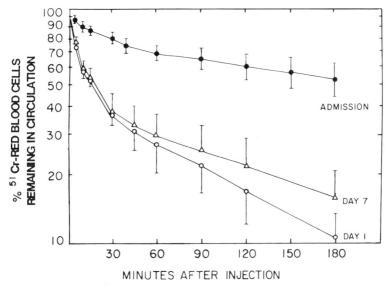

Fig 4–5.—Clearance of ^{51}Cr-labeled heated autologous erythrocytes in 3 patients with acute falciparum malaria without detectable splenomegaly, tested on admission and 1 and 7 days after institution of chemotherapy. (Courtesy of Looareesuwan S, Ho M, Wattanagoon Y, et al: N Engl J Med 317:675–679, Sept. 10, 1987.)

were found (Fig 4–5). Erythrocyte clearance rates returned to normal in most patients in both groups after about 6 weeks.

In malaria patients, splenic clearance of labeled erythrocytes is enhanced in those with splenomegaly but not in those without splenomegaly. However, when malaria patients without splenomegaly are treated with antimalarial drugs, splenic clearance rates increase to the levels observed in malaria patients with splenomegaly.

▶ The spleen is more than a very big lymph node: it performs critical filtration functions that must be under mediator or pharmacologic control, as suggested by this study. I'm not sure where this leads us just yet, but that the study was well done under difficult conditions in sick patients is a credit to the investigators.—G.T. Keusch, M.D.

Acid-Vesicle Function, Intracellular Pathogens, and the Action of Chloroquine Against *Plasmodium falciparum*
Krogstad DJ, Schlesinger PH (Washington Univ School of Medicine)
N Engl J Med 317:542–549, Aug 27, 1987   4–11

Most mammalian cells contain vesicles with an acid pH that serve to transport macromolecules to the cell interior after binding to cell-surface receptors. Other components of the acid-vesicle system include endosomes, which initially sort the internalized macromolecules; lysosomes; and the Golgi complex. The chief functions of the acid-vesicle system are

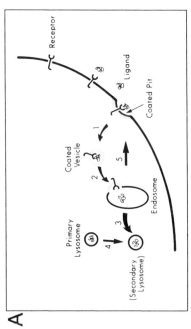
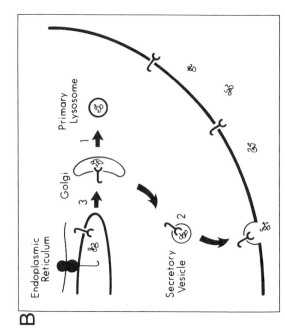

Fig 4–6.— Receptor-mediated endocytosis (**A**) and lysosomal-enzyme targeting (**B**). The normal eukaryotic cell contains a network of acid vesicles, including endosomes, coated pits, lysosomes, and the Golgi complex. **A**, ligands are internalized by receptor-mediated endocytosis and are bound by specific receptors, which form coated pits (*1*). Contents of coated vesicles are then routed (*2*) to the endosome (*3*), where initial sorting takes place and from which both receptors and other membrane components (*4*) are returned to the surface of the cell (*5*). **B**, targeting of proteases and other acid hydrolases from the endoplasmic reticulum to the lysosome (*1*) takes place by means of a process analogous to receptor-mediated endocytosis in which the enzyme is the ligand. After the mannose-6-phosphate recognition site is added to the enzyme in either the endoplasmic reticulum or the Golgi complex (*3*), the enzyme is bound by receptors that direct its targeting to the lysosome (*2*). These receptors are similar to those in the plasma membrane that are responsible for the internalization of extracellular proteins containing the mannose-6-phosphate recognition site. (Courtesy of Krogstad DJ, Schlesinger PH: *N Engl J Med* 37:542–549, Aug 27, 1987.)

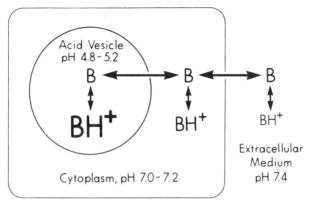

Fig 4–7.—Alteration of the acid-vesicle system by weak bases. Under usual conditions (extracellular pH of approximately 7.4), eukaryotic cells maintain a cytoplamic (internal) pH of about 7.0–7.2. The intracellular acid-vesicle system generally has a pH of 4.8–5.2. Weak bases are typically permeable to plasma membranes and vesicle membranes in their uncharged form *(B)*, but are much less so in their charged (protonated) form *(BH+)*. As a result, concentrations of the uncharged form are equal in all compartments, including the extracellular space, the cytoplasm, and the acid vesicle. The charged form is concentrated in the acid vesicle, which results in progressive entry of the uncharged form to replenish the weak base that has been lost to protonation. The vesicle becomes hyperosmotic, and free water enters to correct the osmotic disequilibrium, producing the swelling of the vesicle that is seen in both mammalian cells and plasmodia on exposure to chloroquine and other weak bases. The sizes of the letters provide qualitative indications of the concentration of uncharged and charged forms of the weak base in each compartment. (Courtesy of Krogstad DJ, Schlesinger PH: N Engl J Med 37:542–549, Aug 27, 1987.)

receptor-mediated endocytosis and lysosomal-enzyme targeting (Fig 4–6). Weak bases are the simplest molecules that alter the function of the acid-vesicle system (Fig 4–7).

Dysfunction of the acid-vesicle system usually damages eukaryotic organisms. Cells treated with ammonium chloride or chloroquine to raise the vesicle pH secrete newly synthesized acid hydrolases extracellularly, rather than routing them to lysosomes. Many genetic defects also result in abnormal acid-vesicle function (table). Several intracellular pathogens survive within macrophages, partly because of an ability to prevent acidification or fusion of the phagosome with the lysosome. Chloroquine, which is used to treat malaria, raises the pH of the parasite vesicle in vitro; this action may be responsible for inhibiting parasite growth.

Weak bases may be used clinically to raise the acid-vesicle pH, as in the use of chloroquine to treat rheumatoid disease or malaria and the prevention of influenza A with amantadine. In addition, toxins could be delivered by the acid-vesicle systems of specific cells. If the means by which some organisms prevent acidification of the macrophage phagosome or its fusion with the lysosome were understood, it might be possible to reverse the process and thereby permit killing of the organisms by macrophages.

▶ Ever since it was recognized that one of the important components in lysosomes were enzymes that worked best at acidic pH, biologists have wondered about the mechanisms for maintaining the acid pH and the overall function of

Examples of Acid-Vesicle Dysfunction*

Mechanism	Example	Effects Observed	Reference No.
Insufficient number of receptors	Familial hypercholesterolemia	Impaired internalization of LDL, resulting in excess synthesis of LDL	57
Defective internalization of ligand bound to receptor	Familial hypercholesterolemia	Impaired internalization of LDL, resulting in excess synthesis of LDL	58
	Myotonic muscular dystrophy	Impaired internalization of ligands such as lysosomal enzymes, growth factors, and transferrin	59
Lack of the M6P recognition site on degradative enzymes after post-translational processing	I-cell disease, Type III mucolipidosis, Type III pseudomucolipidosis	Acid vesicles without degradative enzymes; no functional lysosomes	60
Inhibition of phagosome acidification and/or fusion with the lysosome	Toxoplasma, legionella, chlamydia, and nocardia	Persistent survival in the macrophage phagosome	61–65
Alkalinization of the macrophage vesicle	Malaria chemoprophylaxis with chloroquine	Reduced antibody response to diploid-cell rabies vaccine	56

*LDL, low-density lipoprotein; M6P, mannose-6-phosphate.
(Courtesy of Krogstad DJ, Schlesinger PH: *N Engl J Med* 37:542–549, Aug 27, 1987.)

the acidity. This review highlights some of these functions, including receptor-mediated endocytosis and recycling, targeting of enzymes to primary lysosomes, and the uptake of compounds into these acidic compartments. Because some of the organisms that can persist intracellularly seem to do so in compartments that do not become deleteriously acidified, consideration has been given to increasing the acidic environment around these organisms as an antimicrobial strategy.

Similarly, the uptake and concentration of chloroquine, which is a weak base that concentrates in acidic compartments into the vesicle-containing malaria parasites, are thought to be major antimicrobial mechanisms for this agent. Similar antimicrobial agent uptake into acidic compartments such as clindamycin has been advocated for the ability of this agent to kill intracellular bacteria.—M.S. Klempner, M.D.

Torsade de Pointes During Administration of Pentamidine Isethionate
Wharton JM, Demopulos PA, Goldschlager N (San Francisco Gen Hosp Med Ctr; Univ of California, San Francisco)
Am J Med 83:571–576, September 1987   4–12

Pentamidine isethionate, a diamidine compound, is used in treating a number of parasitic diseases, notably *Pneumocystis carinii* pneumonia. Pentamidine has been previously associated with sudden death, but there are no reported cases of pentamidine-associated arrhythmias. Two cases

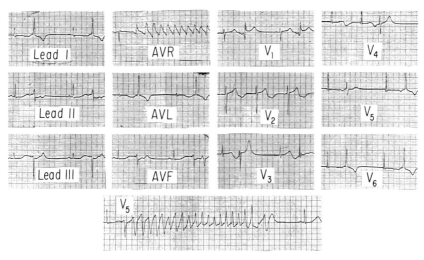

Fig 4-8.—Twelve-lead electrocardiogram (ECG) recorded after an episode of syncope in patient 2 on the day 13 of treatment with pentamidine isethionate. The QT interval is markedly prolonged, and there are pronounced T wave abnormalities, most marked in the precordial leads. Ventricular bigeminy is present in most leads. Two nonsustained runs of polymorphic ventricular tachycardia are noted in lead aVR and in the lead V5 rhythm strip. The recording speed is 25 mm/second. (Courtesy of Wharton JM, Demopulos PA, Goldschlager N: Am J Med 83:571–576, September 1987.)

of torsade de pointes occurring during prolonged administration of pentamidine are reported.

Two adult patients with acquired immunodeficiency syndrome (AIDS) were under pentamidine treatment for *P carinii* pneumonia. After 20 and 12 days of pentamidine therapy, both patients experienced lightheadedness and dizziness. Electrocardiograms (ECGs) for both patients showed repeated bursts of nonsustained, polymorphic ventricular tachycardia (torsade de pointes), as well as marked Q–T interval prolongation, pronounced precordial T-wave abnormalities, and ventricular bigeminy (Fig 4–8). Mild hypomagnesemia was present in both patients, but despite magnesium replacement, torsade de pointes persisted in 1, and the nonspecific ECG changes remained in both. The Q–T interval prolongation and ECG abnormalities resolved slowly over several days to weeks, paralleling the known elimination kinetics of pentamidine.

These cases are the first to document the proarrhythmic effect of pentamidine isethionate. Pentamidine is avidly bound to tissue; and prolonged therapy presumably results in increasing intramyocardial storage, facilitating its toxicity. As prolonged use of pentamidine is frequently required—particularly in AIDS patients with *P. carinii* pneumonia—patients should undergo serial ECG to monitor possible cardiac toxicity.

▶ This paper taught me 2 things. First, that torsade de pointes is a cardiac arrhythmia and not a nouvelle cuisine beef dish. Second, that pentamidine can be associated with this arrhythmia, which may underlie the occasional sudden deaths occurring in subjects receiving the drug. The suggestion to monitor

ECGs is reasonable, and attention to serum magnesium levels (reduced in some receiving pentamidine) may reduce the risk of arrhythmia, though no clear-cut relationship has been established.—G.T. Keusch, M.D.

Similarity of Cruzin, an Inhibitor of *Trypanosoma cruzi* Neuraminidase, to High-Density Lipoprotein
Prioli RP, Ordovas JM, Rosenberg I, Schaefer EJ, Pereira MEA (New England Med Ctr Hosps, Inc, Boston; Human Nutrition Research Ctr on Aging at Tufts Univ)
Science 238:1417–1419, Dec 4, 1987   4–13

Recently, an inhibitor of the *Trypanosoma cruzi* neuraminidase was isolated from human plasma and named cruzin. Purified cruzin was found to be very specific for *T. cruzi* neuraminidase. Cruzin inhibits trypanosome desialylation of the cells but not of soluble glycoconjugates, and it is equally effective when the enzyme is in a soluble form or on the outer membrane of living parasites. Initial attempts to match cruzin with a known human plasma component by using commercially available antiserums to individual plasma proteins were not successful. Thus, the sequence of the first 20 amino acids of the major protein component of cruzin was determined, and matching sequences in a protein and nucleic acid sequence data base were sought.

The sequence proved identical in 18 of 20 positions with the amino

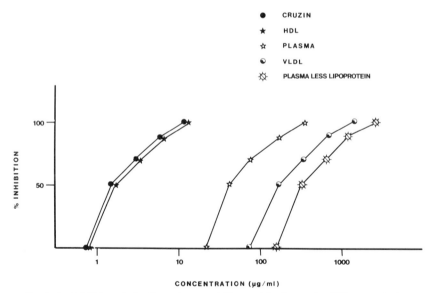

Fig 4–9.—Inhibition of the *T. cruzi* neuraminidase activity by cruzin, HDL, normal plasma, very-low-density lipoprotein, and plasma depleted of lipoproteins. The results are from a representative experiment. The amount of protein required to account for 50% inhibition did not vary more than 20% in each case. (Courtesy of Prioli RP, Ordovas JM, Rosenberg I, et al: *Science* 238:1417–1419, Dec 4, 1987.)

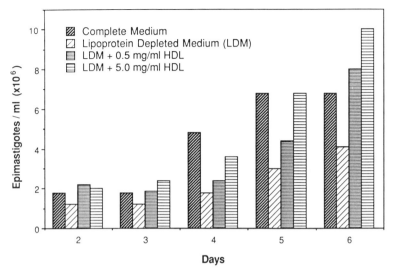

Fig 4–10.—Effect of HDL on the growth of *T. cruzi* epimastigotes (strain MV-13). Parasites were grown for the indicated time in a complete medium containing 10% fetal calf serum, in lipoprotein-depleted medium (LDM), and in LDM reconstituted with human HDL at the indicated concentrations. The results shown are the average of duplicate tubes and representative of 4 experiments (SD less than 20% of the mean). (Courtesy of Prioli RP, Ordovas JM, Rosenberg I, et al: *Science* 238:1417–1419, Dec 4, 1987.)

terminus of human apolipoprotein A-I (apoA-I), the major protein component of plasma high-density lipoprotein (HDL). This similarity suggested that cruzin contained apoA-I and was HDL. This possibility was tested with amino acid homology, sodium dodecyl sulfate-polyacrylamide gel electrophoresis, immunoblot analysis, and isoelectric focusing. Cruzin purified by ion exchange chromotography and HDL isolated by density gradient ultracentrifugation inhibited *T. cruzi* neuraminidase to the same degree (Fig 4–9). Cruzin or HDL restored to normal the reduced multiplication rate of *T. cruzi* epimastigotes grown in a medium depleted of lipoproteins, which suggests that it may be important for the survival of the parasite in nature (Fig 4–10).

A specific inhibitor of the neuraminidase of the protozoan parasite *T. cruzi* was shown to be similar to HDL. The results of this study suggest that HDL may be one of the factors underlying the pathogenesis of Chagas' disease.

▶ The pathogenesis of Chagas' disease has remained a mystery, occurring long after infection with *Trypanosoma cruzi* and at a time when few parasites are detectable. Similarly, why only an occasional patient of the many infected with *T. cruzi* should become ill with chronic disease has been unclear. In this study, a serum factor, identified as HDL, is described as an inhibitor of *T. cruzi* neuraminidase (NA). Neuraminidase is thought to be a virulence factor, but paradoxically, inhibition of NA enhances infection in vitro. It may be that HDL modulation of NA plays a role in selecting those at risk of Chagas' disease, and the high HDL patient may be the one. Although it is too early to prove, Brazilians who are safe from coronary artery disease because they have high HDL levels may be at risk of Chagas' disease.—G.T. Keusch, M.D.

Encystation and Expression of Cyst Antigens by *Giardia lamblia* In Vitro
Gillin FD, Reiner DS, Gault MJ, Douglas H, Das S, Wunderlich A, Sauch JF
(Univ of California, San Diego, Med Ctr; Environmental Protection Agency, Cincinnati)
Science 235:1040–1043, Feb 27, 1987   4–14

Giardiasis, an important cause of human intestinal disease, is transmitted by ingestion of the cyst of *Giardia lamblia*. The process of encystation of this organism was investigated using the suckling mouse model.

Cysts were found initially in every section of the intestine, but with time they accumulated in the large intestine. A cyst-specific polyclonal rabbit serum that was developed reacted with fresh unfixed cysts. Because large numbers of cysts appear initially in the jejunum, where trophozoites are exposed to bile, these parasites were exposed to 16 mM of glycodeoxycholate (GdC) with or without 100 μM of oleic acid.

In the presence of GdC alone, the mean rate of encystation was 8%; when oleic acid was added the mean rate was 9%. Without any additions, there was a mean rate of encystation of 0.15%. Six bile salts were then tested, and all stimulated encystation. However, the kinetics of stimulation were significantly faster in the presence of primary bile salts than with secondary bile salts. These studies should facilitate attempts to carry out the life cycle of *G. lamblia* in vitro, allowing studies of cysts uncontaminated by fecal material.

▶ Clinical interest in the cyst of *Giardia* is because of its role in disease transmission. No cyst means dead-end infection. Research interest centers on the signals for stage transformation and differentiation in the protozoan. This study shows the way toward in vitro production of cysts, an essential step in the study of the biochemistry and regulation of cyst formation. A particularly nice study with beautiful pictures of cysts formed in vitro that are environmentally stable and capable of reinfection of animals has recently been published (see Schupp DG et al: *Gastroenterology* 95:1–10, 1988).—G.T. Keusch, M.D.

5 Mycobacterial Infections

Conservative Treatment of Tuberculosis of the Thoracic and Lumbar Spine in Adults and Children
Moon M-S, Kim I, Woo Y-K, Park Y-O (Catholic Univ Med College, Kang-Nam St-Mary's Hosp, Seoul, South Korea)
Int Orthop 11:315–322, December 1987   5–1

The management of spinal tuberculosis in different parts of the world ranges from immobilization with antituberculous chemotherapy to various forms of surgical treatment combined with drug therapy. Spinal tuberculosis is still prevalent in Korea. The authors report the results of conservative treatment in a group of patients with spinal tuberculosis who were treated on an outpatient basis with triple antituberculosis chemotherapy.

The study population included 27 children, 13 boys and 14 girls, aged 1–15 years, and 48 adults, 21 men and 27 women, aged 16–60 years, who were diagnosed with thoracic or lumbar tuberculosis. Adults were treated with a combination of isoniazid (INH), ethambutol, and rifampicin; children received *p*-aminosalicylic acid (PAS) instead of ethambutol. Bed rest or bracing was recommended only for patients with severe pain and advanced vertebral destruction. Duration of chemotherapy was 1.5 years. Patients were followed up at regular intervals for at least 3 years. Evacuation of large abscesses was carried out as necessary, but no other operations were performed.

Triple chemotherapy was successful in 71 (95%) patients. Four patients with persistent active disease required operation. Intercorporeal bony fusion had occurred in 24% of the patients after 18 months of treatment and in 36% of the patients after 36 months of treatment. Eight children and 21 adults showed increases in the kyphotic angle of 5 degrees or less. Five children and 3 adults had increases in the kyphotic angle of 20 degrees or more, but all had involvement of more than 3 vertebral bodies. Lumbar kyphosis in a child was decreased after 18 months of treatment. Although surgical treatment plus chemotherapy produces earlier bony fusion and arrests the progress of kyphosis, conservative ambulant chemotherapy alone will save lives and eradicate the disease when appropriate treatment facilities are not readily available.

▶ Wow! Seventy-five patients with Potts disease in a single contemporary series! Results of conservative therapy dependent on chemotherapy and little else were excellent, with a greater than 95% rate of cure. The major problem, increase in lumbar kyphosis, occurred only in patients with more than 3 vertebrae involved. Whereas a combination of surgical fusion and chemotherapy permits earlier responses, it is not necessary and may not be possible in developing countries where the disease is common.—G.T. Keusch, M.D.

Mycobacterium chelonae Wound Infections After Plastic Surgery Employing Contaminated Gentian Violet Skin-Marking Solution
Safranek TJ, Jarvis WR, Carson LA, Cusick LB, Bland LA, Swenson JM, Silcox VA (Ctrs for Disease Control, Atlanta)
N Engl J Med 317:197–201, July 23, 1987   5–2

Eight patients having cosmetic plastic surgery by a single surgeon in a 7-month period developed surgical wound infections caused by rapidly growing mycobacteria. Six patients had documented infection with *Mycobacterium chelonae*, subspecies *abscessus*, and 2 had infections presumed to be caused by this organism. All the patients underwent face-lift surgery or augmentation mammoplasty in the surgeon's office. Seven of 8 breast implants had to be removed. The only clinical feature in the face-lift and blepharoplasty cases was a skin eruption.

The source of infection proved to be a gentian violet skin-marking solution. Patients having face-lift surgery or mammoplasty were more likely to be infected than those having blepharoplasty. Postoperative use of antibiotics and of steroids also were risk factors. *Mycobacterium chelonae*, subspecies *abscessus*, was isolated from the gentian violet stock and from 5 of the 8 infected patients. The same organism was present in stock at the pharmacy supplying the solution. Cases of infection ceased when a sterile skin-marking agent was substituted for the contaminated material.

Infection by rapidly growing mycobacteria may be a serious complication of cosmetic surgery. It is important to be aware that solutions used for skin marking are a potential source of wound contamination. Only sterile skin marking agents should be used in surgery.

▶ The atypical mycobacteria certainly do pop up in some of the most unusual places, and the consequences are often disastrous. In addition to this report of *Mycobacterium chelonae* causing postoperative wound infections as a result of inoculation from contaminated gentian violet, there have been other reports implicating the atypical mycobacteria in breast implants, cardiac valves, wound-dressing material, processed hemodialyzers, and corneal implants. In almost all cases, these contaminated materials have resulted in clinically significant infections, and they should heighten our vigilance, specifically toward the mycobacteria when we deal with patients exposed to artificial devices.—M.S. Klempner, M.D.

Pulmonary Disease Caused by *Mycobacterium malmoense*
Alberts WM, Chandler KW, Solomon DA, Goldman AL (Univ of South Florida College of Medicine; James A Haley Veterans Hosp, Tampa, Fla)
Am Rev Respir Dis 135:1375–1378, June 1987   5–3

Mycobacterium malmoense was first described in 1977 as a new pathogenic, nonphotochromogenic mycobacterial species. The original 4 cases of pulmonary disease caused by this species were in Malmo, Sweden. Almost 60 patients with pulmonary disease caused by *M. malmoense* have been described, all but 1 of whom have lived in England, Wales, Scotland, or Sweden. The first and only case of pulmonary disease caused by this organism in the United States was documented in 1984. Four more cases in this country were recently encountered.

Mycobacterium malmoense was isolated from the pulmonary material of 4 patients, all of whom were women aged 32–72 years. Two patients had repeatedly positive smears and cultures, along with radiographic progression of pulmonary disease in the absence of another pathogen. These two patients thus were diagnosed as having pulmonary mycobacteriosis. In the third patient, isolation of the organism may represent colonization. In the fourth patient, the organism was isolated on 2 occasions. It is not yet definite that the pulmonary process in these 2 patients was caused by mycobacterial disease.

Pulmonary disease caused by *M. malmoense* is uncommon, especially in the United States, but may be becoming more prevalent. This is probably due to a true increase in prevalence but may also be due to increased identification as experience with the organism increases. The correct treatment of disease caused by this pathogen is currently not known.

▶ Mycobacterium malmoense is a mesophilic, nonchromogenic, microaerophilic atypical mycobacterium resembling *M. avium-intracellulare* except for its ability to hydrolyze Tween 80. It causes pulmonary disease, and it appears to be actually increasing in prevalence in the U.S. We should therefore be on the lookout for *M. malmoense* among patients with acquired immunodeficiency syndrome. Drug sensitivity varies, but most should be susceptible to INH, ethambutol, and rifampin. But even given for prolonged periods of time, these drugs might not reliably respond to treatment of pulmonary disease (see Banks et al: *Tubercle* 66:197–203, 1985).—G.T Keusch, M.D.

Mycobacterium marinum Infection of the Hand and Wrist: Results of Conservative Treatment in Twenty-Four Cases
Chow SP, Ip FK, Lau JHK, Collins RJ, Luk KDK, So YC, Pun WK (Univ of Hong Kong at Queen Mary Hosp)
J Bone Joint Surg [Am] 69–A:1161–1168, October 1987   5–4

Superficial cutaneous infections of the hand with *Mycobacterium marinum* usually respond to conservative treatment, rarely requiring surgical intervention. However, infections with *M. marinum* of the deep structures of the hand are often more destructive and more resistant to treatment. A combination of surgical débridement and antimycobacterial therapy has been used to control such infections. Nevertheless, inadequate débridement, extensive scarring, and breakdown of the wound have been commonly encountered after surgical débridement. In light of this, a prospective study was undertaken to assess the outcome of a more conservative approach to treatment.

The study population included 16 men and 8 women, aged 13–82 years, who presented with *M. marinum* infections involving the deep structures of the hand and wrist. Sixteen patients were professional fishermen, while 3 patients sold fish. Swelling at the infection site was the most common clinical sign; but patients also had lost gripping power and range of motion in the hand, as a result of long delays between onset of symptoms and diagnosis. After a diagnosis of *M. marinum* infection had been confirmed by biopsy, patients were treated with daily administration of 600 mg of rifampicin and 15–25 mg/kg of ethambutol. The hand and wrist were immobilized for at least 2 weeks following biopsy.

Eleven patients had good results with no complications, 3 patients had delayed healing of the wound, and 10 patients did not respond to conservative treatment and required 1 or more surgical débridements. At follow-up, 21 (87%) of the 24 patients had recovered function of the treated hand equal to that of the other hand.

Persistent pain, a discharging sinus, and a history of prior local steroid injection are unfavorable prognostic indicators. Early radical débridement is recommended when these prognostic factors are present.

6 Infections in the Compromised Host

Prevention of Fungal Sepsis in Patients With Prolonged Neutropenia: A Randomized, Double-Blind, Placebo-Controlled Trial of Intravenous Miconazole
Wingard JR, Vaughan WP, Braine HG, Merz WG, Saral R (Johns Hopkins Hosp)
Am J Med 83:1103–1110, December 1987   6–1

Fungal sepsis is a major problem in patients with prolonged neutropenia, and results of treatment have been disappointing. The authors evaluated the use of miconazole, with empirical antibiotic therapy, in a placebo-controlled study of patients who were given cytotoxic drug therapy that was expected to produce neutropenia for 2 weeks or longer. A total of 208 treatment courses in 180 patients were evaluated. Most of the patients had leukemia or had received bone marrow transplants (Table 1).

Conventional antibiotic therapy with carbenicillin, gentamicin, and trimethoprim-sulfamethoxazole was used. Miconazole was given by infusion in a dose of 5 mg/kg every 8 hours.

Only 1 miconazole-treated patient developed fungal sepsis, compared

TABLE 1.—Characteristics of Patients

	Placebo	Miconazole
Entries (number of patients)	111	97
Age, in years (median with range)	33	35
	(6–75)	(7–74)
Underlying disease or therapy		
Acute leukemia		
Initial therapy	21	29
Prior therapy	20	27
Bone marrow transplant		
Syngeneic	9	6
Allogeneic	33	35
Other malignancy		
Initial therapy	6	2
Prior therapy	8	12
Duration of neutropenia, in days	23	21
(median with range)	(3–87)	(1–71)
Granulocyte transfusions (number of patients)	30	27

(Courtesy of Wingard JR, Vaughan WP, Braine HG, et al: Am J Med 83:1103–1110, December 1987.)

TABLE 2.—Study Outcomes

	Placebo*	Miconazole*	p Value
Fungal sepsis			
Overall	8 of 111	1 of 97	p = 0.03
Among those not receiving granulocyte transfusions	7 of 81	0 of 70	p = 0.01
Death due to fungal sepsis	4	0	p = 0.08
Number of days in study before trial of amphotericin B for persistent unexplained fever (median)	8	10	p = 0.02

*Number of patients.
(Courtesy of Wingard JR, Vaughan WP, Braine HG, et al: Am J Med 83:1103–1110, December 1987.)

with 8 placebo-treated patients (Table 2). Four of the latter patients died. Fungal isolates showed no evidence of resistance to polyenes or imidazoles, and *Aspergillus* infections were not more frequent in patients who were given miconazole. This was also true for 121 later patients who received miconazole on an unblinded basis. Bacterial sepsis developed in 10% of the placebo group and in 8% of the miconazole-treated patients.

Intravenous infusions of miconazole help prevent fungal sepsis in patients with prolonged neutropenia. Significant toxicity did not develop, and there was no increase in *Aspergillus* infections among patients who were given miconazole.

▶ As we have moved into the era of empiric antifungal and, in some cases, antiviral therapy for neutropenic patients with unexplained fever, we are recapitulating many of the same issues of empiric antibiotic therapy that we have faced over the past 20 years. Since antifungal therapy is administered at the onset of fever, one can question whether the drug is actually being given in a preventive manner or whether one is treating low-grade infection. In any event, only intravenous amphotericin begun empirically at the onset of unexplained fever has been shown to reduce the incidence of invasive fungal infections in patients with prolonged neutropenia (see Pizo PA et al: Am J Med 72:101–111, 1982).

Because there is substantial toxicity associated with empiric amphotericin, these authors have sought an alternative in the use of empiric parenteral miconazole therapy. They did observe a decrease in the number of episodes of fungal sepsis, and there also was a decrease in the number of deaths due to fungal sepsis. It is not clear to me whether overall mortality was affected, but as best as I can tell, they did not see any decrease in this variable.

It is also noteworthy that one of the reasons for termination of the study drug (miconazole or placebo) was persistent or recurrent unexplained fever after 6 days. This resulted in the empiric administration of amphotericin B and was required in 66% of the miconazole-treated patients and in 56% of the placebo-treated group. Thus, a large proportion of the patients in whom they were trying to avoid giving amphotericin ultimately received this antibiotic. It is not clear whether amphotericin B therapy that followed miconazole therapy was in any way more or less deleterious. Whereas miconazole might be added to the armamentarium of empiric antibiotics for patients with prolonged neutropenia, this study is not compelling for a strong preference of this agent over empiric amphotericin.—M.S. Klempner, M.D.

Amphotericin B or Ketoconazole Therapy of Fungal Infections in Neutropenic Cancer Patients
Fainstein V, Bodey GP, Elting L, Maksymiuk A, Keating M, McCredie KB (Univ of Texas MD Anderson Hosp and Tumor Inst at Houston)
Antimicrob Agents Chemother 31:11–15, January 1987   6–2

The incidence of fungal infections among neutropenic cancer patients has been increasing over recent years. It is often difficult to diagnose fungal infections antemortem for this group of patients. For this reason, it has become accepted practice to treat neutropenic patients with persistent fever that does not respond to antibacterial agents empirically with antifungal agents. A prospective, randomized trial was conducted to compare the efficacy of the antifungal agents amphotericin B and ketoconazole in the treatment of confirmed or suspected fungal infections in neutropenic cancer patients.

The study population included 172 neutropenic cancer patients who were treated for a total of 192 febrile episodes. The patients were randomly assigned to be treated with either ketoconazole or amphotericin B. Only patients who had received antifungal therapy for at least 4 days were included in the tabulation of the results.

Of 192 febrile episodes, 34 episodes were subsequently excluded from evaluation. Of 158 patients with evaluable episodes, 83 (53%) were

TABLE 1.—Response by Site of Infection

Infection	Amphotericin B		Ketoconazole	
	Total	No. responding (%)	Total[*]	No. responding (%)
Disseminated	3	0 (0)	4	0 (0)
Fungemia	12	7 (58)	8	3 (38)
Pneumonia	20	13 (65)	15	7 (47)
Esophagitis	9	7 (78)	14	9 (64)
Soft tissue	3	2 (67)	1	1 (100)
Other localized[†]	4	2 (50)	7	6 (86)
All	51	31 (61)	49	26 (53)

[*]Eleven episodes subsequently responded to amphotericin B.
[†]Includes hepatitis, urinary tract infection, dental abscess, sinusitis, synovitis, osteomyelitis, and mucositis.
(Courtesy of Fainstein V, Bodey GP, Elting L, et al: *Antimicrob Agents Chemother* 31:11–15, January 1987.)

TABLE 2.—Response According to Infecting Fungal Species

Organism	Amphotericin B		Ketoconazole	
	Total	No. responding (%)	Total	No. responding (%)
C. albicans	7	2 (29)	8	3 (38)
C. tropicalis	8	5 (63)*	8	0 (0)*
Candida	2	1 (50)	4	2 (50)
Aspergillus	4	0 (0)	2	0 (0)
Mucor	1	1 (100)		
Miscellaneous †	4	1 (25)	1	1 (100)

*P = .03.
†Includes *Trichosporon glabrata* (2 strains), *T. cutaneum* (1 strain), *Cryptococcus neoformans* (1 strain), and *T. cutaneum* plus *Candida tropicalis* (1 strain).
(Courtesy of Fainstein V, Bodey GP, Elting L, et al: Antimicrob Agents Chemother 31:11–15, January 1987.)

treated with amphotericin B, and 75 (47%), with ketoconazole. The duration of treatment ranged from 4 to 56 days, for an average of 9.3 days. Overall effectiveness of amphotericin B and ketoconazole was about the same. Response rates for localized fungal infections were similarly low with both drugs (Table 1). Equivalent but much higher response rates were found with both drugs for "probable" and "possible," as opposed to "documented," fungal infections. Neither agent was effective against disseminated fungal infection. Amphotericin B was effective in 5 of 8 *Candida tropicalis* infections, whereas ketoconazole was ineffective in all 8 infections treated (Table 2).

▶ Neither amphotericin B nor ketoconazole was impressive in its effect on documented disseminated fungal infection in neutropenic cancer patients, and each agent was only modestly effective in documented localized fungal infection. Amphotericin B is to be preferred over ketoconazole if there is a suspicion of aspergillosis or mucormycosis on infection by *Candida tropicalis*.

Eight patients had to discontinue treatment with ketoconazole because of severe nausea and vomiting. For 7 patients, the dosage of amphotericin B had to be reduced because of fever and bronchospasm. Overall, 39% of patients receiving ketoconazole for more than 2 weeks experienced hepatotoxicity. As might be expected, renal toxicity was much more frequent among recipients of amphotericin B (41%) than of ketoconazole (9%).—M.J. Barza, M.D.

Diagnosing Bacterial Respiratory Infection by Bronchoalveolar Lavage
Kahn FW, Jones JM (William S Middleton Mem Veterans Hosp, Madison, Wis; Univ of Wisconsin Med School)
J Infect Dis 155:862–869, May 1987

The diagnosis of bacterial pneumonia in immunocompromised hosts remains a problem. In a prospective study, 57 patients with potential res-

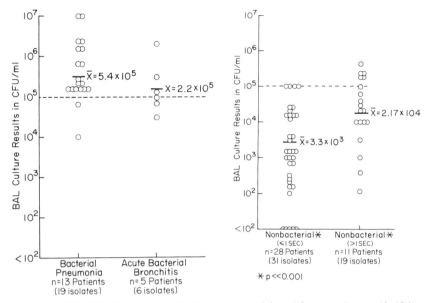

Fig 6–1 (left).—The BAL culture results from patients with bacterial pneumonia (n = 13, 19 isolates) or bronchitis (n = 5, 6 isolates). *Short bold lines* represent the mean cfu/ml. For patients with bacterial pneumonia, mean was 5.4×10^5; for patients with bronchitis, 2.2×10^5. *Dashed line* represents dividing point between positive and negative results.

Fig 6–2 (right).—The BAL quantitative culture results from study patients with nonbacterial respiratory disease, divided into those with ≤ 1% SECs (n = 28, 31 isolates) and those with > 1% SECs (n = 11, 19 isolates) in the BAL cell differential ($P < .001$, *). *Short bold lines* represent mean cfu/ml. For ≤ 1% SECs, mean was 3.3×10^3; for >1% SECs, 2.17×10^4. *Dashed line* represents dividing point between positive and negative results.

(Courtesy of Kahn FW, Jones JM: *J Infect Dis* 155:862–869, May 1987.)

piratory infection, most of whom were immunocompromised, and 18 "control" patients without evidence of respiratory infection underwent fiberoptic bronchoscopy and bronchoalveolar lavage (BAL) to evaluate for the presence of bacterial lower-respiratory-tract infection. The BAL specimens were cultured quantitatively for aerobic bacteria and were Giemsa-stained for cell differential to distinguish between oropharyngeal contaminants and bacterial isolates.

For the control patients, BAL specimens with ≤ 1% squamous epithelial cells (SECs) had $<10^5$ colony-forming units (CFU) per milliliter, whereas those with >1% SECs had $>10^5$ CFU/ml. Three of 5 patients fulfilling the criteria for diagnosis of acute bacterial bronchitis had an organism isolated at $>10^5$ cfu/ml (Fig 6–1). A cutoff of $>10^5$ cfu/ml in a BAL specimen containing ≤ 1% SECs was evaluated for its accuracy in diagnosing lower-respiratory-tract infection in 57 immunocompromised patients with potential respiratory infection (Fig 6–2).

Polymorphonuclear leukocytes were readily identified, and potential lower-respiratory-tract pathogens were recovered in concentrations $>10^5$ CFU/ml in all 13 patients with bacterial pneumonia and 3 of 5 patients with acute bacterial bronchitis; none of these patients had 1% SECs in their BAL sample. No patients without evidence of bacterial infection and with ≤ 1% SECs had >10^5 CFU/ml in BAL cultures. Thus, in accepting isolates with >10^5 CFU/ml in a specimen having ≤ 1% SECs as significant, BAL had a diagnostic sensitivity of 100% for bacterial pneumonia and 88% for all lower-respiratory-tract infections and a specificity of 100%.

Quantitative bacterial culture of BAL specimens, combined with analysis of the BAL cell differential, can be incorporated into a protocol for BAL analysis to obtain useful information in the diagnosis of bacterial respiratory infection.

Bronchoalveolar Lavage for Diagnosing Acute Bacterial Pneumonia
Thorpe JE, Baughman RP, Frame PT, Wesseler TA, Staneck JL (Univ of Cincinnati)
J Infect Dis 155:855-861, May 1987

It is difficult to assess bacterial pneumonia on the basis of microbiologic sputum studies, as the quality of sputum specimens is so often poor. Bronchoalveolar lavage (BAL) via a flexible fiberoptic bronchoscope has gained wide acceptance as a diagnostic tool. This 2-part study was done to determine the diagnostic value of microbiologic assessment of BAL fluid retrieved from patients with acute bacterial pneumonia.

During the first part of the study, gram staining, semiquantitative aerobic culture, and other laboratory tests were performed on BAL fluid retrieved from 92 patients with various clinical diagnoses. Based on clinical findings, patients were divided into 5 groups. One of the groups included 4 men and 11 women, aged 15 to 84 years, who were suspected of clinically active and progressive bacterial pneumonia, as determined by chest radiographs. Seven of 15 patients had been treated unsuccessfully with antibiotics.

Clinically active bacterial pneumonia was confirmed by Gram stain and bacterial culture of BAL fluid in 13 of 15 patients. On the basis of sensitivity studies of the isolated bacteria, the patients were either started on antibiotic treatment or changed over to an antibiotic to which the isolated bacteria were sensitive.

In the second phase of the study, BAL fluid studies were done in 59 immunocompromised patients, aged 21 to 79 years, with underlying illnesses including acquired immunodeficiency syndrome, renal transplantation, leukemia, lymphoma, and other carcinomas, who all had radiographically confirmed pulmonary infiltrates. A microbial diagnosis was confirmed in 39 of 59 patients. On the basis of BAL fluid analysis, 8 (21%) of 39 patients were diagnosed with acute bacterial pneumonia, which resolved with appropriate antibiotic therapy.

The BAL gram stain has a distinct advantage over sputum or transtracheal aspirate gram stains in the diagnosis of patients with suspected bacterial pneumonia, as it can differentiate active pneumonia from bronchitis or resolving pneumonia. Because BAL was tolerated well, even by very ill patients, this approach is strongly recommended for patients who are ill enough to benefit from accurate identification of the causative agent of their pneumonia.

▶ I was struck by several things as I read these 2 papers (Abstracts 6–3 and 6–4). First was the remarkable similarity of their conclusions. Both say that bronchoalveolar lavage fluid that contains >10^5 CFU/ml is an excellent predictor of those patients with acute bacterial pneumonia and correctly identifies the organism in all cases. Second, both studies show that the absolute number or percentage of neutrophils in the BAL is not a good predictor of acute bacterial pneumonia, but the finding of >1% squamous epithelial cells in the BAL specimen is a good indication that the specimen is contaminated from above.

In Abstract 6–4, gram stain of the BAL was shown to accurately predict acute bacterial pneumonia with 1 or more organisms seen per oil immersion field. There was also a striking similarity in the high incidence of bacterial pneumonia among the immunocompromised patients in both of these papers. In Abstract 6–3, 18 of the 57 study patients were found to have bacterial pathogens by BAL and 8 of the 39 patients had bacterial pneumonia by BAL in Abstract 6–4. These represent an incidence of 22% to 31%.

In a large series from the Mayo Clinic, Martin et al. (*Mayo Clin Proc* 62:549–557, 1987) and Stover et al. (*Ann Intern Med* 101:1–7, 1984) found an incidence of acute bacterial pneumonia in immunocompromised hosts evaluated with BAL of between 1% and 6%. I suspect this represents differences in the patients selected and what was being looked for. All of these studies attest to the relative safety of bronchoalveolar lavage, and this technique should certainly be employed in immunocompromised patients who have unexplained pulmonary infiltrates.—M.S. Klempner, M.D.

Staphylococcus aureus **Bacteremia in Patients With Hematological Malignancies and/or Agranulocytosis**
Espersen F, Frimodt-Møller N, Thamdrup Rosdahl V, Jessen O, Faber V, Rosendal K (Rigshospitalet, Copenhagen)
Acta Med Scand 222:465–470, 1987
6–5

Generally, patients with *Staphylococcus aureus* bacteremia are treated for 2–6 weeks with antistaphylococcal agents because of the frequent occurrence of endocarditis. However, a shorter duration of therapy has been proposed for patients with acute leukemia because of the low incidence of endocarditis associated with staphylococcal bacteremia. To verify further, the incidence and mortality of endocarditis in 479 patients with hematologic malignancies, agranulocytosis, or both, and *S. aureus* bacteremia were compared to those of 5,774 other patients with *S. aureus* bacteremia.

The incidence of endocarditis was significantly lower among patients with hematologic malignancies, agranulocytosis, or both, than among other patients (0.4% vs 4.7%). An unknown portal of entry was significantly more common among patients with hematologic malignancies, agranulocytosis, or both (Table 1), and these patients had a higher mor-

TABLE 1.—Portal of Entry in Patients With *Staphylococcus aureus* Bacteremia

	Hematologic malignancy or agranulocytosis		Other patients		Total	
	n	%*	n	%	n	%
Unknown	334	70	2 756	48	3 253	52
Lungs	73	15	757	13	877	14
Operation etc.	48	10	1 743	30	1 832	29
Skin	32	7	504	9	561	9

*In some patients, several portals were possible.
(Courtesy of Espersen F, Frimodt-Møller N, Thamdrup Rosdahl V, et al: *Acta Med Scand* 222:465–470, 1987.)

TABLE 2.—Mortality in Patients With *Staphylococcus aureus* Bacteremia

	n	Died	%
Hematological malignancy	438	217	50
Acute lymphocytic leukemia	57	16	28
Chronic lymphocytic leukemia	59	29	49
Acute myelocytic leukemia	94	47	50
Chronic myelocytic leukemia	27	16	59
Other leukemia	25	14	56
Lymphomas	84	36	43
Multiple myeloma	70	50	71
Waldenström's macroglobulinemia	10	3	30
Polycythemia vera/myelofibrosis	12	6	50
Agranulocytosis	41	19	46
Other patients	5 774	1 880	33
Total	6 253	2 116	34

(Courtesy of Espersen F, Frimodt-Møller N, Thamdrup Rosdahl V, et al: *Acta Med Scand* 222:465–470, 1987.)

tality than other patients (Table 2). Mortality was highest among patients with multiple myeloma and lowest among patients with acute lymphocytic leukemia.

Patients with hematologic malignancies, agranulocytosis, or both only rarely develop endocarditis complicating *S. aureus* bacteremia, thus justifying a shorter course of antibacterial therapy than usually recommended. However, the higher mortality among these patients may indicate that empiric antibiotic regimens for granulocytic patients should include a specific antistaphylococcal agent.

▶ I chose this paper because of the extraordinary number of patients that it draws on. Since 1956, there has been a nationwide registration of patients with staphylococcal infections, and nearly all those with *S. aureus* strains isolated from blood cultures in Denmark are referred to the authors' department. Therefore, a total of 6,253 cases of *S. aureus* bacteremia constitute the cohort on which this study is based. The authors make the observation that in patients with hematologic malignancies, the incidence of endocarditis after S. aureus bacteremia is less than one tenth of that seen among other patients who experience S. aureus bacteremia. Their conclusion that a shorter course of antistaphylococcal antibiotic than the usually prescribed 2–6 weeks is justified. For more information on this extraordinary number of patients with S. aureus bacteremia, readers are referred to the Scandinavian Journal of Infectious Diseases S41:19–26, 1983.—M.S. Klempner, M.D.

Clostridium difficile **Diarrhea in Critically Ill Burned Patients**
Grube BJ, Heimbach DM, Marvin JA (Univ of Washington)
Arch Surg 122:655–661, June 1987　　　　　　　　　　　　　　　　6–6

Patients with serious burns are frequently given antibiotics. One potentially life-threatening complication that can develop is antibiotic-associated pseudomembranous colitis, which has been attributed to *Clostridium difficile*. To determine the incidence and outcome of this infection, data on 112 burn patients in an intensive care unit (ICU) were analyzed prospectively.

Diarrhea occurred in 20 patients. These patients had larger burns, had longer ICU stays, underwent more surgical procedures, and received more antibiotic therapy than those who did not become diarrheic. Forty-two episodes of diarrhea occurred in these 20 patients. In 11, none of the diarrhea specimens contained *C. difficile*; the 9 others had at least 1 episode of *C. difficile*-associated diarrhea. There was no significant difference in burn size, length of hospital stay, number of operations, or age between the 2 groups. When nonspecific episodes were compared with *C. difficile*-caused episodes, no difference in temperature, albumin levels, or total days of antibiotic administration preceding diarrhea could be discovered. Vancomycin hydrochloride was used to treat *C. difficile* diarrhea. The 2 recurrences also responded to vancomycin.

In this series of 112 burn patients in the ICU, the total incidence of diarrhea was 17%. Among diarrheic patients there was a 45% incidence of *C. difficile* diarrhea. Because clinical signs and symptoms were not helpful in diagnosis, a positive culture or toxin titer was necessary. Treatment with vancomycin led to rapid resolution.

▶ Though common, the *C. difficile* diarrhea in these severely burned patients responded readily to proper treatment. Clinical suspicion and the availability of culture, toxin titer, or both were key to early diagnosis.—G.T. Keusch, M.D.

Infections After Liver Transplantation: An Analysis of 101 Consecutive Cases
Kusne S, Dummer JS, Singh N, Iwatsuki S, Makowka L, Esquivel C, Tzakis AG, Starzl TE, Ho M (Graduate School of Public Health, Univ of Pittsburgh)
Medicine 67:132–143, 1988　　　　　　　　　　　　　　　　　　　　6–7

Infections were monitored in 101 consecutive patients who had liver transplantation during 1984–1985 and lived longer than 72 hours. Patients received cefotaxime and ampicillin for 5 days after operation, and oral mycostatin was given until discharge to prevent *Candida* infection. Immunosuppression was induced with cyclosporine and steroids. The patients, with a mean age of 39 years, were followed for periods averaging 394 days.

All but 17% of patients had infection after liver transplantation, and two thirds had severe infections. Twenty-three of 26 deaths were associated with infection. The most frequent severe infections were cytomegalovirus disease, abdominal abscess, and bacterial pneumonia. Most severe infections occurred within 2 months after operation. All severe fungal infections occurred in patients who were in the operating room longer than 12 hours. Patients given larger amounts of red cells and fresh frozen plasma had higher rates of bacterial and fungal infections than did other patients.

Many patients have serious infections after orthotopic liver transplantation, although rates have declined in recent years. Fungal infections remain a serious clinical problem and may require the earlier empirical treatment of recipients at high risk of such infection.

Toxoplasmosis in Two Renal Transplant Recipients From a Single Donor
Mason JC, Ordelheide KS, Grames GM, Thrasher TV, Harris RD, Dang Bui RH, Mackett MCT (Loma Linda Univ Med Ctr)
Transplantation 44:588–592, October 1987
6–8

Acute toxoplasmosis is a well-documented hazard in immunosuppressed patients that has contributed significantly to infectious complications in organ transplantation recipients. The occurrence of acute toxoplasmosis in 2 patients who received renal allografts from a single donor is described.

Woman, 48, had a history of polycystic renal disease. Immunosuppression was achieved by intravenously administered cyclosporine and methylprednisolone. The immediate postoperative period was complicated by acute tubular necrosis. Pseudomembranous colitis was diagnosed 18 days after surgery. She was leukopenic and continued to be febrile, despite antimicrobial therapy. She eventually deteriorated to bradycardia, refractory hypotension, electromechanical dissociation, and cardiac arrest. At autopsy, myocarditis due to cysts of *Toxoplasma* were documented. Similar cysts were seen in the lungs, hepatocytes, and bone marrow. One serum specimen 25 days posttransplant showed an IgG titer of 1:256 and an IgM titer of 1:512 to *T. gondii*.

Girl, 16, had proteinuria and received a renal allograft from the same donor as for patient 1. Immunosuppression in this patient was similar to that for the first patient. She was oliguric in the early postoperative period and her serum creatinine level increased to 10.5 mg/dl. She developed a generalized tonic-clonic seizure 9 days after surgery. The seizure was controlled, and she was discharged.

Two days later, she was rehospitalized for malaise, fever, and arthralgias. Fever and chills persisted for almost 3 weeks. *Toxoplasma* IgG antibody was 1:2,048 and IgM was 1:4,096. A needle biopsy specimen of the allograft showed acute rejection and transplant glomerulopathy. Transplant nephrectomy was performed and active toxoplasmosis was treated. *Toxoplasma gondii* was isolated from blood at day 52 posttransplant. The patient had acute myositis that could not be conclusively attributed to toxoplasmosis. After anti-toxoplasma therapy for 8 weeks, all clinical manifestations had resolved.

Acute toxoplasmosis was documented in both these recipients. The possibility of reactivation existed in patient 1, but her increased IgM immunofluorescent antibody titer of 1:512 suggests a new infection. Patient 2 was serologically negative at 2 weeks and serologically positive at 8 weeks after transplantation, at which time *Toxoplasma* was isolated from her blood. Evidence suggests that the donor had recent acute infection, probably within 2–9 months of her death and subsequent transplantation. The transmission of *Toxoplasma gondii* by the allografts is the most plausible explanation for acute toxoplasmosis in these 2 patients.

▶ This is an interesting report that provides some presumptive evidence of toxoplasmosis transmission by the donor kidney. The second case is the more clear-cut example of primary toxoplasma infection; the first may be an example of reactivation. These examples are reminiscent of *Toxoplasma* transmission from cardiac transplantation and raise issues of screening and prophylaxis in the renal transplant setting (see the 1988 YEAR BOOK OF INFECTIOUS DISEASES, p 160).—D.R. Snydman, M.D.

7 Human Immunodeficiency Virus (HIV) Infection

Epidemiology

Risk of Transmitting the Human Immunodeficiency Virus, Cytomegalovirus, and Hepatitis B Virus to Health Care Workers Exposed to Patients With AIDS and AIDS-Related Conditions
Gerberding JL, Bryant-LeBlanc CE, Nelson K, Moss AR, Osmond D, Chambers HF, Carlson JR, Drew WL, Levy JA, Sande MA (San Francisco Gen Hosp; Univ of California, San Francisco; Mount Zion Hosp and Med Ctr, San Francisco; Univ of California, Davis)
J Infect Dis 156:1–8, July 1987

Transmission of the human immunodeficiency virus (HIV) by sexual contact with infected individuals, direct inoculation of contaminated blood products, and perinatal exposure in infants born to infected mothers is well documented. The virus has been isolated from blood, semen, tears, saliva, breast milk, vaginal secretions, and cerebrospinal fluid. Similarities between transmission of HIV and that of hepatitis B virus (HBV) has caused concern that health care workers with occupational exposures to infected patients and body fluids are at risk for becoming infected. A prospective cohort study was done to assess the risk of occupational transmission of HIV, HBV, and cytomegalovirus (CMV) to health care personnel with intensive exposure to HIV-infected patients.

The 270 health care workers studied included physicians, nurses, laboratory assistants, and phlebotomists. Sixty percent were women; mean age was 33 years. Any participant with additional risk factors for infection, such as homosexuality, was excluded from the study. One hundred sixty-seven subjects performed or assisted with procedures on patients with acquired immunodeficiency syndrome (AIDS) or AIDS-related complex (ARC) at least once a week. Accidental exposures to HIV, such as percutaneous needle-stick injuries, were frequent in this cohort: 35% sustained a total of 342 such exposures.

None of the 270 subjects had antibody to AIDS-associated retrovirus (ARV) or human T-cell leukemia/lymphoma virus type III (HTLV-III) by Western blot or immunofluorescence assay, although 1.5% had initial reactivity to HTLV-III by enzyme-linked immunosorbent assay. Of the 175 subjects followed-up for 10 months, none developed antibody to HIV. None reported symptoms of ARC or AIDS on a self-administered questionnaire. There was no evidence of increased risk of acquiring CMV or

HBV. More than 2,400 health care workers exposed to HIV have been enrolled in studies and have been tested for antibody to HIV.

This study demonstrated that a large group of health care workers with intensive exposure for a prolonged time to patients with AIDS or ARC were at minimal risk for HIV, CMV, and HBV transmission from occupational exposure. The subjects in this study—health care workers at San Francisco General Hospital—represent one of the most highly exposed cohorts of health care workers in the world.

▶ There have been a number of cohorts of hospital employees who have been exposed to HIV. There are several features of this report that make it worthy of mention. One is that the authors also surveyed seroconversion rates to hepatitis B and cytomegalovirus in addition to HIV. Two, compliance with recommended isolation procedures for HIV was evaluated by questionnaire. The authors document that between 4% and 5% of their employees surveyed for 10 months seroconverted to hepatitis B or CMV, yet none of the 175 HIV-seronegative individuals seroconverted to HIV. The lack of seroconversion to HIV is reassuring and consistent with the less than 1% risk demonstrated to date (see the 1988 YEAR BOOK OF INFECTIOUS DISEASES, pp 185–187).

The rates of HBV seroconversion are somewhat high. In our own cohort of 650 hospital employees followed for more than a year we found 0.75% seroconverted per year. The authors did not employ a control group, but I wonder whether poor compliance (25%) with appropriate infection control practices is reflected in the high rate of HBV seen in the group.

The results reported below (Abstract 7–2) in dental professionals are also consistent with the low HIV nosocomial transmission risk; this despite poor adherence to infection control techniques. Fortunately, gloves, gowns, goggles, and masks are becoming routine in the dental office, if Woody Allen's quote in *Hannah and Her Sisters* is reflective of reality.—D.R. Snydman, M.D.

Low Occupational Risk of Human Immunodeficiency Virus Infection Among Dental Professionals

Klein RS, Phelan JA, Freeman K, Schable C, Friedland GH, Trieger N, Steigbigel NH (Montefiore Med Ctr, New York; Albert Einstein College of Medicine; Ctrs for Disease Control, Atlanta)

N Engl J Med 318:86–90, Jan 14, 1988

Because of the similar epidemiologic features of human immunodeficiency virus (HIV) and hepatitis B and the recognized increased occupational risk of hepatitis B infection among health care workers, a study was conducted to determine the occupational risk for HIV infection of dental health professionals, a group among health care workers at greatest risk of acquisition of hepatitis B infection. A total of 1,309 dental professionals, including 1,132 dentists, 131 dental hygienists, and 46 dental assistants, completed questionnaires on behavior, type, duration, and location of their dental practice, infection-control practices, and estimated numbers of potential occupational exposures to HIV. Serum samples were tested for antibodies to HIV by enzyme immunoassay and to hepatitis B surface antigen (unvaccinated subjects).

Approximately half the participants worked in locations where many cases of acquired immunodeficiency syndrome (AIDS) have been reported. Twenty-one percent of unvaccinated subjects had antibodies to hepatitis B surface antigen. Despite frequent accidental parenteral inoculations with instruments used in treating patients (94%), infrequent adherence to recommended infection-control practices, and frequent occupational exposure to patients with AIDS (15%) and persons at increased risk for HIV infection (72%), only 1 dentist had serum antibodies to HIV. The absence of a history of behavioral risk factors for AIDS in this dentist and his wife suggests that occupational exposure was the likely mode of transmission of HIV. If this assumption was correct, the observed risk among all subjects was 1 in 1,309 (95% confidence interval, 0 to 0.004), the risk in all subjects practicing in a location with many cases of AIDS was 1 in 673 (95% confidence interval, 0 to 0.008), and the risk in all dentists practicing in these locations was 1 in 523 (95% confidence interval, 0 to 0.011).

Dental professionals are at low occupational risk for HIV infection. Since most AIDS patients or those at increased risk for it cannot be detected reliably, strict adherence to recommended infection-control guidelines for dental professionals should be recommended with the idea that all patients have the potential to transmit the infection.

AIDS and Antibodies to Human Immunodeficiency Virus (HIV) in Children and Their Families
Martin K, Katz BZ, Miller G (Yale Univ School of Medicine)
J Infect Dis 155:54–63, January 1987   7–3

Because children are the reservoir of human immunodeficiency virus (HIV) infection for future generations, antibodies to HIV were studied by a sensitive and specific immunoblotting method in 14 children having symptoms of acquired immunodeficiency syndrome (AIDS) or AIDS-related complex. Immunoblots blocked with milk proved to be more sensitive than those blocked with gelatin or the enzyme-linked immunosorbent assay in the serodiagnosis of HIV infection.

In all cases but 1, 1 or both parents abused intravenous drugs. Sixteen of 17 parents of affected children were positive for antibody to HIV, as was 1 of 8 siblings living in the same household (table). All siblings had been infected by and acquired antibodies to Epstein-Barr virus. The affected children were less likely than their HIV-infected parents to have decreased numbers of circulating T4 cells. Their sera recognized fewer HIV polypeptides on Western blots.

The HIV is not merely an opportunistic pathogen in immunodeficient persons, because antibody is regularly present in children with AIDS and their parents but not in children who are immunosuppressed after liver allografting. Intravenous drug abuse is the chief risk factor in families of

Summary of Frequency of Antibody Detection by Immunoblotting to HIV and EBV Polypeptides in 14 Families

Population group	No. of persons	No. with AIDS/ARC	No. of sera	No. positive for antibody to	
				HIV	EBV
Affected children	14	14	13	13	12
Mothers	14	1	12	12	12
Fathers	5	1	5	4	5
Siblings of index case	8	1	8	1	8
Immunosuppressed controls	6	0	6	0	4

(Courtesy of Martin K, Katz BZ, Miller G: J Infect Dis 155:54-63, January 1987.)

children with AIDS in Connecticut. Infection appears not to be readily transmitted by contact with saliva, respiratory secretions, urine, or feces in or outside households. Antibodies may influence the spread of virus within an infected host. It is possible that a more severe course of HIV infection in children compared with that in their parents is related to a decreased antibody response to the virus.

Acquired Immunodeficiency Syndrome in Children: Report of the Centers for Disease Control National Surveillance, 1982 to 1985
Rogers MF, Thomas PA, Starcher ET, Noa MC, Bush TJ, Jaffe HW (Ctrs for Disease Control, Atlanta; New York City Dept of Health)
Pediatrics 79:1008–1014, June 1987   7–4

Of more than 20,000 cases of acquired immunodeficiency syndrome (AIDS) reported to the Centers for Disease Control since 1981, 307 have been in children younger than 13 years. As in adults, the annual incidence of AIDS in children has increased. Just over three fourths of affected children had mothers known to be infected with human immunodeficiency virus or to be at increased risk of infection. Most of these mothers were intravenous drug users or the sex partners of drug users. About one fifth of children with AIDS had received transfusions of blood or blood products.

Nearly three fourths of cases were from New York, New Jersey, California, and Florida. *Pneumocystis carinii* pneumonia was the most frequent opportunistic disease, occurring in 53% of children. Only 11 children had Kaposi's sarcoma. Eighty percent of children were diagnosed before age 3 years. The estimated mean incubation period in perinatally acquired cases was 17 months but has risen over time. Slightly more boys than girls were affected. The median survival time is less than 1 year, and 68% of patients are known to have died.

The number of children with AIDS reported in 1985 is more than double that reported in 1984. The prognosis for affected children is poor. All health personnel should continue to report cases of AIDS to local or state health departments so that new modes of transmission may be identified and epidemiologic trends discerned.

Human T-Lymphotropic Virus Type 4 and the Human Immunodeficiency Virus in West Africa

Kanki PJ, M'Boup S, Ricard D, Barin F, Denis F, Boye C, Sangare L, Travers K, Albaum M, Marlink R, Romet-Lemonne J-L, Essex M (Harvard School of Public Health; Dakar Univ, Senegal; Centre Hospitalier Regional et Universitaire Bretonneau and UER Pharmaceutical Sciences, Tours, France; Centre Hospitalier Regional et Universitaire Dupuytren, Limoges, France)
Science 236:827–832, May 15, 1987   7–5

A new human T-lymphotropic virus (HTLV-4) that is related to but distinct from human immunodeficiency virus (HIV) was detected in Senegal. This virus does not appear to be associated with immunodeficiency. Serum samples were obtained from 4,248 individuals in 6 West African countries from 1985 to 1987. These samples were analyzed for reactivity to HTLV-4 and HIV by radioimmunoprecipitin-gel electrophoresis and immunoblotting.

Evidence of infection with HTLV-4 was observed in persons from 5 of these 6 West African countries. The highest level of infection was found in healthy sexually active individuals. The prevalence of HTLV-4 infection was low but was seen among 2.2% of patients hospitalized with disease.

The presence of both of these viruses indicates the need to develop assays to distinguish between them. Further study of HTLV-4 may enhance understanding of acquired immunodeficiency syndrome.

▶ This study (Abstract 7–5) indicates that HTLV-4 and HIV are both present in West Africa. The studies reported here show that in some West African countries HTLV-4 is more common than HIV.

There is serologic evidence of the presence of HTLV-4 in West Africa during the mid-1970s. The biology of HTLV-4 (Abstract 7–6), lymphadenopathy-associated virus type 2, and HIV needs to be explored in prospective studies among many different populations.— D.R. Snydman, M.D.

Human Immunodeficiency Virus Type 2 Infection Associated With AIDS in West Africa

Clavel F, Mansinho K, Chamaret S, Guetard D, Favier V, Nina J, Santos-Ferreira M-O, Champalimaud J-L, Montagnier L (Inst Pasteur, Paris; Hosp de Egas Moniz and Faculta de Farmacia, Lisbon)
N Engl J Med 316:1180–1185, May 7, 1987   7–6

These authors have previously reported the isolation of a new retrovirus, called human immunodeficiency virus type 2 (HIV-2), from two West African patients with acquired immunodeficiency syndrome (AIDS).

This virus was related to, but distinct from, HIV-1. The authors describe evidence for infection of 30 West African patients with HIV-2.

A clinical syndrome indistinguishable from AIDS was observed in 17 of the 30 patients. Seven of these patients died. All patients had antibodies in their serum that reacted with HIV-2 by indirect immunofluorescence and by immunoprecipitation assays. In some cases, these antibodies cross-reacted with HIV-1. In 11 cases, HIV-2 was isolated from the patients' lymphocytes. This virus did not hybridize with an HIV-1 probe.

Some cases of AIDS in West Africa appear to be caused by HIV-2, a virus that is related to but distinct from HIV-1. Large-scale, prospective seroepidemiologic studies will be necessary to determine the extent of the spread of this virus.

Unsuspected Human Immunodeficiency Virus in Critically Ill Emergency Patients
Baker JL, Kelen GD, Sivertson KT, Quinn TC (Johns Hopkins Hosp, Baltimore; Natl Insts of Health, Bethesda, Md)
JAMA 257:2609–2611, May 15, 1987

Current information suggests that transmission of the human immunodeficiency virus (HIV) from patients to health care workers is rare. Nevertheless, some health personnel have developed seropositivity to HIV following needle-stick injuries or ungloved contact with body fluids of patients with AIDS. As the number of unsuspected asymptomatic carriers of HIV may approach 2 million, the risk—particularly to emergency service personnel—is significant. To determine the prevalence of unsuspected HIV in emergency patients, a study was conducted to test serum samples from critically ill or injured patients without history of HIV infection who were triaged to a critical care unit.

Patients who had blood drawn for any procedure were included in the study. The researchers evaluated specimens by enzyme-linked immunoassay for HIV antibodies. Specimens initially positive were examined again, and those that were repeatedly reactive were evaluated by Western blot analysis.

Three percent of patients were seropositive for HIV antibody by both enzyme-linked immunoassay and Western blot analysis. The seropositive patients were all trauma victims between the ages of 25 and 34 years who were bleeding and required multiple invasive procedures. This group represented 16% of the trauma patients in their age group. History of intravenous (IV) drug use did not assist in identifying potential seropositives.

First-line health care personnel, police, and firemen should use infection-control procedures when responding to the needs of bleeding patients. At minimum, these people should wear gloves when exposed to blood, and they should be extremely careful when inserting IV lines in the field. A caregiver who is injured should be doubly cautious in order to avoid blood-to-blood exposure.

▶ As one might expect, the prevalence of HIV infection among trauma victims is higher than the prevalence among first time blood donors or military recruits (Abstract 7-7). Another study (Abstract 7-8) also establishes an alarmingly high rate of HIV seropositivity among patients attending a clinic for sexually transmitted diseases. The 3% and 5% figures cited here and the 2% figure for HIV seropositivity in parturient patients reported by Landesman below (Abstract 7-9) are strikingly similar. Many of the patients in these studies do not admit to identifiable risk factors. Therefore, it is incumbent for all hospital personnel to take precautions when confronted with any bleeding trauma victim. The Centers for Disease Control will be initiating a sentinel hospital survey to establish HIV seroprevalence among hospitalized patients.— D.R. Snydman, M.D.

Human Immunodeficiency Virus Infection Among Patients Attending Clinics for Sexually Transmitted Diseases
Quinn TC, Glasser D, Cannon RO, Matuszak DL, Dunning RW, Kline RL, Campbell CH, Israel E, Fauci AS, Hook EW III (Natl Inst of Allergy and Infectious Diseases; Johns Hopkins Univ; Baltimore City Health Dept; Ctrs for Disease Control; Maryland Dept of Health and Mental Hygiene, Baltimore)
N Engl J Med 318:197-203, Jan 28, 1988   7-8

Infection by human immunodeficiency virus (HIV) now is highly prevalent in the United States. Screening for HIV antibody has not proved very useful for monitoring infection in some populations that may be at increasing risk or among those who do not consider themselves to be at risk. The authors anonymously screened 4,028 persons attending inner-city clinics for sexually transmitted diseases in Baltimore. Positive tests for HIV antibody were obtained in 5.2% of the study population.

Two thirds of the group were men. Behavior placing a patient at risk of HIV infection was acknowledged by 24% of men and by 15% of women. Frequency of HIV occurrence was higher among men and blacks. Rates for all clinic patients increased steadily with age. Seropositivity of HIV was significantly increased among men participating in homosexual or bisexual activity and among those using parenteral drugs. Rates for women were higher among parenteral drug users. On multivariate regression analysis, seropositivity in men was independently associated with increasing age and black race, homosexual activity or parenteral drug use since 1978, a history of syphilis, and a reactive serologic test for syphilis. Predictive factors for women included parenteral drug use and being a sex partner of a bisexual man or parenteral drug user.

If HIV testing in clinics is limited to subjects who perceive or acknowledge high-risk behavior, many infected men and women will not be tested. Screening and counseling should be offered to all patients attending sexually transmitted disease clinics.

Serosurvey of Human Immunodeficiency Virus Infection in Parturients: Implications for Human Immunodeficiency Virus Testing Programs of Pregnant Women

Landesman S, Minkoff H, Holman S, McCalla S, Sijin O (State Univ Health Science Ctr of New York at Brooklyn; New York Univ)
JAMA 258:2701–2703, Nov 20, 1987

Perinatal transmission of the human immunodeficiency virus (HIV) is recognized, but the seroprevalence rates of HIV in women of reproductive age have not been studied. The HIV seroprevalence was determined in childbearing women drawn from a population with a known high incidence of acquired immunodeficiency syndrome.

Cord blood samples were obtained for serologic study from women who delivered at Kings County Hospital Center, which provides medical care for a large inner-city minority population, including a sizable Haitian community. Demographic data, risk factor data, and serologic findings were available for 602 women. Of 602 samples tested, 12 (2.0%) were positive for HIV on both enzyme-linked immunosorbent assay and Western blot analysis. Seven of the 12 seropositive women had risk factors for HIV acquisition as defined by the Centers for Disease Control and confirmed by interview. Routine HIV testing of pregnant women is not available at this hospital, yet the HIV seroprevalence rate of 2.0% is several times higher than that of many other diseases for which screening is already in place. There is an obvious need for routine HIV antibody testing of pregnant women in areas having significant seroprevalence rates of HIV infection.

▶ Infection with HIV among parturients is the major mode of transmission for pediatric AIDS. This is the first published study illustrating a very high prevalence of HIV infection in a high-risk population. Another study recently published shows similar findings (Hoff R et al: *N Engl J Med* 318:525–530, 1988) and underscores the need for counseling and screening among high-risk populations of parturients. The delivery of such individuals also poses a potential infection control problem. Minkoff (*JAMA* 258:2714–2717, 1987) has nicely reviewed this subject recently.— D.R. Snydman, M.D.

Prevalence of Antibody to Human Immunodeficiency Virus and Hepatitis B Surface Antigen in Blood Samples Submitted to a Hospital Laboratory: Implications for Handling Specimens

Handsfield HH, Cummings MJ, Swenson PD (Seattle–King County Dept of Public Health; Harborview Med Ctr, Seattle; Univ of Washington School of Medicine)
JAMA 258:3395–3397, Dec 18, 1987

Laboratory workers and other health care professionals who handle clinical specimens are at increased risk for infection with hepatitis B virus (HBV). Most hospitals and many clinicians routinely use warning labels to denote potentially infectious specimens to protect these workers. The prevalence of hepatitis B surface antigen (HBsAg) and antibody to human immunodeficiency virus (HIV) in blood specimens submitted to an urban teaching hospital's laboratory was analyzed and correlated with the presence of biohazard labeling.

Specimens from 506 patients were analyzed. Hepatitis B surface antigen, HIV antibody, or both were found in 6.3%, 3%, and 8.7% of specimens, respectively. Biohazard labels were present on 67% of 15 specimens with HIV antibody and on 28% of 32 specimens containing HBsAg. Among 473 specimens that were not labeled, HIV antibody was found in 1.1% and HBsAg was found in 4.9%. Either or both of these markers were present in 5.7% of the specimens.

This investigation detected prevalences of 3% and 6.3% of HIV antibody and HBsAg, respectively, in blood specimens from 506 patients. Although the presence of biohazard labels was associated with an increased probability of finding either HBsAg or antibody to HIV, the absence of such a label was not a reliable indication of a noninfectious specimen. Thus, regardless of whether biohazard labels are used, all clinical and laboratory personnel should be vaccinated against hepatitis B and should handle all specimens as though they were infected. By fostering complacency in the handling of unlabeled specimens, the use of biohazard labels may actually increase the risk that health care workers will be exposed to HIV and hepatitis B virus.

Human Immunodeficiency Virus Transmission by Organ Donation: Outcome in Cornea and Kidney Recipients
Schwarz A, Hoffman F, L'age-Stehr J, Tegzess AM, Offermann G (Klinikum Steglitz, Berlin; Robert Koch Institut, Berlin; Univ Hosp, Groningen, the Netherlands)
Transplantation 44:21–24, July 1987   7–11

Human immunodeficiency virus (HIV) or its antibody can be present in many body fluids, and transmission of HIV with transfusion of blood or blood products, artificial insemination, and renal transplantation has been reported. The authors studied the outcome in 4 cornea and 3 kidney transplants from 2 HIV-infected donors. One of the donors was an intravenous drug abuser. The HIV was transmitted to 2 kidney recipients, who developed acute illness shortly after transplantation and had antibodies 50 days afterwards. None of the cornea recipients had clinical signs of infection, and the 3 tested lacked antibody to HIV.

All organ donors now are tested for HIV antibodies. Members of HIV risk groups, such as homosexual men and intravenous drug abusers should be excluded from donation regardless of the results of HIV testing. A test done during the incubation period could be negative at the time of donation, and polytransfused donors could have false-negative results. Patients with fatal neurologic disorders of unknown cause also should be excluded from organ donation, to avoid transmission of neurotropic viruses.

▶ The lack of transmission of HIV by cornea transplantation in the 3 cases cited herein should not be interpreted as sufficient evidence to prove lack of HIV infectivity by this route. Careful screening of all transplant donors for HIV, hepatitis B, and Jakob-Creutzfeldt disease is essential.— D.R. Snydman, M.D.

▶ ↓ There is a real but very small risk of HIV infection from HIV-antibody-negative blood. As the authors state in an appendix to this paper, the rate is approximately 26 per million transfusion units. At issue is whether HIV antigen screening will be cost-effective. Many of the donors in this study were retrospectively identified to have been from high-risk groups. Educational efforts should continue to be emphasized as one of our highest priorities.— D.R. Snydman, M.D.

Transmission of Human Immunodeficiency Virus (HIV) by Transplantation: Clinical Aspects and Time Course Analysis of Viral Antigenemia and Antibody Production
Bowen PA II, Lobel SA, Caruana RJ, Leffell MS, House MA, Rissing JP, Humphries AL (Med College of Georgia)
Ann Intern Med 108:46–48, January 1988   7–12

Several cases of transmission of HIV infection via organ transplantation are known. The patient described below had transmission by a renal allograft.

Man, 30, required 56 units of blood and blood products after sustaining massive head injuries in a vehicular accident. After brain death was declared and human immunodeficiency virus (HIV) antibody testing was negative by the enzyme-linked immunosorbent assay (ELISA) method, multiple organs were harvested. One of the kidneys was offered to a man with diabetes, hypertension, and end-stage renal disease. A positive result for HIV by ELISA later was found in pretransfusion serum and was confirmed by Western blot analysis, and a homosexual history of the donor was elicited. The allograft was left in place, and the recipient had a transient rise in HIV antigen levels, followed by a more sustained increase. Antibody to HIV was detected 51 days after transplantation, but there was no clinical evidence of HIV infection within 15 months of transplantation. The patient was immunosuppressed with antilymphocyte serum, azathioprine, and prednisone. When acute rejection occurred, anti-T3 monoclonal antibody and cyclosporin A were administered.

The sustained rise in antigen levels in this patient was ascribed to viral replication. Antigen had been undetectable since day 40 after transplantation. Potential cadaver organ donors should have testing for HIV antibody in pretransfusion sera or in sera taken several hours after massive transfusion. It is possible that cyclosporine blocks the entry of circulating virus into CD4-positive cells, reducing the chance of a severe deficiency of helper cells developing.

Transmission of Human Immunodeficiency Virus (HIV) by Blood Transfusions Screened as Negative for HIV Antibody
Ward JW, Holmberg SD, Allen JR, Cohn DL, Critchley SE, Kleinman SH, Lenes BA, Ravenholt O, Davis JR, Quinn MG, Jaffe HW (Ctrs for Disease Control, Atlanta; Denver Disease Control Service; American Red Cross Blood Service at Atlanta, Los Angeles, Miami; et al)
N Engl J Med 318:473–478, Feb 25, 1988   7–13

Since 1985, all blood donations in the United States have been screened for antibodies to human immunodeficiency virus (HIV). However, instances of HIV transmission by antibody-negative blood donations do occur, as not all infected donors are identified by testing. This study was done to determine why 7 donors with HIV infection were screened as negative for HIV antibodies and to assess the 13 recipients who were HIV-seropositive after receiving blood from these donors.

All 7 donors were found to be infected with HIV, including 5 homosexual men who admitted to high-risk activities, 1 man who refused to come to the blood center but in a telephone interview denied any activities associated with HIV transmission, and 1 heterosexual woman who reported sexual contact with an intravenous drug user. Most HIV-infected donors were probably not identified because they had been infected too recently and were still negative for HIV at the time of blood donation according to available antibody tests.

Twelve recipients had no identifiable risk factor for HIV infection other than the blood transfusions they had received, but 1 recipient admitted to having had multiple homosexual partners during the 12 years preceding his transfusion. At follow-up 8–20 months after transfusion, 3 recipients had developed HIV-related illnesses, and 1 recipient, a 66-year-old woman, had died of AIDS within 1 year after transfusion. It is concluded that there is a small but identifiable risk of HIV infection for recipients of screened blood.

The San Francisco Men's Health Study: III. Reduction in Human Immunodeficiency Virus Transmission Among Homosexual/Bisexual Men, 1982–86
Winkelstein W Jr, Samuel M, Padian NS, Wiley JA, Lang W, Anderson RE, Levy JA (Univ of California, Berkeley; Children's Hospital, San Francisco; California Dept of Health Services, Sacramento; Cancer Research Inst, Univ of California, San Francisco)
Am J Public Health 77:685–689, June 1987   7–14

The San Francisco Men's Health Study (SFMHS), begun in 1984, is a study of the epidemiology and natural history of acquired immunodeficiency syndrome in a cohort of single men, aged 25 to 55 years, recruited by sampling from a 6-km square area in San Francisco where the epidemic has been most intense. Using this cohort, rates of seroprevalence and seroconversion to the human immunodeficiency virus (HIV) and factors affecting these rates were investigated.

The cohort consisted of 1,034 men; the study period was 1982 until mid-1986. Data were collected twice a year through a long questionnaire. Subjects were also given physical examinations, and a variety of specimens were taken for long-term storage. Prevalence of infection among homosexual and bisexual subjects increased from an estimated 22.8% in the last half of 1982 to 48.6% between July and December 1984. Prevalence remained stable at about 50% in the subsequent year and a half. Annual infection rates, which were measured by seroconversion among seronegative subjects, decreased from an estimated 18.4% per year from 1982 to 1984 to 5.4% and 3.1% during the first and second halves of 1985, respectively, and 4.2% in the first half of 1986.

The prevalence of high-risk activities, defined as more than 10 sexual partners in the 6 months before each examination period and 2 or more partners with whom insertive or receptive anal/genital contact with ejaculation occurred, was estimated without regard to HIV serostatus from the total experience of the cohort. For each of the 3 high-risk activities studied, declines of 60% or more occurred during the 24 months of study—July 1984 to June 1986.

This study demonstrated a relatively rapid increase in the prevalence of HIV seropositivity early in the epidemic, which is consistent with theories of infectious disease spread by contact. The declines noted later in the study were associated with reductions of 60% or more in the prevalence of high-risk sexual practices linked to both acquiring and disseminating infection by the human immunodeficiency virus.

▶ It has been well recognized that two high-risk activities (increased numbers of sexual partners and receptive anal intercourse) are associated with increased HIV seroconversion rates in gay men. Many of us have stressed that education will continue to be a major part of public health efforts to prevent the spread of HIV. Others have argued that there is no evidence to support the idea that such education will work. Although it is possible that the decrease over time in seroconversion rates noted in this study was due to other factors, I believe these data strongly support the concept that education led to changes in high-risk behavior and subsequent decrease in spread of HIV.—S.M. Wolff, M.D.

Long-Term Evaluation of HIV Antigen and Antibodies to p24 and gp41 in Patients with Hemophilia

Allain J-P, Laurian Y, Paul DA, Verroust F, Leuther M, Gazengel C, Senn D, Larrieu M-J, Bosser C (Abbott Labs, North Chicago, Ill; Hopital de Bicetre, Kremlin-Bicetre, France; Centre pour hemophiles Air et Soleil, La Queue les

Yvelines, France; Hopital Necker-Enfants Malades, Paris; Centre pour hemophiles L'Espoir, St Alban Leysse, France)

As many as half of all hemophilia patients may test positive for antibodies to human immunodeficiency virus (HIV). This study was designed to investigate the relationship between HIV antigenemia and the development of symptoms of HIV infection.

The study group was made up of 96 patients, 84 with hemophilia A and 12 with hemophilia B. Follow-up was possible in 93 patients, and these were given clinical, hematologic, immunologic, and virologic evaluations every 4 to 10 months over a 3-year period. Serum samples were tested for HIV antigen, antibody to p24, and antibody to gp41. Results of the tests divided the patients into 4 groups. Group 1 was made up of 8 patients who tested positive for HIV antigen at the start of the study. In group 2, 14 patients became positive during the study. Group 3, with 8 subjects, tested negative for HIV antigen with a low anti-p24 titer. The 66 patients in group 4, also with a negative HIV antigen, showed a high anti-p24 titer.

Patients in each group were analyzed by the Walter Reed staging method. At the start, 86% to 100% in each group were at stage 1 or 2. By the end of the study, 3 years later, the percentage fell to 25, 29, 88, and 73, respectively, for groups 1 to 4. Eleven of the 16 patients who had demonstrated immunodeficiency during the study were from groups 1 and 2. Another significant finding was that thrombocytopenia (a platelet count at or below $100 \times 10^3/\mu l$) developed in 43% of patients with low anti-p24 titers but only in 1.6% of those with high titers.

Hemophilia patients who are HIV-antigen-positive are at greater risk for AIDS and for other HIV-related clinical complications. The decline of p24 antibody and the introduction of HIV antigen predicts the development of these complications and signals a poor outlook for the patient.

► Teleologically, it seems to me that if you have detectable serum HIV antigen levels, then the degree of infection with the virus would be greater. Dr. Allain and his colleagues present evidence that supports such reasoning. Ultimately, detection of antigen will most likely prove to be more useful than antibody tests.—S.M. Wolff, M.D.

Survival With the Acquired Immunodeficiency Syndrome: Experience With 5833 Cases in New York City
Rothenberg R, Woelfel M, Stoneburner R, Milberg J, Parker R, Truman B (New York City Dept of Health; New York State Dept of Health; Ctrs for Disease Control, Atlanta)

Sufficient data are now available to allow initial estimates of the probability of surviving with the acquired immunodeficiency syndrome (AIDS) for 5 years. The pattern of survival among AIDS patients was analyzed among 5,833 persons in New York City in whom AIDS was diagnosed before January 1986. The percentage of homosexual men with AIDS was 58.3%; of intravenous (IV) drug users, 28.5%; and of persons who were both homosexual and IV drug users, 5.7%.

The crude mortality ratio in the cohort was 66.8%. The spectrum of survival in New York City was bounded by 665 persons who died at the time of diagnosis of AIDS and the 1 person who survived for 8.9 years, the spectrum in between being of considerable heterogeneity. The cumulative probability of survival was 48.8% ± 0.7% at 1 year and 15.1% ± 1.8% at 5 years (Fig 7–1). The most favorable survival rate was observed in the group composed of white homosexual men aged 30 to 34 years old who presented with Kaposi's sarcoma only. This group was used as the reference group in assessing the effect of 5 variables: sex, race or ethnic background, age, probable route of acquiring AIDS (risk group), and manifestation of AIDS at diagnosis.

Proportional-Hazards-Model Coefficients for Each Study Variable

Variable	Referent	Coefficient* ±SE	P Value
Sex			
Women	Men	0.158±0.060	0.008
Race or ethnic background			
Black	White	0.159±0.056	0.004
Hispanic		0.154±0.060	0.008
Age			
<30	30–34	0.073±0.050	0.147
35–39		0.119±0.047	0.011
≥40		0.290±0.044	<0.001
AIDS manifestations at diagnosis			
Kaposi's sarcoma and *P. carinii* pneumonia	Kaposi's sarcoma alone	0.655±0.077	<0.001
Kaposi's sarcoma and another disease		0.761±0.093	<0.001
P. carinii pneumonia alone		0.664±0.056	<0.001
P. carinii pneumonia and another disease		0.844±0.065	<0.001
One other disease alone		0.814±0.067	<0.001
Two other diseases alone		0.920±0.091	<0.001
Risk group			
Homosexuality and intravenous drug abuse	Homosexuality	0.131±0.074	0.078
Intravenous drug abuse		−0.031±0.083	0.711
Other risk factor		0.154±0.136	0.258
Interaction of variables			
Black — intravenous drug abuse	No interaction	−0.104±0.093	0.259
Black — other risk factor		−0.383±0.160	0.016
Hispanic — intravenous drug abuse		−0.120±0.098	0.224
Hispanic — other risk factor		−0.033±0.185	0.858
P. carinii pneumonia — drug abuse		0.147±0.070	0.037

*A coefficient is the logarithm of the relative risk of death at any time, as compared with the value in the referent group. A value of 0 implies an identical risk of death, whereas a positive (or negative) coefficient implies an increased (or decreased) risk.
(Courtesy of Rothenburg R, Woelfel M, Stoneburner R, et al: N Engl J Med 317:1297–1302, Nov 19, 1987.)

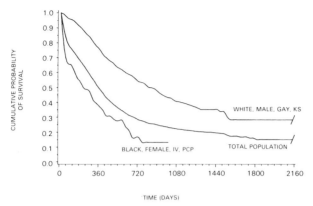

Fig 7–1.—Survival in a cohort of 5,833 patients with AIDS (diagnosed in New York City through December 1985) and in 2 subgroups. Number of subjects surviving at 1 year was 2,494; at 2 years, 754; at 3 years, 233; at 4 years, 77; and at 5 years, 16. In subgroup with "more favorable" survival—white homosexual men with Kaposi's sarcoma (KS)—corresponding value at time 0 was 688 subjects; at 1 year, 476; at 2 years, 203; at 3 years, 72; at 4 years, 24; and at 5 years, 6. In subgroup with "less favorable" survival—black women with IV drug use and *Pneumocystis carinii* pneumonia *(PCP)*—total follow-up has been less than 3 years; 101 subjects were alive at time 0, 31 at 1 year, and 5 at 2 years. The curves for the total population and for white homosexual men with KS are truncated at 2,160 days. Both extend unchanged to 3,240 days. (Courtesy of Rothenburg R, Woelfel M, Stoneburner R, et al: *N Engl J Med* 317:1297–1302, Nov 19, 1987.)

The range in mortality was greater than 3-fold, depending on these variables. Women and subjects with conditions other than Kaposi's sarcoma or *Pneumocystis carinii* pneumonia had the poorest early prognosis. The 1-year cumulative probability of survival more than doubled among patients with *P. carinii* pneumonia alone, but not among subjects without *P. carinii* pneumonia. A proportional hazards model showed that the manifestations of disease at diagnosis were the single largest adverse influence on survival (56.3% of the excess risk) (table). This was followed in importance by age (12.2%), race or ethnicity (10.6%), risk-group (8.4%), and sex (8.0%), with 4.5% of the risk attributable to interactions between variables. Increasing age, female sex, and black or Hispanic ethnicity were important independent factors that adversely affected survival.

It is perhaps too soon to know whether AIDS is universally fatal. There appears to be a spectrum of severity of disease, and long-term survival appears possible.

Diagnostic Tests

Long Latency Precedes Overt Seroconversion in Sexually Transmitted Human-Immunodeficiency-Virus Infection
Ranki A, Valle S-L, Krohn M, Antonen J, Allain J-P, Leuther M, Franchini G, Krohn K (Natl Cancer Inst, Bethesda, Md: Helsinki Univ; Aurora Municipal Hosp, Helsinki; Univ of Tampere, Finland; Abbott Labs, North Chicago, Ill)
Lancet 2:589–593, Sept 12, 1987

The diagnosis of human immunodeficiency virus (HIV) infection is based on the demonstration of antibodies to the viral proteins by enzyme-linked immunosorbent assay (ELISA). More rigorous testing for HIV antibodies with the Western blot antibody test against HIV core protein revealed low-level serologic evidence of HIV infection in serum samples that were negative or borderline-positive by conventional ELISA. Second-generation antibody assay methods, including Western blotting and p24 antigen assay, were used to measure antibodies to recombinant HIV proteins or the presence of viral antigen in serum samples.

In a cohort of 235 Finnish homosexual or bisexual men, there were initially 23 HIV-seropositive men, in 9 of whom seroconversions occurred during 24–36 months of follow-up. All stored serum samples from these 23 men were studied retrospectively, as were serum samples obtained from 25 seronegative sexual partners of HIV-seropositive men, 9 other seronegative homosexual men who had at least 1 enlarged lymph node of unknown origin, 14 randomly selected symptom-free seronegative individuals, and 100 heterosexual Finnish controls.

All 9 men in whom seroconversion occurred had free HIV antigen, low-titer antibodies to recombinant structural or nonstructural proteins, or both, 6–14 months before seroconversion (Fig 7–2). Five of the 25 seronegative exposed partners and 2 of the 23 other seronegative homosexual subjects had persistent signs of latent HIV infection for 16–34 months. However, none of these latently infected patients had antibodies diagnostic of human T-cell lymphotropic virus, type 1 (HTLV-1) or HIV-2 infection. No signs of HIV infection were found among the 110 heterosexual controls. Extensive use of newer techniques that can detect latent HIV infection (e.g., the p24 antigen assay or Western blotting) in at-risk groups may show that latent HIV infection is more common than previously thought.

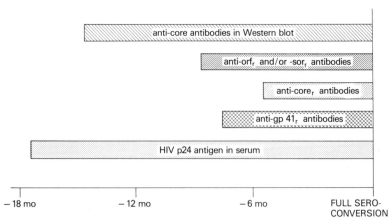

Fig 7–2.—Range of appearance of serologic markers for HIV infection in 9 seroconverters. (Courtesy of Ranki A, Valle S-L, Krohn M, et al: *Lancet* 2:589–593, Sept 12, 1987.)

Compulsory Premarital Screening for the Human Immunodeficiency Virus: Technical and Public Health Considerations
Cleary PD, Barry MJ, Mayer KH, Brandt AM, Gostin L, Fineberg HV (Harvard Univ)
JAMA 258:1757–1762, Oct 2, 1987

It is estimated that in 1991, 54,000 Americans may die of acquired immunodeficiency syndrome (AIDS). Many state legislatures are considering mandatory premarital AIDS screening in an effort to reduce the incidence of new infections. The authors examined whether this program would be an effective way to achieve this goal.

In 1 year, universal premarital screening would detect fewer than 0.1% of HIV-infected individuals and would cost in excess of $100 million. Approximately 1,200 people who had not already transmitted the virus to their partner would be detected per year. There would be more than 350 false positive results, and more than 100 individuals would receive false negative results (table). Fewer than 250 infected births would be prevented by screening each year.

Mandatory premarital screening in this population, with a low prevalence of infection, is a relatively ineffective method of preventing transmission of AIDS and a relatively inefficient use of resources. The more resources that are devoted to such marginally effective programs, the fewer resources will be available to develop effective public health programs. The choice of program should be motivated by epidemiology rather than political considerations.

▶ This paper and the one by Meyer and Pauker (N Engl J Med 317:238–241, 1987) illustrate the problem engendered by false positive results in a population with a low a priori probability of infection. Why is this concept so difficult for the Reagan administration, William Bennett, and the Illinois State legislature?— D.R. Snydman, M.D.

▶ ↓ Measurements of HIV antigen look promising as a means of assessing

Expected EIA Results and Western Blot Test Performance in 1 Year of a Premarital Screening Program*

	HIV Infection	No HIV Infection	Total
Enzyme Immunoassay			
Positive	1325	7648	8973
Negative	23	3816372	3816395
Total	1348	3824020	3825368
Western Blot			
EIA-positive, positive Western blot	1219	382	1601
EIA-positive, negative Western blot	106	7266	7372
Not tested (EIA-negative)	23	3816372	3816395
Total	1348	3824020	3825368

*EIA, enzyme immunoassay; HIV, human immunodeficiency virus.
(Courtesy of Cleary PD, et al: JAMA 258:1757–1762, Oct 2, 1987.)

efficacy of antiviral therapy and predicting the development of AIDS in a cohort of infected individuals. The 3 papers below (Abstracts 7–19 to 7–21) all report on such correlates. It may be that the level of antigenemia is a measure of the number of HIV-infected cells capable of expressing antigen.—D.R. Snydman, M.D.

Human Immunodeficiency Virus (HIV) Antigenemia (p24) in the Acquired Immunodeficiency Syndrome (AIDS) and the Effect of Treatment with Zidovudine (AZT)

Jackson GG, Paul DA, Falk LA, Rubenis M, Despotes JC, Mack D, Knigge M, Emeson EE (Univ of Illinois College of Medicine; Abbott Labs, North Chicago, Ill)

Ann Intern Med 108:175–180, February 1988

The enzyme-linked immunoassay was used to assess changes in human immunodeficiency virus (HIV) antigenemia during treatment with zidovudine (azidothymidine) in 16 patients with acquired immunodeficiency syndrome (AIDS) or severe AIDS-related complex. Half the patients were randomized to receive 250 mg of zidovudine every 4 hours in a double-blind trial lasting about 20 weeks. Surviving placebo recipients then were offered treatment with 200 mg every 4 hours.

Antigenemia was found in 12 of the 16 patients. Three of 4 antigen-negative patients had serum anti-p24 antibody. Three of 5 placebo-treated patients with a high level of antigenemia died in a cumulative time of 17.5 patient-months. Antigen levels declined by more than 90% in the first 4–5 weeks of zidovudine therapy. Fewer patients had high symptom scores during active treatment, and both symptom scores and antigenemia increased when the dose was lowered because of toxicity. High antigen levels correlated with CD4 cell counts, but cell counts decreased when the drug dose was lowered. The HIV cultures were nearly always positive in patients with antigenemia, regardless of the level of antigen.

Treatment with zidovudine had a confirmed antiviral effect in these cases. Monitoring HIV antigenemia can help in evaluating patients with HIV infection and in assessing the efficacy of antiviral chemotherapy.

Effect of Zidovudine on Serum Human Immunodeficiency Virus Antigen Levels in Symptom-Free Subjects

de Wolf F, Lange JMA, Goudsmit, J, Cload P, de Gans J, Schellekens PTA, Coutinho RA, Fiddian AP, van der Noordaa J (Univ of Amsterdam; Municipal Health Service, Amsterdam; Wellcome Research Labs, Beckenham, England)

Lancet 1:373–376, Feb 20, 1988

The nucleoside analogue zidovudine (AZT) has delayed death and lowered the risk of opportunistic infection in selected patients with acquired immunodeficiency syndrome (AIDS) or AIDS-related complex. However, toxicity makes the selective use of zidovudine appropriate. The authors evaluated low-dose AZT therapy in 18 homosexual men who were asymptomatic but had long-standing human immunodeficiency virus (HIV) antigenemia. Groups of 6 patients received the drug in doses of 250 mg every 6 hours, 500 mg every 6 hours, and 500 mg every 12 hours. Some patients also received acyclovir for varying periods.

Serum HIV antigen levels declined significantly in 13 cases, 9 of which had declines to below cutoff values. The antigen level rose in only 1 instance. A positive result in HIV testing of cerebrospinal fluid in 1 patient converted to negative after 12 weeks of treatment. Acyclovir therapy did not appear to influence serum antigen levels. In 7 untreated men, serum antigen levels increased or remained the same during follow-up. Counts of $CD4^+$ cells increased in 14 of 18 treated men and in 1 of 7 untreated subjects. No patient in either group had progressive disease during the observation period. Enlarged lymph nodes regressed in treated men. Side effects were infrequent and mild. No patient had severe leukopenia or neutropenia, though cell counts did decline in most subjects.

Frequent dosing apparently is not necessary for AZT to inhibit HIV replication. Larger placebo-controlled trials are warranted in subjects with HIV antigenemia who are at high risk of progressing rapidly to AIDS.

Risk of AIDS-Related Complex and AIDS in Homosexual Men With Persistent HIV Antigenaemia
de Wolf F, Goudsmit J, Paul DA, Lange JMA, Hooijkaas C, Schellekens P, Coutinho RA (Univ of Amsterdam; Municipal Health Service, Amsterdam; Abbott Labs, North Chicago, Ill; Netherlands Red Cross Blood Transfusion Service, Amsterdam)
Br Med J 295:569–572, Sept 5, 1987   7–21

The development of acquired immunodeficiency syndrome (AIDS) in patients infected with human immunodeficiency virus (HIV) appears to be associated with the presence of HIV antigen and a decrease in HIV core antibodies in serum. The incidence of HIV antigenemia and clinical disease was determined over an average of 19.3 months in 198 HIV antibody seropositive and 58 HIV antibody seroconverted homosexual men.

Of the 198 seropositive men, 40 were antigen-positive and remained positive at follow-up. Of the remainder, 20 became antigen-positive during follow-up. Eight of the 58 seroconverters became antigen-positive during follow-up. The end point attack rate of HIV antigenemia was 14.3% in this series of patients. In 25 of the HIV antigen-negative men, AIDS-related complex was diagnosed. It was also diagnosed in 14 of the HIV antigen-positive men. The diagnosis of AIDS was made in 15 patients. The end point attack rate of AIDS was 23.9% in the antigen-positive group and 1.3% in the antigen-negative group (Fig 7–3).

The incidence of HIV antigen positivity increases over time in

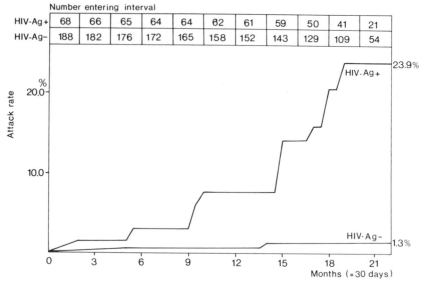

Fig 7–3.—Acquired immunodeficiency syndrome life-table attack rates in HIV antibody/HIV antigen seropositive and HIV antibody seropositive/HIV antigen seronegative homosexual men (October 1984–October 1986). (Courtesy of de Wolf F, Goudsmit J, Paul DA, et al: *Br Med J* 295:569–572, Sept 5, 1987.)

HIV-infected homosexual men. The attack rate of AIDS is significantly higher among antigen-positive men than among antigen-negative men.

Clinical Manifestations

Seronegative Secondary Syphilis in a Patient Infected with the Human Immunodeficiency Virus (HIV) with Kaposi Sarcoma: A Diagnostic Dilemma
Hicks CB, Benson PM, Lupton GP, Tramont EC (Walter Reed Army Med Ctr, Washington, DC)
Ann Intern Med 107:492–495, October 1987   7–22

Negative serology delayed the diagnosis of secondary syphilis in a human immunodeficiency virus (HIV)-infected patient. When spirochetes were demonstrated in a stained skin biopsy, successful treatment was possible.

Man, 31, presented with adenopathy and oral candidiasis and was found to be HIV antibody-positive. Kaposi's sarcoma was evident 2 months later. After about 1 year, negative VDRL and fluorescent treponemal antibody-absorbed test results (FTA-ABS) were obtained. Chills, fever, and orthostasis developed 3 months afterward. Symptoms resolved but recurred 1 month later, and a diffuse erythematous maculopapular eruption was present on the trunk and proximal extremities. Repeat serology was negative even after serum dilution. Warthin-Starry staining of a skin biopsy specimen showed spirochetes in the epidermis and dermis accompanying a moderately dense infiltrate of lymphocytes, histiocytes, and plasma cells. A VDRL, done 20 days after a negative test, was positive at a titer of 1:8, and the FTA-ABS was reactive. Intramuscular benzathine penicillin was given. A Jarisch-Herxheimer reaction occurred, but the patient did well clinically.

The altered immunity of HIV-infected patients may lead to atypical presentations of secondary syphilis. Even in normal hosts, the dermatologic features are quite variable. If the clinical picture is appropriate, treatment can be based on silver staining. A definitive diagnosis of syphilis requires special immunofluorescence staining or antigen detection. Higher doses of penicillin, given for a longer time, may be required to be sure of curing an immunosuppressed patient.

Neurologic Relapse After Benzathine Penicillin Therapy for Secondary Syphilis in a Patient With HIV Infection
Berry CD, Hooton TM, Collier AC, Lukehart SA (Univ of Washington School of Medicine)
N Engl J Med 316:1587–1589, June 18, 1987   7–23

Benzathine penicillin failed in the treatment of secondary syphilis in a homosexual man who was seropositive for human immunodeficiency virus (HIV).

Man, 26, homosexual, with a history of multiple sexual partners and heroin abuse, complained of malaise and a diffuse maculopapular rash. The serum VDRL titer was 1:256 and the fluorescent treponemal-antibody absorption test was reactive. Secondary syphilis was diagnosed, and the patient was given 2.4 million units of benzathine penicillin intramuscularly. Results of monthly follow-up examinations were unremarkable. Five months after treatment, the patient was found in a stuporous state, with right hemiparesis, hemianopia, and aphasia. Results of the enzyme-linked immunosorbent assay and Western blot assay were positive for HIV. The VDRL serum titer was 1:256, and the CSF titer was 1:4. Crystalline penicillin G was administered intravenously for 14 days. All 4 of the patient's sexual contacts were nonreactive on VDRL. Therefore, the patient's illness was believed to represent relapse rather than reinfection.

Despite an initial response to benzathine penicillin, the described patient presented several months later with meningovascular syphilis and irreversible neurologic damage. It is likely that this relapse resulted from failure of the penicillin to reach treponemicidal levels in the CSF. The role of HIV infection and immunosuppression in the syphilitic relapse in this patient is not known.

Relation of Oral Hairy Leukoplakia to Infection With the Human Immunodeficiency Virus and the Risk of Developing AIDS
Greenspan D, Greenspan JS, Hearst NG, Pan L-Z, Conant MA, Abrams DI, Hollander H, Levy JA (Univ of California, San Francisco, School of Medicine, the AIDS Clinical Research Ctr)
J Infect Dis 155:475–481, March 1987   7–24

Hairy leukoplakia (HL) is a lesion of the oral mucosa that has been detected in immunosuppressed homosexual men. The relationship between HL and infection with human immunodeficiency virus (HIV), as well as the development of acquired immunodeficiency virus (AIDS), was investigated in 155 patients with HL.

All 155 patients were immunosuppressed homosexual men. Serum samples were obtained from 101 of these patients who did not have AIDS. Of these, antibodies to HIV were detected in 100 samples. Of the 28 patients tested, HIV could be recovered from peripheral blood mononuclear cells of 22 patients. Of the 155 patients, 12 had AIDS initially. Acquired immunodeficiency syndrome developed in 43 more patients over the next 31 months. Survival analysis demonstrated that the probability of developing AIDS for patients with HL was 48% by 16 months and 83% by 31 months.

Oral HL appears to be highly predictive of AIDS. The men in this study developed AIDS at the highest rate reported for any AIDS-associated condition.

Diagnosis of Human Immunodeficiency Virus Infection in Seronegative Homosexuals Presenting With an Acute Viral Syndrome
Kessler HA, Blaauw B, Spear J, Paul DA, Falk LA, Landay A (Rush-Presbyterian–St. Luke's Med Ctr, Chicago; Abbott Labs, North Chicago)
JAMA 258:1196–1199, Sept 4, 1987   7–25

The early events in human immunodeficiency virus (HIV) infection are not well understood. The authors report on the diagnosis of acute HIV infection in 4 seronegative patients at high risk for HIV infection. An enzyme immunoassay (EIA) that detects HIV antigen (HIV-Ag) in the serum was used for this diagnosis.

The clinical syndrome of these patients was characterized by fever, rash, myalgias-arthralgias, and pharyngitis. All symptoms resolved spontaneously within 8–12 days. All patients were initially negative for serum HIV antibody; all have subsequently seroconverted. During the acute illness, HIV was isolated from 2 patients. Initial serum samples were positive for HIV-Ag. Serum samples then became negative for HIV-Ag and positive for HIV antibody.

Serum HIV-Ag detection by EIA could become a rapid and simple diagnostic test for acute HIV infection. It could also be useful in defining the early natural history of this disease. Assessment of the sensitivity of this test will require more extensive testing.

Congestive Cardiomyopathy and Illness Related to the Acquired Immunodeficiency Syndrome (AIDS) Associated With Isolation of Retrovirus From Myocardium
Calabrese LH, Proffitt, MR, Yen-Lieberman B, Hobbs RE, Ratliff NB (Cleveland Clinic Found)
Ann Intern Med 107:691–692, November 1987   7–26

Cardiac manifestations in patients with the acquired immunodeficiency syndrome (AIDS) have generally reflected opportunistic infections of the myocardium itself or direct involvement with malignancies. A case is presented of an AIDS patient with congestive cardiomyopathy in whom the retrovirus itself was cultured from a subendomyocardial biopsy.

Case.—Man, 32, homosexual, with a 4-year history of AIDS-related complex, presented with progressive shortness of breath, orthopnea, and severe peripheral edema. Chest roentgenogram revealed greatly enlarged cardiac silhouette and congestive heart failure. Cardiac study revealed a markedly dilated right ventricle with moderate hypokinesis and a moderately dilated left ventricle with normal systolic function. A right ventricular transvenous endomyocardial biopsy was performed. Electron microscopy showed extensive degenerative changes in numerous myocytes. Virologic culture with the human immunodeficiency virus (HIV)-phytohemagglutinin-stimulated lymphoblasts showed syncytial cells and detectable reverse transcriptase activity. The HIV antigen was detectable by an antigen capture assay.

An underlying HIV infection should be considered in all high-risk persons presenting with dilated cardiomyopathy of unknown cause. These results warrant further investigation.

▶ The culture findings from this study are in accord with a previous study (Cohen IS et al: Congestive cardiomyopathy in association with the acquired immunodeficiency syndrome. *N Engl J Med* 315:628–630, 1986) demonstrating a congestive cardiomyopathy in patients with AIDS. These studies raise the possibility of a direct cardiac effect from HIV infection.—D.R. Snydman, M.D.

Neurologic Manifestations of AIDS
McArthur JC (Johns Hopkins Univ School of Medicine)
Medicine (Baltimore) 66:407–437, November 1987   7–27

As experience with the spectrum of human immunodeficiency virus (HIV) has widened, it has become apparent that the nervous system is frequently involved, often before the full development of acquired immunodeficiency syndrome (AIDS). The most frequent disorder is a progressive dementia, occurring in 50% to 70% of patients with AIDS. Recognition of the frequency of nervous system invasion by HIV is important in planning treatment.

A group of 186 patients with HIV infection were referred for neurologic evaluation. More than half met the criteria for AIDS; 12% had no

TABLE 1.—Neurologic Complications in 186 Patients With HIV Infection

Central Nervous System	Number (%)	Peripheral Nervous System	Number (%)
Viral infections		Inflammatory demyelinating neuropathy	11 (6)
AIDS-related dementia	30 (16)	Sensory neuropathy	26 (14)
CMV encephalitis	3 (2)	Cranial neuropathies	4 (2)
CMV retinitis	9 (5)	Multiple mononeuropathies	2 (1)
HIV-related meningitis	13 (17)	Herpes zoster myeloradiculitis	8 (4)
Progressive multifocal leukoencephalopathy	1 (.5)	Miscellaneous	
Intracranial mass lesions		Cryptococcal meningitis	11 (6)
Cerebral toxoplasmosis	15 (8)	Neurosyphilis (treated)	1 (.5)
Primary CNS lymphoma	7 (4)	Metabolic encephalopathy	5 (3)
Undefined mass lesions	6 (3)	Cerebrovascular accident	1 (.5)
Systemic lymphoma	1 (.5)		

(Courtesy of McArthur JC: *Medicine (Baltimore)* 66:407–437, November 1987.)

constitutional symptoms but did have neurologic complaints. A total of 165 HIV-related neurologic complications were identified in 120 patients (Table 1). Most patients were homosexual or bisexual males, were intravenous drug users, or had mixed-risk factors.

Progressive dementia was identified in 30 patients; of these, 20 had early acute respiratory disease (ARD) (Table 2). Memory loss was found in 80% of patients with early ARD. Apathy and depressive symptoms were noted in 15% and 30% of patients, respectively. Ten patients had late AIDS-related dementia and were incapable of independent functioning. All these patients had neurologic deficits including diffuse hyperreflexia, hypertonia, impaired rapid alternating movements, and release signs. Psychomotor retardation, incontinence, and mutism developed in the late stages.

The course of the dementia was unpredictable, and no specific prognostic factors were identified. There is evidence linking unchecked viral replication within the brain and progressive dementia, but the basic pathogenic mechanisms have yet to be identified.

The study demonstrates that HIV enters the CNS during the earliest stages of infection. This finding has major implications for antiviral agents that have to penetrate brain parenchyma to clear the virus adequately. Treatment for other neurologic complications such as myelopathies, peripheral neuropathies, opportunistic CNS infections, and CNS neoplasms is available in some instances, but it is generally not curative and is often poorly tolerated. Further research will focus on better understanding of the pathogenic mechanisms, earlier and more specific detection of these conditions, and development of improved therapeutic agents.

▶ There have been several reviews of the neurologic manifestations of AIDS in

TABLE 2.—Clinical Presentation in 30 Patients With AIDS-Related Dementia

	Early ARD (N = 20) Number (%)	Late ARD (N = 19) Number (%)
Symptoms		
Memory loss	16 (80)	14 (74)
Behavioral change	6 (30)	2 (11)
Depressive symptoms	6 (30)	3 (16)
Apathy	3 (15)	11 (58)
Delirium	3 (15)	8 (42)
Psychosis	1 (5)	2 (11)
Motor complaints	5 (20)	4 (21)
Signs*		
Normal examination	7 (39)	0 (0)
Abnormal MMS†	6 (33)	13 (72)
Psychomotor slowing	2 (11)	7 (39)
Hyperreflexia	9 (50)	14 (78)
Hypertonia	4 (22)	6 (33)
Release signs	4 (22)	7 (39)
Impaired rapid movements	4 (22)	5 (28)
Myelopathy	2 (11)	7 (39)

*Examination performed on 18 with early ARD and 18 with late ARD.
†Mini-Mental Status examination: score less than 26/30.
(Courtesy of McArthur JC: Medicine (Baltimore) 66:407–437, November 1987.)

the past year. I commend this one to the reader and also another (Gabuzda DA, Hirsch MS: Ann Intern Med 107:383–391, 1987).—D.R. Snydman, M.D.

Evidence for Early Central Nervous System Involvement in the Acquired Immunodeficiency Syndrome (AIDS) and Other Human Immunodeficiency Virus (HIV) Infections: Studies with Neuropsychologic Testing and Magnetic Resonance Imaging
Grant I, Atkinson JH, Hesselink JR, Kennedy CJ, Richman DD, Spector SA, McCutchan JA (Univ of California, San Diego; San Diego VA Med Ctr, La Jolla, Calif)
Ann Intern Med 107:826–836, Dec 1987

Patients with acquired immunodeficiency syndrome (AIDS) are known to develop serious neuropsychologic complications. The involvement of the brain with human immunodeficiency virus (HIV) infection can bring about cognitive dysfunction and dementia. Both neuropsychologic testing and magnetic resonance imaging (MRI) were used to define the presence of brain disease and the degree of impairment in AIDS patients.

The 55 homosexual men who entered the study were divided into 4 groups according to clinical symptoms and the results of immunologic tests. Fifteen patients, group A, met the criteria for AIDS as set by the Centers for Disease Control. The 13 patients in group B had AIDS-related complex. Sixteen patients who were seropositive for HIV but did not meet the criteria for groups A and B were classified as group C, and 11 men who tested negative for HIV antibody made up the control group D. All patients underwent 8 standard tests designed to measure cognitive ability, mental flexibility, and memory. Magnetic resonance imaging of the central nervous system, because of its expense, was limited to groups A and B. Immunologic studies were also performed.

Group A patients scored significantly lower than the other 3 groups on a test measuring speed of information processing. Group A also performed most poorly on several other tests, and those in groups B and C tended to score lower than the controls. When a patient was characterized as definitely impaired on at least 1 test and probably impaired on 2 or more, that patient's neuropsychologic condition was judged abnormal. By this standard, 87% of group A and 54% of group B showed abnormal findings. Magnetic resonance imaging detected abnormalities in 69% of group A and 50% of group B. The two sets of results gave an agreement rate of 74%. Previous substance abuse in patients was not related to abnormal findings.

Some patients with AIDS who show no symptoms of mental deterioration and have normal findings on computed tomographic scans of the brain do, nevertheless, present evidence of neurologic disease through cognitive evaluation and MRI. It is postulated that HIV is principally responsible for this deterioration in AIDS patients who are free of other brain disease, though the process remains to be documented.

▶ There are many frightening aspects of the AIDS epidemic. To me, one of the most frightening is the fact that we have only 7 years' experience with the disease so that long-term consequences of HIV infection are still to be documented. It is easy to postulate that with CNS involvement of the magnitude noted early in the course of HIV infection, one might expect much more serious and possibly widespread changes with time: not a pleasant thought.— S.M. Wolff, M.D.

Early Predictors of In-Hospital Mortality for *Pneumocystis carinii* Pneumonia in the Acquired Immunodeficiency Syndrome
Kales CP, Murren JR, Torres RA, Crocco JA (St Vincent's Hosp and Med Ctr, New York)
Arch Intern Med 147:1413–1417, August 1987   7–29

Known predictors of a poor outlook in patients with *Pneumocystis carinii* pneumonia include failure to respond to sulfamethoxazole/trimethoprim therapy and the need for mechanical ventilation. However, both occur relatively late during the hospital stay. The authors analyzed 145 patients with *P. carinii* pneumonia at a center serving a large homosexual population in an attempt to predict hospital mortality early in the course of disease. All had biopsy-proven disease. In 85% of cases, the only risk factor was male homosexuality or bisexuality.

Mortality was 19% for the 124 first admissions with *P. carinii* pneumonia. The mean duration of symptoms at admission was 3 weeks. Survival could not be related to any particular symptom or its duration. Patients with abnormal lung findings had a higher mortality, but the presence of bilateral interstitial infiltrates was not a factor. Patients with leukocytosis had increased mortality, as did those with an abnormal Pa_{CO_2}. Patients with another pulmonary infection in addition to *P. carinii* pneumonia had a mortality of 50%, compared to 18% for those with *P. carinii* pneumonia alone. Five of 17 patients with cutaneous Kaposi's sarcoma died.

Adverse predictors in patients with *P. carinii* pneumonia include multiple admissions, leukocytosis, compromised blood gases, and a low serum albumin. Patients with multiple pulmonary infections, including *P. carinii* pneumonia, have a very high mortality. Neither the total T4 count nor the T4/T8 ratio influenced hospital mortality in the present series.

Assessment of Therapy for *Toxoplasma* Encephalitis
The TE Study Group (Natl Inst of Allergy and Infectious Diseases, Bethesda, Md; Palo Alto Med Found, Palo Alto, Calif; Univ of Miami; M.D. Anderson Hosp, Houston; Norwalk Hosp, Norwalk, Conn; et al)
Am J Med 82:907–914, May 1987   7–30

Among patients with acquired immunodeficiency syndrome (AIDS), *Toxoplasma* encephalitis (TE) occurs as a life-threatening infection. The

TE study group was established to review the available data and address clinical issues.

Toxoplasma encephalitis was confirmed in 68 patients between January 1, 1978, and March 1984. The initial symptoms were headache, disorientation, seizures, and hemiparesis. The median survival after therapy initiation was 4 months. Of the 61 patients who received therapy, 92% died. Patients described as alert survived longer than those described as stuporous. The use of corticosteroids was neither harmful nor beneficial. Pyrimethamine and sulfonamide therapy generated adverse reactions (e.g., leukopenia) in 60% of the patients. Clinical relapse occurred in 50% of the patients discharged from the hospital.

The overall prognosis for TE patients is poor, although those who are alert tend to survive longer than those who are not alert. Patients with AIDS and TE have a high rate of adverse reactions to therapy and of relapse. There is a need for better TE therapy.

▶ The response is so poor that one is tempted to try to make an early diagnosis in patients at risk (AIDS, toxoantibody-positive) by prospective surveillance of antibody titers and perhaps head computed tomographic scanning or magnetic resonance imaging. The idea would be to begin treatment before CNS symptoms occur. This will not be easy but perhaps necessary, since this paper does not bode well for waiting to treat those clinically affected.— G.T. Keusch, M.D.

Therapy

The Efficacy of Azidothymidine (AZT) in the Treatment of Patients with AIDS and AIDS-Related Complex: A Double-Blind, Placebo-Controlled Trial
Fischl MA, Richman DD, Grieco MH, Gottlieb MS, Volberding PA, Laskin OL, Leedom JM, Groopman JE, Mildvan D, Schooley RT, Jackson GG, Durack DT, King D, the AZT Collaborative Working Group (Univ of Miami; Univ of California, San Diego; St Luke's–Roosevelt Hosp Ctr, New York; Univ of California, Los Angeles; Univ of California, San Francisco; et al)
N Engl J Med 317:185–191, July 23, 1987   7–31

Azidothymidine (AZT) is a thymidine analogue that inhibits the replication of human immunodeficiency virus in vitro by inhibiting the reverse transcriptase of the virus. A double-blind trial of oral AZT therapy was carried out in 282 patients with acquired immunodeficiency syndrome (AIDS) manifested by *Pneumocystis carinii* pneumonia alone, or with advanced AIDS-related complex (ARC). Subsets of patients stratified by the number of T cells with CD4 surface markers were assigned to receive 250 mg AZT or placebo orally every 4 hours over 24 weeks.

Nineteen placebo recipients and one AZT-treated patient died during the study. The latter patient died of disseminated cryptococcosis. Eight of the placebo patients died of *P. carinii* pneumonia. Survival was improved in both AIDS and ARC patients. No opportunistic infections occurred in

ARC patients after 6 weeks of AZT treatment. Ten placebo patients and 6 given AZT therapy developed Kaposi's sarcoma.

Performance scores and body weight increased significantly in AZT-treated patients, and a persistent increase in CD4 cells was observed in patients with ARC. Skin-test anergy was reversed more often in AZT recipients (29% vs. 9% of those receiving placebo). Administration of AZT reduces mortality and the occurrence of opportunistic infections in patients with AIDS or ARC.

The Toxicity of Azidothymidine (AZT) in the Treatment of Patients with AIDS and AIDS-Related Complex: A Double-Blind, Placebo-Controlled Trial
Richman DD, Fischl MA, Grieco MH, Gottlieb MS, Volberding PA, Laskin OL, Leedom JM, Groopman JE, Mildvan D, Hirsch MS, Jackson GG, Durack DT, Nusinoff-Lehrman S, AZT Collaborative Working Group (Univ of California, San Diego; Univ of Miami; St Luke's–Roosevelt Hosp Ctr, New York; Univ of California, Los Angeles; Univ of California, San Francisco, et al)
N Engl J Med 317:192–197, July 23, 1987   7–32

Toxicity of orally administered azidothymidine (AZT) was studied in a double-blind trial in 282 patients with acquired immunodeficiency syndrome (AIDS) or AIDS-related complex. Azidothymidine was given to 145 patients, while 137 received placebo.

Significant clinical benefit was documented (see Abstract 7–31), but 84% of AZT recipients and 72% of placebo recipients reported adverse clinical events. The only symptoms reported significantly more often by AZT-treated patients were nausea, myalgia, and insomnia. Most AZT recipients developed macrocytosis, and about one fourth had anemia, with hemoglobin values below 7.5 gm/dl. About one fifth of AZT-treated patients and 4% of the placebo group required multiple red-cell transfusions. Neutropenia developed in 16% of AZT recipients and in 2% of the placebo group. Hematologic abnormalities were more frequent among patients with low lymphocyte counts or anemia initially and those given acetaminophen.

Because of its toxicity AZT must be administered cautiously to patients with AIDS or AIDS-related complex. However, when carefully managed, the drug can be given to some patients for extended periods with some toxicity and, in certain patients, therapeutic benefit.

▶ Azidothymidine was developed 25 years ago but was never used clinically. Screening of agents for anti-HIV activity led to the present trial, within 5 years of the description of the first AIDS cases. Applications for its clinical use passed through the Food and Drug Administration in record time (it is amazing what can be done when necessary). Although expensive and toxic, AZT significantly prolongs life: a major advance, but only the beginning in what will prove to be a long and difficult battle to find curative agents for HIV infection.—S.M. Wolff, M.D.

Azidothymidine Associated With Bone Marrow Failure in the Acquired Immunodeficiency Syndrome (AIDS)
Gill PS, Rarick M, Brynes RK, Causey D, Loureiro C, Levine AM (Univ of Southern California School of Medicine; Los Angeles County Univ of Southern California Med Ctr, Los Angeles)
Ann Intern Med 107:502–505, October 1987

Azidothymidine (AZT) is a thymidine analogue used to treat patients with acquired immunodeficiency syndrome (AIDS) and *Pneumocystis carinii* pneumonia. Anemia is a major side effect, usually seen after prolonged drug use. Four patients developed severe pancytopenia and marrow aplasia following AZT treatment for AIDS. They were among 74 patients given the drug for the indication of AIDS and *P. carinii* pneumonia. Low hemoglobin levels and platelet and granulocyte counts were noted 12 to 17 weeks after the start of AZT therapy. Three patients had markedly hypocellular bone marrow, and 1 was moderately affected. Partial recovery was noted after 4–5 weeks in 3 cases, but 1 patient had not as yet recovered in more than 6 months after AZT was withdrawn.

Azidothymidine appears to have its chief toxic effect on the bone marrow. Anemia usually is observed after 6 weeks of treatment, and it usually resolves when the dose is reduced. Some patients, however, develop pancytopenia due to markedly lowered marrow production. Azidothymidine should be used cautiously in patients with AIDS, and the hemoglobin and cell counts should be closely monitored. Marrow recovery may be long delayed. Patients with terminal illness may be especially disposed to marrow suppression by AZT. Other drugs that may suppress the bone marrow should not be used in conjunction with AZT.

▶ These cases illustrate the tenuous nature of AZT therapy in HIV infection. Fatal bone marrow aplasia is a definite risk, and marrow recovery may not occur following completion of therapy.—D.R. Snydman, M.D.

Aerosolised Pentamidine as Sole Therapy for *Pneumocystis carinii* Pneumonia in Patients With Acquired Immunodeficiency Syndrome
Montgomery AB, Debs RJ, Luce JM, Corkery KJ, Turner J, Brunette EN, Lin ET, Hopewell PC (San Francisco Gen Hosp Med Ctr; Cancer Research Inst, School of Medicine, School of Pharmacy, Univ of California, San Francisco)
Lancet 2:480–482, Aug 29, 1987

The standard therapy for *Pneumocystis carinii* pneumonia is either trimethoprim-sulfamethoxazole administered intravenously (IV) or orally or pentamidine isethionate given intravenously or intramuscularly. The agents are equally effective against first episodes of *P. carinii* pneumonia in patients with acquired immunodeficiency syndrome (AIDS). Nevertheless, the frequency with which they cause adverse reactions necessitates changing from 1 drug to the other. Aerosolized pentamidine has been shown to yield high concentrations of pentamidine in bronchoalveolar lavage specimens, thus presumably within alveoli, with little or no pulmonary clearance or systemic drug uptake for at least 24 hours. Aerosolized pentamidine as the sole therapy was tested in an open trial of 15 patients.

Patients accepted into the study had serum creatinine levels less than or equal to 2 mg/dl; no more than 48 hours of empirical therapy for *P. carinii* pneumonia; and arterial Po_2 of at least 50 mm Hg while breathing ambient air. Treatment consisted of inhalations of pentamidine aerosol once a day for 21 days. The specially designed nebulizer system held 600 mg of pentamidine isethionate dissolved in 6 ml of sterile water. Thirteen patients exhibited objective and subjective improvement during treatment. Ten patients improved clinically in the first week of therapy; 3 improved during the second week. One patient, who was also being treated for tuberculosis, died of progressive respiratory failure. Intravenous (IV) trimethoprim-sulfamethoxazole was initiated in this patient and was continued until his death 6 days later. The last patient was put on IV trimethoprim-sulfamethoxazole because he required mechanical ventilation for acute neurologic and respiratory deterioration 20 hours after the first dose of aerosolized pentamidine. In patients successfully treated, mean Pa_{O_2} and vital capacity were 67.9 mm Hg and 50.8%, respectively, before therapy and 80.1 mm Hg and 67.9%, respectively, after therapy. Serum pentamidine concentrations tended to be low in all patients. No systemic side effects occurred. The only local side effect was cough, occurring in 12 patients.

Aerosolized pentamidine is safe and effective in treating mild to moderate *P. carinii* pneumonia in patients with AIDS. The overall efficacy rate was 87%, equal to or better than that of trimethoprim-sulfamethoxazole, parenteral pentamidine, or trimethoprim-dapsone.

▶ Despite the lack of controlled trials, aerosolized pentamidine has become the treatment of choice for AIDS patients with *P. carinii* pneumonia, especially in those patients whose bone marrow is already marginal from AZT therapy or HIV infection itself. This study and the one cited below are the only ones published to date. We await further comparative trials with more hypoxic individuals in order to see whether efficacy and relative lack of systemic toxicity hold up.—D.R. Snydman, M.D.

Inhaled or Reduced-Dose Intravenous Pentamidine for *Pneumocystis carinii* Pneumonia: A Pilot Study
Conte JE Jr, Hollander H, Golden JA (School of Medicine and Gen Clinical Research Ctr, Univ of California, San Francisco)
Ann Intern Med 107:495–498, October 1987

Conventional treatment for *Pneumocystis carinii* pneumonia involves considerable toxicity and fails in one fourth of cases. Inhaled pentamidine might provide an effective and safer form of treatment. This treatment was evaluated in a prospective series of 22 men with mild *P. carinii* pneumonia. None of these patients deteriorated clinically within 4 days of enrollment. Thirteen patients received pentamidine by nebulizer in a dose of 4 mg/kg over 30–60 minutes; 9 others received 3 mg/kg of pentamidine intravenously in a 2-hour infusion once daily.

Nine of 10 evaluable patients given pentamidine by inhalation responded satisfactorily. Three patients later were treated successfully for recurrent *P. carinii* pneumonia. Eight of 9 patients treated intravenously also had a satisfactory outcome. Two patients given inhaled pentamidine developed neutropenia. Two of those treated intravenously had major toxicity.

Inhaled or reduced-dose pentamidine may be an effective and relatively safe treatment for mild *P. carinii* pneumonia and may be suitable for outpatient use. High concentrations of the drug are achieved in bronchoalveolar lavage fluid by this route, and very little inhaled drug is absorbed into the systemic circulation. The best dosage regimen remains to be determined.

Trimetrexate for the Treatment of *Pneumocystis carinii* Pneumonia in Patients With the Acquired Immunodeficiency Syndrome
Allegra CJ, Chabner BA, Tuazon CU, Ogata-Arakari D, Baird B, Drake JC, Simmons JT, Lack EE, Shelhamer JH, Balis F, Walker R, Kovacs JA, Lane HC, Masur H (Natl Cancer Inst; Natl Inst of Allergy and Infectious Diseases; George Washington Univ Med Ctr)
N Engl J Med 317:978–985, Oct 15, 1987   7–36

Pneumocystis carinii (PC) pneumonia is now recognized as the most frequent pulmonary infection and the most common cause of death in acquired immunodeficiency syndrome (AIDS) patients. Trimetrexate, a potent inhibitor of dihydrofolate reductase from PC, was used as an antipneumocystis agent in 49 patients with AIDS and pneumocystis pneumonia. Reduced folate leucovorin was used simultaneously to protect host tissues from the toxic effects of the antifolate.

Group I comprised 16 patients in whom conventional therapy had failed or was not tolerated; group II was 16 patients who had histories of sulfonamide intolerance or inefficacy and were treated primarily; group III was 17 patients with no known intolerance to sulfa drug who were given trimetrexate, leucovorin, and sulfadiazine. In group I, 69% of the patients responded to the treatment, and the same proportion survived. Group II patients showed a 63% response rate and 88% survived. In group III, 71% met all criteria for response and 77% survived. Toxicity was minimal (transient neutropenia, thrombocytopenia) and abated when the drug was stopped. Trimetrexate with leucovorin is an effective and safe treatment for pneumocystis pneumonia in patients with AIDS.

▶ Not enough data are available to suggest that trimetrexate will replace conventional therapy for *Pneumocystis* pneumonia, but the need for better, less toxic therapies is clear. There is no doubt in my mind that one of the beneficial side effects of the AIDS epidemic will be the development of new and better agents for a variety of conditions.—S.M. Wolff, M.D.

Effect of Recombinant Human Granulocyte–Macrophage Colony-Stimulating Factor on Myelopoiesis in the Acquired Immunodeficiency Syndrome
Groopman JE, Mitsuyasu RT, DeLeo MJ, Oette DH, Golde DW (New England Deaconess Hosp, Boston; Harvard Med School; Sandoz Research Inst, East Hanover, NJ; Univ of California, Los Angeles, School of Medicine)
N Engl J Med 317:593–598, Sept 3, 1987   7–37

Recombinant human granulocyte-macrophage colony-stimulating factor (GM-CSF) has in vitro biologic activity identical to that of natural GM-CSF initially purified from a T-lymphoblast cell line. In addition to stimulating proliferation of myeloid precursor cells, recombinant GM-CSF has several in vitro actions on mature effector cells, including inhibition of neutrophil migration; potentiation of tumoricidal capacity of monocytes-macrophages; enhancement of antibody-dependent cellular cytotoxicity; augmentation of neutrophil oxidative metabolism, chemotaxis, and phagocytosis; and inhibition of replication of the human immunodeficiency virus in a monocytoid cell line. Defects in host defense that are reflected as quantitative or functional abnormalities of lymphocytes, monocytes, and neutrophils have been described in patients with acquired immunodeficiency syndrome (AIDS), and such abnormalities may contribute to the high incidence of opportunistic infections and neoplasms in these patients. Leukopenia is a common finding in patients with AIDS and is often the toxic effect limiting doses of drugs used in the treatment of opportunistic infections and neoplasms, as well as antiviral agents. The authors investigated the safety and hematologic effects of recombinant GM-CSF in leukopenic patients with AIDS.

Thirteen of the 16 patients had histories of opportunistic infection, and during the study, 10 patients continued to receive treatment or prophylaxis for cryptococcal infection, oral candidiasis, *Mycobacterium tuberculosis*, or herpesvirus infection. Each patient first was administered a single dose of recombinant GM-CSF intravenously; 48 hours later, a 14-day continuous intravenous infusion of the agent was initiated. The doses used were 1.3×10^3 (n = 4), 2.6×10^3 (n = 4), 5.2×10^3 (n = 4), 1.0×10^4 (n = 3), 2.0×10^4 (n = 1) units/kg of body weight per day. Dose-dependent increases in circulating leukocytes and increases in circulating neutrophils, eosinophils, and monocytes resulted from administration of recombinant GM-CSF. The peak leukocyte count ranged from $4,575 \pm 2,397$ cells/µl at the lowest dose to 48,700 in the patient receiving the highest dose. Low-grade fever, myalgia, phlebitis, and flushing were seen in some patients; there were no life-threatening adverse effects.

These findings demonstrate that recombinant human GM-CSF is well tolerated and biologically active in leukopenic patients with AIDS. Methods of increasing the number and function of circulating leukocytes may reduce morbidity and mortality in these and other patients with leukopenia.

Treatment of Cytomegalovirus Retinopathy With Ganciclovir
Holland GN, Sidikaro Y, Kreiger AE, Hardy D, Sakamoto MJ, Frenkel LM, Winston DJ, Gottlieb MS, Bryson YJ, Champlin RE, Ho WG, Winters RE, Wolfe PR, Cherry JD (Univ of California, Los Angeles, School of Medicine)
Ophthalmology 94:815-823, July 1987

Cytomegalovirus (CMV) retinal infection may occur in immunosuppressed patients and is the most frequent opportunistic eye infection in patients with acquired immunodeficiency syndrome (AIDS). The authors evaluated an experimental antiviral drug, ganciclovir, in 40 patients having AIDS and CMV retinopathy. The drug has in vitro activity against human CMV. Patients received a 10 to 14-day course of treatment with 2.5 mg/kg every 8 hours or 5 mg/kg every 12 hours, followed by maintenance therapy, usually with 5 mg/kg daily 5 days a week by infusion.

All but 1 of 32 evaluable patients had initial responses to treatment, and 88% had complete responses (table). Acuity improved by more than 2 Snellen lines in 15% of patients and decreased by this amount in 12%. Disease consistently was reactivated in patients who did not receive additional treatment or were given maintenance therapy only after a delay. Neutropenia was frequent during initial treatment and also developed during maintenance therapy. Ten eyes developed rhegmatogenous retinal detachment.

Ganciclovir is useful in treating CMV retinopathy in patients with AIDS through reducing or delaying visual loss. Nevertheless, most treated patients in this study lost vision by reactivation of lesions during interruption of treatment, progression despite treatment, or retinal detachment. Ganciclovir might be more effective in preserving vision in patients who require immunosuppressive drug therapy only for a limited time.

▶ This paper represents observations in a large number of AIDS patients with cytomegalovirus retinitis treated with DHPG (ganciclovir) and carefully followed. The initial promise of this drug has been amply documented in this and other reports which confirm that patients with CMV retinitis routinely experience at least a transient improvement in sight or delay in the natural progression of CMV retinitis when they are treated with DHPG. Indeed, this paper goes a long way to describe the natural history of CMV retinitis in the treated patient.

Several things have changed even since the publication of this report. Many patients are now receiving both DHPG and azidothymidine, which was not possible under the initial protocols. It will be necessary to assess the efficacy of DHPG in this setting. Moreover, recent reports have demonstrated that the human immunodeficiency virus (HIV) can be isolated from retinal tissue, which may mean that some of the "CMV retinitis relapses" may represent HIV. It may also be possible to use DHPG via the intravitreal or subconjunctival route,

Treatment of CMV Retinopathy With Ganciclovir:
Summary of Results

Treatment	No. of Patients (%)	
Initial treatment		
Response		
Complete	28/32*	(88)
Incomplete	3/32*	(9)
None	1/32*	(3)
Vision after initial treatment		
Improved†	5/34‡	(15)
Stable	25/34‡	(73)
Decreased†	4/34‡	(12)
Reactivation after cessation of treatment	10/10§	(100)
Maintenance therapy		
Reactivation of disease		
With interruption of maintenance therapy	9/9‖	(100)
While receiving maintenance therapy	9/18¶	(50)
Adverse reactions		
Patients with neutropenia**		
During initial treatment	12/40	(30)
During maintenance therapy	10/26	(38)
Infected eyes with rhegmatogenous retinal detachment		
During maintenance therapy	10/42	(24)

CMV, cytomegalovirus.
*Patients who completed at least 1 week of treatment and for whom photographic documentation of response is available.
†Improvement or decrease indicates greater than 2-line change in acuity on Snellen chart.
‡Patients whose visual acuity was measured at the end of treatment.
§Patients who did not receive maintenance therapy or for whom the start of maintenance therapy was delayed longer than 1 week.
‖Patients whose maintenance therapy was interrupted for a period of 1 week or longer, and who were examined during interruption of therapy.
¶Patients with complete response to initial treatment and who received uninterrupted maintenance therapy for at least 3 weeks.
**Absolute neutrophil count < 1,000/mm^3.
(Courtesy of Holland GN, Sidikaro Y, Kreiger AE, et al: *Ophthalmology* 94:815–823, July 1987.)

and the efficacy of such regimens has yet to be fully evaluated.—M.S. Klempner, M.D.

Regression of Oral Hairy Leukoplakia After Orally Administered Acyclovir Therapy

Resnick L, Herbst JS, Ablashi DV, Atherton S, Frank B, Rosen L, Horwitz SN (Mount Sinai Med Ctr, Miami Beach, Fla; Univ of Miami School of Medicine; National Cancer Inst)
JAMA 259:384–388, Jan 15, 1988

Oral hairy leukoplakia is an early manifestation of human immunodeficiency virus (HIV) infection and is highly predictive of the development of acquired immunodeficiency syndrome (AIDS). The affected epithelial cells appear to be permissively infected by Epstein-Barr virus (EBV). Acyclovir, which inhibits EBV replication in vitro and in vivo, was given to 13 patients having oral hairy leukoplakia and no evidence of active AIDS-related opportunistic infection. The open-label trial involved oral treatment with 800 mg every 6 hours over 20 days.

Five of the 13 patients—all HIV-seropositive men—had diagnoses of AIDS, and 3 others had AIDS-related complex. Five of 6 patients who received oral acyclovir had regression of the lesion, and 3 of them had complete responses. Six of 7 untreated patients had no clinical change, while 1 had progression of the leukoplakia. No serious adverse reactions occurred. No patient developed opportunistic infection during the study. Positive immunofluorescence studies at baseline converted to negative after acyclovir therapy. Repeat biopsies in patients with complete clinical responses showed normal-appearing mucosa. Titers of EBV antibody did not change significantly with treatment.

Infection with EBV appears to produce oral hairy leukoplakia. The epithelial tissue of the tongue may be an aberrant site of EBV replication in HIV-infected patients. Alternately, it may be a site of natural infection that remains latent for a time or a preferred site for coinfection by human papillomavirus. When acyclovir halts EBV replication, normal-appearing epithelium regenerates.

▶ As is true of most infections in patients with AIDS, relapse was the rule after discontinuation of treatment. In this study hairy leukoplakia recurred within 7 weeks after discontinuation of acyclovir therapy in all 5 patients who initially responded.—M.J. Barza, M.D.

▶ ↓ A number of groups are working under the assumption that blocking the T4 receptor to inhibit HIV attachment may slow down HIV replication or prevent infection. Such an approach might be especially useful to prevent needle-stick or perinatal transmission. However, all the studies to date have been in vitro neutralization studies, and one can only speculate about the toxicity such an approach may engender (see also *Nature* 7:78–81, 82–84, 84–86, 1988).—D.R. Snydman, M.D.

Neutralisation of HIV Isolates by Anti-Idiotypic Antibodies Which Mimic the T4 (CD4) Epitope: A Potential AIDS Vaccine

Dalgleish AG, Thomson BJ, Chanh TC, Malkovsky M, Kennedy RC (Northwick Park Hosp, Harrow, England; Southwest Found for Biomedical Research, San Antonio, Tex)
Lancet 2:1047–1049, Nov 7, 1987   7–40

All human immunodeficiency virus (HIV) isolates tested appear to use T4 antigen, or CD4, as a receptor, and in vitro infection is blocked by anti-CD4 antibodies. The authors raised polyclonal anti-idiotypic antibodies in mice against anti-Leu3a, a murine monoclonal antihuman CD4 antibody that blocks the in vitro binding of HIV to the CD4 molecule. Binding to recombinant HIV envelope antigens was examined.

Sera containing anti-idiotypic antibody specifically recognized the envelope glycoproteins of HIV and the specific HIV binding site to CD4 in different isolates. Three different isolates of HIV-1 and an isolate of HIV-2 were neutralized in vitro. The anti-idiotypes did not recognize OKT4, an anti-human T4 antibody that does not inhibit HIV binding to CD4.

This anti-idiotypic antibody approach may prove to be useful in the management of HIV-infected patients. Immunization of newly HIV-positive patients who are not yet anergic to neoantigens might induce an anti-idiotypic response to anti-CD4. In AIDS patients who may not respond to immunization with monoclonal antibody, a monoclonal antibody idiotype that mimics CD4 could be used in passive immunotherapy.

8 Sexually Transmitted Diseases

High Prevalence of Papillomavirus-Associated Penile Intraepithelial Neoplasia in Sexual Partners of Women With Cervical Intraepithelial Neoplasia

Barrasso R, De Brux J, Croissant O, Orth G (Institut A Fournier, Institut de Pathologie et de Cytologie Appliquée and Institut Pasteur, Paris)
N Engl J Med 317:916–923, Oct 8, 1987   8–1

To determine whether neoplastic cervical lesions are associated with papillomavirus infection of sexual partners, the male sexual partners of 294 women with flat condylomas and 186 women with cervical intraepithelial neoplasia were examined by colposcope before and after the application of 5% acetic acid. In 309 men, condylomata acuminata, papules, and macules were observed. In 204 of these men, papules and macules were detected only after application of acetic acid. Condylomas were observed in 121 partners of women with condylomas but in only 10 partners of women with cervical intraepithelial neoplasia.

Intraepithelial neoplastic lesions were observed in 61 partners of women with cervical intraepithelial neoplasia, but in only 4 partners of women with condylomas. Papillomavirus DNA was detected in 60% of the lesions assayed. In penile intraepithelial neoplastic lesions, human papillomavirus types 16 and 33 were detected. In condylomatous lesions, human papillomavirus types 6, 11, and 42 were detected. Unknown papillomaviruses were detected in 15% of the specimens. Cervical carcinomas and precancerous lesions in women may be associated with genital papillomavirus infection of their male sexual partners.

▶ As the authors point out, lesions were occasionally found in sites other than the penis, including the distal urethra and the anal canal, thus emphasizing the need for urethroscopy and proctoscopy in a complete evaluation.—D.R. Snydman, M.D.

Chlamydia trachomatis Infection and Pregnancy Outcome

Sweet RL, Landers DV, Walker C, Schachter J (Univ of California, San Francisco)
Am J Obstet Gynecol 156:824–833, April 1987   8–2

Chlamydia trachomatis is the most common sexually transmitted disease in the United States. The infection can be transmitted from pregnant women to their infants. However, the extent to which this infection adversely affects pregnancy has not yet been established. In a prospective study, 270 pregnant women with endocervical C. trachomatis were compared to 270 pregnant control subjects matched for age, race, and socioeconomic status.

In the entire group harboring C. trachomatis, 10% had premature membrane rupture, 11% had preterm delivery, 4% had amnionitis, 4.3% had intrapartum fever, 14.5% had infants small for gestational age, 6% had postpartum endometritis, and 1.8% had babies with neonatal sepsis. In the subset of women with C. trachomatis-specific IgM, which suggests recent or invasive infection, preterm delivery and premature rupture of the membranes occurred in 19%, as compared to 8% of IgM-negative infected women.

Chlamydia trachomatis infection alone does not appear to have an adverse effect on pregnancy. There is a subset of infected women with IgM seropositivity who have a significantly increased risk of premature rupture of membranes and premature delivery. Screening for C. trachomatis is endorsed as a method of preventing the vertical transmission of infection from mother to infant.

▶ Colonization of the birth canal has previously been shown to be predictive of colonization and infection in the neonate. The present study has focused upon the antepartum and immediate peripartum complications that may be attributed to infection by C. trachomatis. Although colonization of the endocervix was not predictive of problems in labor and delivery, there was an increased incidence of premature delivery among women with an elevated IgM titer to C. trachomatis. In any event, the authors favor routine screening for colonization by C. trachomatis during pregnancy because appropriate treatment reduces perinatal transmission of infection to the neonate.—M.J. Barza, M.D.

Single-Dose Ceftriaxone for Chancroid
Bowmer MI, Nsanze H, D'Costa LJ, Dylewski J, Fransen L, Piot P, Ronald AR (Mem Univ, St John's, Newfoundland; Univ of Manitoba, Winnipeg; Univ of Nairobi, Kenya; Natl Inst, Antwerp, Belgium)
Antimicrob Agents Chemother 31:67–69, January 1987   8–3

Alternative treatments for chancroid are sought because of the antimicrobial resistance of strains of *Hemophilus ducreyi*. Ceftriaxone, which is quite active against *H. ducreyi* in vitro, was given in 3 single-dose intramuscular regimens to 182 males with chancroid who had positive ulcer cultures. These were negative for *Treponema pallidum*. Ceftriaxone was given in doses of 0.25, 0.5, and 1 gm.

Twenty-eight percent of patients failed to return for adequate follow-up. All but 1 of 50 patients treated with 1 gm of ceftriaxone were cured. The 0.5-gm dose cured 43 of 44 men, and the 0.25-gm dose, 37 of 38 patients. Two patients, both given the 1-gm dose, had recurrences of ulceration. Buboes responded equally well to all drug doses. The injections were well tolerated. All isolates produced β-lactamase, and all were susceptible to 0.003 mg or less of ceftriaxone per liter.

A single 250-mg intramuscular dose of ceftriaxone is an effective treatment for chancroid. Further studies will be needed to determine whether the treatment is similarly effective in patients with incubating or infective syphilis.

▶ These authors have previously shown that a single dose of trimethoprim-sulfametrole or of trimethoprim combined with rifampin are also highly effective in the treatment of chancroid; however, the recent emergence of trimethoprim-resistant strains of *H. ducreyi* in Thailand has led to the need for alternative treatments of which this is an excellent example. Ciprofloxacin has recently been reported to be highly effective given orally in a single dose (Bodhidatta L et al: *Antimicrob Agents Chemother* 32:723–725, 1988). The authors recommend that a dark-field examination and a serologic test for syphilis be done before treatment, because ceftriaxone treatment could conceivably cause the dark-field examination to become negative without curing syphilis in extragenital sites.—M.J. Barza, M.D.

9 Nosocomial Infections

Prospective Study of Replacing Administration Sets for Intravenous Therapy at 48- vs 72-Hour Intervals: 72 Hours Is Safe and Cost-Effective
Maki DG, Botticelli JT, LeRoy ML, Thielke TS (Univ of Wisconsin Med School)
JAMA 258:1777-1781, Oct 2, 1987   9-1

Intravenous (IV) therapy has become an essential feature of health care but carries a risk of bloodstream infection. A prospective study was carried out to determine the safety of replacing IV delivery systems every 72 hours instead of every 48 hours for 487 patients.

During 4 months of study, cultures were obtained from 710 IV sets replaced at 48-hour intervals and from 664 sets replaced at 72-hour intervals. The prevalence of contamination in the sets replaced after 72 hours was 1.5%, and the prevalence of contamination from those replaced after 48 hours was 0.8%. This difference was not significant. Contamination

Studies of Replacing Intravenous Administration Sets at Periodic Intervals as an Infection Control Measure

Authors (Year Published)	Location of Patients	Type of Infusions	No. of Sets Cultured	Prevalence of Contamination in Sets Changed at Intervals				No. of Concordant Bacteremias
				24 h	48 h	72 h	Indefinite	
Buxton et al (1979)	Ward	Mainly peripheral*	2537	0.4	0.6	...	...	0
Band and Maki (1979)	Ward, ICU†	Peripheral	694	0.5	1.0	0.7	...	0
		Central, access‡ and TPN	119	0	0	0	...	0
Gorbea et al (1984)	ICU	Peripheral (62%) and central, access (38%)*	676	2.0	4.0	...	...	0
Josephson et al (1985)	Ward	Peripheral	219	...	0.8	...	0.8	0
Snydman et al (1985)	ICU	Peripheral and central, access‡	1194	...	5.0	4.4	...	0
Present study (1986)	Ward, ICU	Peripheral	878	...	0.2	1.0	...	0
		Central, access	331	...	1.9	1.2	...	0
		Central, TPN	165	...	2.7	4.4	...	0
	Ward	All types	1168	...	0.5	1.4	...	0
	ICU	All types	204	...	3.2	1.8	...	0

*Infusions for total parenteral nutrition (TPN) excluded; contamination rates with different types of infusions not given.
†ICU, intensive care unit.
‡Access refers to a central venous infusion used for administering fluids and blood products and delivering drugs or hemodynamic monitoring, but not TPN.
(Courtesy of Maki DG, et al: JAMA 258:1777-1781, Oct 2, 1987.)

in both groups was due to small numbers of coagulase-negative staphylococci. No contamination was associated with bacteremia (table). Contamination was detected in 0.6% of peripheral venous infusions, 1.5% of central venous access or hemodynamic monitoring IV systems, and 3.6% of total parenteral nutrition IV systems. In the intensive care unit, 2.5% of IV systems were contaminated, while in medical and surgical wards, 0.9% of them were contaminated.

Intravenous contamination is rarely the cause of endemic nosocomial septicemia. Routine replacement of IV sets can be safely carried out at 72-hour intervals, thereby reducing the use of sets by about 35% and permitting annual cost savings of more than $100,000 in a 450-bed hospital.

▶ This study and our own (*Infect Control* 8:113–116, 1987) demonstrate virtually identical data on bacterial contamination of intravenous infusion sets at 48 hours and 72 hours. The current recommendation to change intravenous tubing and burettes at 72 hours is cost-effective from an infection control standpoint.—D.R. Snydman, M.D.

▶ ↓ There have been several reports of *Malassezia furfur* fungemia in infants receiving total parenteral nutrition. In the cases cited below *M. furfur* fungemia complicated total parenteral nutrition administration in 2 adults. The contribution of this pathogen to the patients' deaths is not clear since appropriate studies were not conducted at autopsy. These cases underscore the need for special measures for isolation of fungi if patients are receiving lipid emulsions.—D.R. Snydman, M.D.

Intravenous Catheter-Associated *Malassezia furfur* Fungemia
Garcia CR, Johnston BL, Corvi G, Walker LJ, George WL (Sepulveda VA Med Ctr, Sepulveda, Calif; Wadsworth VA Med Ctr, Los Angeles; Univ of California, Los Angeles, School of Medicine)
Am J Med 83:790–792, October 1987   9–2

The lipophilic yeast *Malassezia furfur* can be part of the normal skin flora and causes the benign rash tinea versicolor. Recently, *M. furfur* has been found to cause serious systemic infections in infants given total parenteral nutrition with lipid emulsions. Two adults managed in this way developed *M. furfur* fungemia.

Case 1.—Man, 62, received total parenteral nutrition (TPN) after a pneumonectomy for lung cancer and subsequent partial small bowel resection for infarction. The TPN was supplemented with intravenous medium-chain triglycerides and 10% lipid solution. A mixed gram-negative and aerobic peritonitis occurred that was treated with antibiotics. Persistent leukocytosis developed with negative blood cultures, but a yeast was eventually found and later identified, by its need for exogenous fatty acids for growth, as *M. furfur*. The patient died from cardiac arrest. Autopsy showed lung cancer but no vasculitis or thromboembolism; special stains for fungi were not performed.

Case 2.—Man, 49, with short bowel syndrome and recurrent aspiration pneumonia, received TPN with 20% lipid solution. He became febrile 2 weeks after antibiotics were stopped. A slow-growing yeast in the blood was identified morphologically as *M. furfur*, and a central venous catheter specimen also was positive. The serum triglyceride was mildly elevated. Parenteral amphotericin B was given for 4 weeks, but recurrent episodes of catheter-related bacteremia and pulmonary aspiration ensued as well as documented *M. furfur* fungemia. The patient died from cardiac arrest. The yeast again was isolated from a catheter specimen, 16 days after Intralipid had been reinstituted. Autopsy showed bilateral pneumonia, but no special fungal stains or cultures were performed.

If blood cultures are done for a patient receiving parenteral lipid emulsion, the laboratory should know that fungemia with a lipophilic organism is a possibility. Isolation will require the use of solid media supplemented with medium- and long-chain fatty acids. The present cases of *M. furfur* fungemia were diagnosed by overlaying sterile olive oil onto Sabouraud agar.

▶ ↓ Cutaneous aspergillosis is an unusual finding (See the 1987 YEAR BOOK OF INFECTIOUS DISEASES, p 114). This report summarizes 9 cases in patients with Hickman catheters. The source of the *Aspergillus* infection in these immunosuppressed patients is not clear but was associated epidemiologically with several operating rooms that had a common air supply. After thorough vacuuming of the air ducts, the epidemic ceased. It is of interest to note that there are no standards for aspergilli in air.—D.R. Snydman, M.D.

Primary Cutaneous Aspergillosis Associated With Hickman Intravenous Catheters
Allo MD, Miller J, Townsend T, Tan C (Johns Hopkins Med Institutions)

Aspergillus rarely is pathogenic in a normal host. However, in an immunocompromised host, invasive *Aspergillus* infection can occur. Nine patients aged 17–74 years (table), with hematologic cancer, contracted primary cutaneous aspergillosis at Hickman intravenous catheter sites. All of these patients were immunocompromised.

Clinical signs of infection included erythema, induration, and necrosis. The diagnosis was confirmed by culture of *Aspergillus flavus*. Treatment consisted of intravenous doses of amphotericin B and flucytosine orally, as well as local wound care. Three patients recovered completely; 3 others required operative débridement and delayed grafting. Two patients died of disseminated aspergillosis, and another died of unrelated causes.

Primary cutaneous aspergillosis can occur at Hickman catheter sites in immunocompromised patients. This serious infection requires prompt diagnosis and treatment. Successful treatment requires resolution of aplasia

Characteristics of 9 Patients With Primary Cutaneous Aspergillosis

Patient No.	Age/Sex	Diagnosis	Site of Lesion	Duration of Leukopenia*	Outcome
1	41/M	Acute myelogenous monocytic leukemia (in remission)	Exit	21 days; WBC 1.2 at discharge	Pulmonary infiltrate; healed cutaneous lesion and normalized chest film
2	17/M	Undifferentiated lymphoblastic lymphoma (in remission)	Exit	22 days; WBC 2.8 at discharge	Healed totally; never had other sites of aspergillosis
3	74/F	Acute erythroblastic leukemia (active)	Exit, entrance, tunnel	20 days; WBC 6.9 at discharge	Wound began granulating and was healing when patient died of unrelated causes; no other site of aspergillosis
4	33/M	Acute myelogenous leukemia (active)	Exit, entrance, tunnel	24 days; WBC 10.4 at discharge	Cavitary lung lesion; both skin and lung lesions healed; skin grafting was required
5	23/M	Acute lymphoblastic leukemia (active)	Exit	25 days; WBC 4.4 at discharge	Pulmonary infiltrates; both skin and lung lesions healed
6	72/F	Acute nonlymphoblastic leukemia (active)	Entrance	46 days; aplastic until death	Cavitary lung lesion; died of pulmonary aspergillosis; unhealed chest-wall lesions; no autopsy
7	50/F	Acute myelogenous leukemia (active)	Exit, entrance, tunnel, catheter tip	29 days; WBC 6.2 at discharge	Cavitary lung lesion; skin lesion healed after skin grafting; pulmonary infiltrates resolved
8	53/M	Acute myelogenous monocytic leukemia	Tunnel	23 days; WBC 6.1 at discharge	Nodular lung infiltrate; skin lesions healed after grafting; pulmonary infiltrates resolved
9	53/M	Aplastic anemia	Exit, catheter tip	35 days; aplastic until death	Bronchoscopic washings grew *A. flavus*; lung and skin lesions never healed; patient died after respiratory arrest; autopsy determined aspergillosis to be the cause of death

*WBC, white blood cell count ($\times 10^{-9}$ per liter).
(Courtesy of Allo MD, Miller J, Townsend T, et al: *N Engl J Med* 317:1105–1108, Oct 29, 1987.)

or leukopenia, catheter removal, intravenously administered amphotericin B, and local wound care.

Diagnosis of Central Venous Catheter-Related Sepsis: Critical Level of Quantitative Tip Cultures
Brun-Buisson C, Abrouk F, Legrand P, Huet Y, Larabi S, Rapin M (Hôpital Henri Mondor and Université Paris Val de Marne, Creteil, France)
Arch Intern Med 147:873–877, May 1987

Catheter-related sepsis is a frequent problem in acutely ill patients. A quantitative tip culture (QTC) technique was designed and assessed prospectively in the diagnosis of clinically important catheter-related sepsis.

Technique.—Catheters were removed and handled aseptically. The distal 5–6 cm was rinsed with 1 ml of sterile water, the tube was vortexed, and 0.1 mL of the suspension was plated on blood agar at 37 C. Results of culture were reported as colony-forming units (CFU) per milliliter.

TABLE 1.—Clinical Characteristics and Risk Factors for Infection of 331 Central Venous Catheterizations in 232 Patients

Classification of Catheters

Risk Factors (No. of Catheters)	Culture Negative	Contaminated, No. (%)	Infected or Colonized, No. (%)	P^* (χ^2 Value)
No. in each group (331)	246	42 (12.7)	43 (13)	...
Site of catheter				
Internal jugular (94)	58	16 (17)	20 (21)	<.005 (10.95)
Subclavian (237)	188	26 (11)	23 (10)	
Catheterization				
Repeated (108)	70	18 (16.6)	20 (18.5)	<.01 (7.59)
First (223)	176	24 (10.7)	23 (10.3)	
Septic focus				
Other (203)	140	33 (16)	30 (14.8)	<.01 (7.88)
No other (128)	106	9 (7)	13 (10)	
Bacteremia				
Exposed (59)	37	6 (10)	16 (27)	<.05 (5.07)
Unexposed (272)	209	36 (13)	27 (10)	
Systemic antimicrobials				
Present (175)	125	24 (13.7)	26 (14.8)	.2 (1.62)
Absent (156)	121	18 (11.5)	17 (10.9)	

*P value (χ^2 test) for comparison between culture-negative and culture-positive catheters (contaminated plus infected or colonized).
(Courtesy of Brun-Buisson C, Abrouk F, Legrand P, et al: *Arch Intern Med* 147:873–877, May 1987.)

TABLE 2.—Organisms Recovered from Quantitative Catheter Tip Culture of 85 Central Venous Catheters

	Catheter Group					Organisms, %	
	Contaminated (n = 42)	Catheter Sepsis (n = 36)		Colonized (n = 7)	Total Organisms	Contaminated	Infected or Colonized
Microbial Isolates		Nonbacteremic	Bacteremic				
Staphylococcus aureus	1	5	13	1	20	2	42
Staphylococcus species (coagulase negative)	34	8	2	...	44	63	22
Pseudomonas aeruginosa	2	1	...	3	6	15	13.5
Acinetobacter species	6	2	...	...	8		
Klebsiella species	3	1	2	...	6		
Proteus species, Providencia species	4	...	...	1	5	15	18.4
Enterobacter cloacae	1	...	2	...	3		
Escherichia coli	...	1	1	1	2		
Candida species	1	1	...	...	2	5	4.5
Other*	2	...	...	1	3		
Total Isolates†	54	18	20	7	99		

*One each Corynebacterium species, enterococcus, and pneumococcus.
†The total number of isolates is 99, because 2 organisms grew from 14 catheters.
(Courtesy of Brun-Buisson C, Abrouk F, Legrand P, et al: Arch Intern Med 147:873–877, May 1987.)

TABLE 3.—Quantitative Culture of 85 Culture-Positive Central Venous Catheter Tips

Catheter Group (No. of Catheters)	Colony Count,* CFU/mL					No. of Isolates†
	10-100	110-500	510-1000	10^3-10^4	$\geq 10^4$	
Contaminated (42)	24	25	0	5	0	54
Colonized (7)	1	2	2	2	...	7
Infected Nonbacteremic (16)	0	1	0	13	4	18
Bacteremic (20)	0	0	0	7	13	20
Total (85)	25	28	2	27	17	99

*The sensitivity of the threshold value of 10^3 colony-forming units per ml (CFU/ml) to diagnose catheter-related infection is 37 (97.3%) of 38, and its specificity is 54 (88%) of 61.

†There are 99 bacterial isolates because 7 contaminated and 7 infected or colonized catheters had 2 bacterial species grow from each (28 isolates, of which 19 were contaminants, and were included in the group "contaminated").

(Courtesy of Brun-Buisson C, Abrouk F, Legrand P, et al: Arch Intern Med 147:873–877, May 1987.)

Quantitative tip culture was performed on 331 central venous catheters (Table 1). No growth was observed from 246 catheters, but 85 yielded colonies. Clinically, 42 catheters were classified as contaminated and 36 were classified as culture-related sepsis. Of these, 20 led to septicemia, 16 were classified as nonbacteremic culture-related sepsis, and 7 were classified as being colonized from a distant septic focus. The risk of infection increased with the duration of catheterization. The risk of contamination also increased with repeated catheterization, use of internal jugular insertion sites, or distant septic foci. Thirty-eight organisms were grown from the 36 infected catheter tips. *Staphylococcus aureus* accounted for 47% of the isolates and caused 65% of the culture-related sepsis (Table 2).

The QTC technique can accurately identify culture-related sepsis. Catheter tips that grew 10^3 colony-forming units per milliliter were associated with clinical infection (Table 3). This assay was 97.5% sensitive and 88% specific for CRS.

The Benefits of Isolator Cultures in the Management of Suspected Catheter Sepsis

Mosca R, Curtas S, Forbes B, Meguid MM (Univ Hosp, State Univ of New York Health Science Ctr, Syracuse)
Surgery 102:718–723, October 1987

When catheter-related sepsis was suspected in patients receiving total parenteral nutrition (TPN), the catheter was removed and the tip was cultured. This led to the unnecessary removal and replacement of many catheters. An alternate method of assessing catheter contamination was established using lysis centrifugation in an Isolator. An 8-month prospective study was undertaken in 138 patients given TPN with 160 catheters to determine the efficacy of this method.

Quantitative blood cultures were obtained both from a peripheral vein and through the catheter while the catheter remained in place. If the catheter culture produced 5 times as many colonies as the peripheral culture did, the catheter was considered the source of sepsis and was removed.

Of the 138 patients, 113 did not have sepsis. The Isolator culture method was used to analyze 26 catheters. The catheter was implicated as the source of sepsis by this method in 8 instances. The catheter was removed, and the patients became afebrile within 24 hours. In 18 cases there was little or no difference between the catheter and peripheral blood cultures. Although 9 of these catheters were removed, there was no clinical improvement. The other 9 catheters remained in situ, and another source of sepsis was identified and treated.

Using the Isolator method, when a catheter was considered contaminated its removal always led to patient improvement. When the catheter was not incriminated, its removal did not lead to improvement in the patient's clinical state. The use of the Isolator method allows determination of catheter-related sepsis in situ.

In Situ Management of Confirmed Central Venous Catheter-Related Bacteremia
Flynn PM, Shenep JL, Stokes DC, Barrett FF (St Jude Children's Research Hosp, Memphis; Univ of Tennessee; LeBonheur Children's Med Ctr, Memphis)
Pediatr Infect Dis J 6:729–734, August 1987

Most catheter-related bacteremia studies are based on the assumption that all bacteremic episodes in patients with central venous catheters are catheter-related. Criteria to diagnose catheter-related bacteremia were developed from analysis of simultaneous quantitative cultures of central venous and peripheral blood in animals infected experimentally. These criteria were then used to confirm catheter-related bacteremia in patients, and a standard management plan to eradicate bacteremia without removing the catheter was evaluated.

Thirty-one patients with suspected central venous catheter-related bacteremia were studied. Bacterial concentrations were significantly larger in the superior vena cava samples compared with femoral vein samples (Table 1). Quantitative and routine qualitative cultures of catheter blood were positive for bacterial growth in 20 of 32 episodes suspected of being catheter-related bacteremia. Only 6 of these episodes were accompanied by positive cultures of peripheral blood. Nineteen of the 20 patients with positive quantitative blood cultures were diagnosed with catheter-related bacteremia. Infecting organisms were isolated from 2 to 7 separate cul-

TABLE 1.—Simultaneous Blood Bacterial Concentrations in Central and Peripheral Veins in Septic Rabbits*

Blood Bacterial concentration (cfu/ml)		SVC/FV†
Superior vena cava	Femoral vein	
2.1×10^6	9.6×10^5	2.19
2.5×10^5	9.0×10^4	2.78
1.2×10^5	4.7×10^4	2.55
1.7×10^6	4.8×10^5	3.54
1.4×10^6	1.2×10^6	1.14
4.0×10^5	2.0×10^5	2.00
1.1×10^5	9.0×10^4	1.22
2.0×10^6	6.9×10^5	2.90
1.7×10^6	1.4×10^6	1.21
1.0×10^7	3.7×10^6	2.70
1.6×10^6	8.0×10^5	2.00

*The blood bacterial concentration was significantly higher in the SVC compared to the concentration in the FV as assessed by the Wilcoxon signed rank test ($P < .01$).
†SVC/FV, ratio of the absolute blood bacterial concentrations in the superior vena cava and femoral vein. The mean SVC/FV is 2.20 ± 0.78 (SD).
(Courtesy of Flynn PM, Shenep JL, Stokes DC, et al: Pediatr Infect Dis J 6:729–734, August 1987.)

tures (Table 2). Antibiotic therapy was given through the catheter—in situ therapy—to 17 patients to assess the feasibility of treating patients with true central venous catheter-related bacteremias without catheter removal. In 11 patients (65%) bacteremia was successfully eradicated, permitting 7 to retain their catheters for a median of 157 days.

These results validate the use of comparative quantitative blood cultures in diagnosing catheter-related bacteremia. In situ therapy was found to offer a rational alternative to catheter removal in patients with catheter-related bacteremia.

▶ Whereas improved management of central venous catheters and a heightened awareness of catheter-related sepsis have led to a decrease in the overall incidence of this complication, it continues to present clinicians with an important diagnostic and therapeutic problem. These 3 papers (Abstracts 9–4 to 9–6) address several of the important issues.

In Abstract 9–4, the authors have addressed the question of separating catheters that are the source of bactermia from those that are colonized. This follows from the time-honored practice of removing central venous catheters based on clinical suspicion of their relationship to bacteremia. A simple quantitative culture of the catheter tip confirmed that those catheters that were the source of bacteremia contained a greater number of organisms than colonized catheters that were not the source of bacteremia. A quantitative tip culture prepared by vortexing the distal 5-to-6-cm catheter segment in 1 ml of sterile water and then quantitatively plating it showed that 1,000 CFU/ml or more was 97.5% sensitive and 88% specific for the diagnosis of catheter-related sepsis.

TABLE 2.—Blood Culture Results, Therapy, and Outcome in 19 Episodes of Documented Catheter-Related Bacteremia*

Patient	Qualitative Culture		Quantitative Culture		Organism	Treatment	Outcome
	Catheter blood	Peripheral blood	Catheter blood (cfu/ml)	Peripheral blood (cfu/ml)			
1	+	NG	7.3×10^4	NG	CNS	Vancomycin	Cure
2	+	+	7.1×10^4	1.0×10^1	CNS	Vancomycin	Cure†
3	+	+	5.7×10^4	1.0×10^3	Staphylococcus aureus	Vancomycin	Cure†
4	+	NG	3.5×10^4	NG	Streptococcus faecalis	Ampicillin/gentamicin; vancomycin/tobramycin	Failure
5	+	NG	8.0×10^2	NG	Bacillus sp.		
	+	NG	3.0×10^2	NG	Klebsiella pneumoniae		
	+	NG	7.0×10^2	NG	Streptococcus faecalis	Ampicillin/tobramycin	Cure†
6	+	+	1.1×10^4	5.0×10^1	Staphylococcus aureus	Vancomycin	Failure‡
7	+	NG	1.4×10^5	NG	Escherichia coli	Ampicillin	Relapse§
8	+	+	1.7×10^5	1.0×10^2	CNS	Vancomycin	Cure‖
9	+	NG	2.0×10^2	NG	CNS	Vancomycin	Cure
10	+	NG	8.8×10^2	NG	Klebsiella pneumoniae	Cephalothin/gentamicin	Cure
11	+	NG	1.2×10^3	NG	Pseudomonas aeruginosa	Piperacillin/gentamicin	Cure
12	+	NG	3.0×10^3	NG	CNS	Vancomycin	Cure
13	+	NG	3.9×10^4	NG	CNS	Cefamandole	Failure¶
14	+	NG	9.0×10^2	NG	Klebsiella pneumoniae	Catheter removal	
15	+	NG	4.0×10^5	NG	Acinetobacter anitratus	Catheter removal	
16	+	NG	3.0×10^2	NG	Acinetobacter lwoffi		
	+	NG	3.0×10^2	NG	Pseudomonas pudita	Ticarcillin/amikacin	Failure**
17	+	+	1.3×10^5	3.0×10^1	Klebsiella pneumoniae	Cefotaxime/amikacin	Cure
18	+	NG	1.0×10^1	NG	Bacillus sp.	Vancomycin/amikacin/ticarcillin	Failure
19	+	NG	2.0×10^1	NG	Klebsiella pneumoniae	Cephalothin/amikacin	Cure

*CNS, coagulase-negative staphylococci; NG, no growth.
†Catheter removed because no longer needed.
‡Tunnel tract infection.
§Relapsed with ampicillin-resistant *Escherichia coli*.
‖Catheter removed as a result of malfunction.
¶Patient intolerant of vancomycin.
**Multiresistant organisms

(Courtesy of Flynn PM, Shenep JL, Stokes DC, et al: *Pediatr Infect Dis J* 6:729–734, August 1987.)

Abstract 9–5 adds an important new dimension to the management of suspected catheter sepsis. In this study, the authors performed quantitative isolator cultures from the central venous catheter and peripheral blood and left the catheters in place. They were uniformly able to distinguish catheters that were the source of sepsis by the finding of a central venous catheter colony count 5 times greater than the peripheral blood colony count. While only 26 catheters were evaluated by this isolator culture method, the uniformity of their results were impressive, and if these results can be confirmed in a larger trial, they would provide a cogent way to decide on the management of these catheters.

Abstract 9–6 goes 1 step further. In children with central venous catheters, these authors also addressed the separation of catheter-related bacteremia by quantitative cultures from the catheter and from a peripheral site. The finding of 5 times more CFU per milliliter in the catheter blood than in peripheral blood appeared to be an accurate predictor of catheter-related sepsis, which is in agreement with Abstract 9–5. It is noteworthy that isolator cultures were not required for the quantitative cultures used in this pediatric study. These authors left catheters that were the source of bacteremia in place, and in 11 of 17 patients, the catheter-related sepsis was successfully treated by antibiotics administered via the central venous catheter.

The 6 patients for whom in situ therapy failed included 1 who could not receive vancomycin for coagulase-negative staphylococci, 2 with multiresistant gram-negative organisms, 2 with *Bacillus* species infection, and 1 with a tunnel tract infection due to *Staphylococcus aureus*. The fact that 4 of the 6 patients with gram-negative catheter-related sepsis were successfully treated with in situ management of the catheter is particularly interesting since many pediatric oncologists have previously claimed to routinely sterilize gram-positive and even candidal infections with antibiotics infused through the catheter but have not done as well with gram-negative infections.

Overall, I think these studies provide adequate documentation that quantitative cultures are useful in determining whether the central venous catheter is the source of bacteremia and provide some confidence that, at least in pediatric patients, in situ management is possible. Whether a similar approach in adults also applies awaits further study.—M.S. Klempner, M.D.

Infections Associated With Transhepatic Biliary Drainage Devices
Szabo S, Mendelson MH, Mitty HA, Bruckner HW, Hirschman SZ (Mount Sinai Med Ctr, New York)
Am J Med 82:921–926, May 1987

Infection now seems to be a major problem with percutaneous biliary drainage. Thirty-eight patients having this procedure were reviewed for infectious complications. A pigtail catheter was used in 11 patients, a Ring catheter/feeding tube in 13, and a Carey-Coons endoprosthesis in 15. All patients but 1 had neoplastic disease. Eleven patients had recently been operated on. Most patients received antibiotics before insertion or manipulation of the biliary device.

Sixteen of the 38 patients had 19 infectious events (Table 1), for a rate

TABLE 1.—Type and Distribution of Biliary Devices

Biliary Device	Total (n = 39)	Number of Devices Infected (n = 17)	Noninfected (n = 22)
Pigtail catheter	11	4	7
Ring catheter/ feeding tube	13	7	6
Endoprosthesis	15	6	9

(Courtesy of Szabo S, Mendelson MH, Mitty HA, et al: Am J Med 82:921–926, May 1987.)

of 0.5 infections per patient. Ten episodes of bacteremia and 8 of cholangitis occurred. The organisms most frequently isolated were *Escherichia coli, Pseudomonas aeruginosa, Klebsiella pneumoniae,* and *Streptococcus fecalis* (Table 2). Cancer of the gallbladder and biliary tree was more frequent in infected than in uninfected patients. Recent cancer surgery also was more frequent in the infected group. The occurrence of infection could not be related to the use of antibiotic prophylaxis.

Infectious complications frequently occur in patients having percutaneous transhepatic biliary drainage and may be a significant cause of morbidity in these patients. Patients with malignancy of the gallbladder or biliary tract and those recently operated on are at the greatest risk.

TABLE 2.—Organisms Isolated From Infected Blood and Bile

Organism	Number of Isolates Blood	Bile
Gram-positive bacteria		
Streptococcus faecium	2	2
Streptococcus faecalis		3
Staphylococcus epidermidis		1
Diphtheroids		1
Gram-negative bacteria		
Escherichia coli	3	1
Pseudomonas aeruginosa	3	3
Proteus mirabilis		1
Klebsiella oxytoca	1	2
Klebsiella pneumoniae		3
Serratia marcescens		1
Hafnia alvei	1	1
Enterobacter cloacae		2
Fungi		
Candida albicans		2
Candida tropicalis		2

(Courtesy of Szabo S, Mendelson MH, Mitty HA, et al: Am J Med 82:921–926, May 1987.

Nosocomial Pneumonia in Intubated Patients Given Sucralfate as Compared With Antacids or Histamine Type 2 Blockers: The Role of Gastric Colonization

Driks MR, Craven DE, Celli BR, Manning M, Burke RA, Garvin GM, Kunches LM, Farber HW, Wedel SA, McCabe WR (Boston Univ School of Medicine; Boston City Hosp)
N Engl J Med 317:1376–1382, Nov 26, 1987   9–8

Hospital-acquired pneumonia often results from gram-negative bacilli that are aspirated from the oropharynx. Retrograde pharyngeal colonization by gastric organisms may contribute to its pathogenesis, particularly when the gastric pH is high. Sixty-one of 130 patients ventilated in an intensive care unit received sucralfate, which does not raise the gastric pH, to prevent stress ulceration. The other 69 patients received antacids, histamine type 2 (H2) blockers, or both.

No bleeding occurred in 74% of sucralfate-treated patients and in 62% of those treated with antacid or H2 blockers. Patients given sucralfate more often had a gastric aspirate with a pH of 4 or below, and they had lower concentrations of gram-negative bacilli in gastric and tracheal aspirates and pharyngeal swabs (Fig 9–1). Pneumonia developed in 11.5% of the sucralfate group and 23.2% of the antacid-H2 group. All patients with colonization had a gastric pH

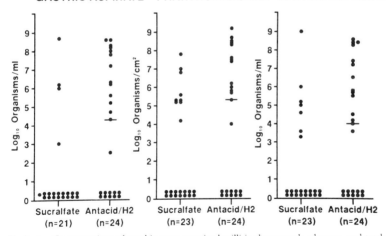

Fig 9–1.—Concentrations of aerobic-gram-negative bacilli in the stomach, pharynx, and trachea of patients receiving sucralfate and patients receiving antacids or histamine type 2 blockers (H2) for prophylaxis against stress-ulcer hemorrhage. Each symbol represents the highest level of colonization in 1 patient during the first 5 days after randomization. The line in each group of symbols represents the median for the antacid-H2 group; the median was 0 for values for all 3 sites in the sucralfate group. No gastric aspirate could be obtained from 2 of the 23 patients in the sucralfate group. Colonization was significantly higher at all 3 sites in patients in the antacid-H2 group than in the sucralfate group ($P <.05$, Wilcoxon rank-sum test, adjusted for ties). (Courtesy of Driks MR, Craven DE, Celli Br, et al: N Engl J Med 317:1376–1382, Nov 26, 1987.)

TABLE 1.—Colonization on Culture of Gastric Aspirates, Pharyngeal Swabs, and Tracheal Aspirates from 47 Study Patients

Organism	Gastric Aspirate		Pharyngeal Swab		Tracheal Aspirate	
	SUCRALFATE (N = 21)	ANTACID–H2 (N = 24)	SUCRALFATE (N = 23)	ANTACID–H2 (N = 24)	SUCRALFATE (N = 23)	ANTACID–H2 (N = 24)
	no. colonized (percent)		no. colonized (percent)		no. colonized (percent)	
Gram-negative bacilli	4 (19.0)	14 (58.3)*	9 (39.1)	14 (58.3)*	7 (30.4)	14 (58.3)*
Enterobacteriaceae†‡	6	18	9	17	5	10
Nonfermenting organisms‡§	0	7	2	7	2	13
Gram-positive cocci	3 (14.3)	13 (54.2)	14 (60.9)	10 (41.7)	9 (39.1)	10 (41.7)
Staphylococcus aureus‡	0§	3	7	3	8	3
Coagulase-negative staphylococci‡	3	9	8	7	2	7
Group D streptococci‡	0	4	2	3	1	2
Candida species	7 (33.3)	10 (41.7)	4 (17.4)	7 (29.2)	2 (8.7)	4 (16.6)
No growth	5 (23.8)	1 (4.2)	0	0	1 (4.3)	3 (12.5)

*Significantly more patients in the antacid-H2 group had colonization with gram-negative bacilli ($P < .05$).
†Includes *Escherichia coli*, *Klebsiella* species, *Enterobacter* species, *Proteus* species, *Morganella morganii*, and *Citrobacter freundii*.
‡Number of isolates from colonized patients.
§Includes *Pseudomonas aeruginosa*, other *Pseudomonas* species, and *Acinetobacter* species.
(Courtesy of Driks MR, Craven DE, Celli BR, et al: N Engl J Med 317:1376–1382, Nov 26, 1987.)

greater than 4 and lower numbers of species of gram-negative bacilli than patients in the antacid-H2 group (Table 1). Mortality was 1.6 times higher in the antacid-H2 group than in the sucralfate group (Table 2).

Drugs that elevate the gastric pH may raise the risk of nosocomial pneumonia in mechanically ventilated patients, through promoting gastric colonization by gram-negative bacilli. It may therefore be best to use an agent that preserves the gastric acid barrier against bacterial overgrowth to prevent stress ulceration.

TABLE 2.—Rates of Pneumonia and Mortality Among Patients in the Intensive Care Unit

	Sucralfate Group (N = 61)	Antacid–H2 Group (N = 69)	Relative Risk	95% Confidence Interval	P Value
	patients affected/patients studied (%)				
Pneumonia					
All patients	7/61 (11.5)*	16/69 (23.2)	2.02	0.89–4.58	0.11
Excluding crossovers	5/55 (9.1)	16/69 (23.2)	2.55	1.00–6.53	0.05
Mortality					
All patients	18/61 (29.5)	32/69 (46.4)	1.57	0.99–2.50	0.07
Excluding crossovers	13/55 (23.6)	32/69 (46.4)	1.97	1.15–3.36	<0.05

*Includes 2 patients in whom pneumonia developed 3 and 8 days after their treatment was switched to antacids.
(Courtesy of Driks MR, Craven DE, Celli BR, et al: N Engl J Med 317:1376–1382, Nov 26, 1987.)

Prevention of Nosocomial Respiratory Syncytial Virus Infections Through Compliance With Glove and Gown Isolation Precautions

Leclair JM, Freeman J, Sullivan BF, Crowley CM, Goldmann DA (Children's Hosp, Boston; Brigham Young and Women's Hosp, Boston; West Roxbury VA Hosp, Boston; Harvard Med School)
N Engl J Med 317:329–334, Aug 6, 1987

Respiratory syncytial virus (RSV) is recognized as the leading cause of nosocomial respiratory virus infection in infants. A study was done to determine whether increased compliance with a policy of glove-and-gown isolation precautions could reduce the high rate of RSV infection on a ward for infants and toddlers.

The longitudinal intervention trial was conducted during 3 RSV seasons, from 1982 to 1985. An intervention to increase compliance was introduced halfway through the second season. The risk of acquiring the nosocomial infection was adjusted for the intensity of nosocomial exposure to the virus by assigning each study week to 1 of 5 strata, defined by the proportion of hospital days on which virus was shed by children on the ward.

Overall, during 7,547 days at risk, 37 patients acquired nosocomial RSV infections. The adjusted relative risk, comparing the infection rate during the time before intervention, when compliance with isolation precautions was observed in 38.5% of patient contacts, with the infection rate in the postintervention period, when compliance more than doubled, was 2.9 (table). The rates of nosocomial RSV infection tended to increase linearly with increasing levels of exposure to patients shedding virus.

Number and Incidence Density of Nosocomial RSV Infections and Number of Patient-Days at Risk Before and After the Intervention With Respect to Compliance With Glove and Gown Precautions, Stratified According to the Level of Exposure to Shed RSV*

% Days RSV Was Shed	Before Intervention		After Intervention	
	NO. INFECTIONS/ NO. DAYS	INCIDENCE DENSITY/ 1000 DAYS	NO. INFECTIONS/ NO. DAYS	INCIDENCE DENSITY/ 1000 DAYS
0	0/1631	0.0	0/811	0.0
1.1–9.9	9/1364	6.6	2/1107	1.8
10.0–19.9	4/580	6.9	5/837	6.0
20.0–29.9	10/365	27.4	3/532	5.6
≥30.0	3/104	28.8	1/216	4.6
Crude overall	26/4044	6.4	11/3503	3.1

*The summary adjusted relative risk of nosocomial RSV infection before intervention as compared with that after intervention was 2.9 (95% confidence interval, 1.5 to 5.7). The summary adjusted risk difference between the 2 periods was 2.7 per 1,000 days (95% confidence interval, 1.0 to 4.3 per 1,000 days).

(Courtesy of Leclair JM, Freeman J, Sullivan BF, et al: N Engl J Med 317:329–334, Aug 6, 1987.)

Nevertheless, the rise in infection rate with increasing exposure was less than one fourth as great in the period after the intervention as in the period before. Glove-and-gown precautions can substantially reduce the nosocomial transmission of RSV, especially with increasing exposure to patients shedding the virus.

▶ This study and another recently published one (Snydman DR et al: *Infect Control Hosp Epidemiol* 9:105–108, 1988) confirm that the use of gown-and-glove precautions reduce the spread of nosocomial RSV. We also employed masks to prevent autoinoculation of staff members, but this measure has been considered somewhat more controversial.—D.R. Snydman, M.D.

Nosocomial Dermatitis and Pruritus Caused by Pigeon Mite Infestation
Regan AM, Metersky ML, Craven DE (Boston Univ School of Medicine, Boston City Hosp)
Arch Intern Med 147:2185–2187, December 1987

Pigeons create many public health problems in urban areas, but reports of pigeon mite infestation and dermatitis in humans are uncommon and not widely appreciated. Past outbreaks have been caused by the avian

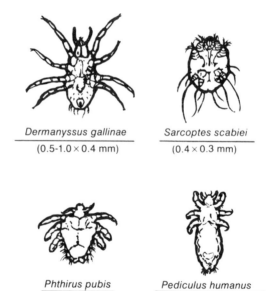

Fig 9–2.—Schematic diagrams demonstrating differences in appearance and size of avian mite *Dermanyssus gallinae* de Geer (ventral view), human mite *Sarcoptes scabiei* (ventral view), crab louse *Phthirus pubis* (dorsal view), and body louse *Pediculus humanus corporis* (dorsal view). (Courtesy of Regan AM, Metersky ML, Craven DE: *Arch Intern Med* 147:2185–2187, December 1987.)

mite *Dermanyssus gallinae*. An outbreak of pigeon mite infestation involving patients and personnel on a medical ward in a municipal hospital was reported.

Two patients, 2 nurses, and 1 physician were affected. The index patient was a 38-year-old man hospitalized for hand cellulitis and consolidation chemotherapy for acute myelocytic leukemia. He developed a diffuse, pruritic erythematous maculopapular rash on his trunk and extremities. The nonburrowing, blood-sucking avian mite *D. gallinae* was found on the patient and his bedding (Fig 9–2). Another patient began to complain of scalp pruritus, and the mites were found on her pillow and bed linen. Mite infestation was also present on the intern and the 2 nurses caring for these patients.

The source of the mites was found to be pigeons roosting on the air conditioners and near the doors connecting the patients' rooms to a sun porch. Control measures included removal of a wooden panel on the sun porch that acted as a shelter for pigeons in inclement weather, cleaning and screening of the porches, and sealing of the cracks around air conditioners and doors. It was hypothesized that condensate from the air conditioners was an important water source for the pigeons. After the control measures were implemented, the mite problem abated.

This outbreak illustrates an unusual cause of nosocomial pruritic dermatitis that could have been misdiagnosed as scabies or pediculosis. Health care personnel working in urban centers should be aware that pigeon mites can cause pruritic dermatitis that may be chronic, recurrent, or unresponsive to ectoparasiticides.

▶ Having grown up in New York City, I am always on the lookout for reasons to support my dislike of dogs (especially their indiscriminate droppings) and pigeons (any and all reasons are OK by me). Here's one more against the old bird: a *blood-sucking* mite infestation of humans with a pigeon parasite that was directly related to pigeon roosts outside the hospital.—G.T. Keusch, M.D.

Nosocomial Infection by Gentamicin-Resistant *Streptococcus faecalis*: An Epidemiologic Study
Zervos MJ, Kauffman CA, Therasse PM, Bergman AG, Mikesell TS, Schaberg DR (Univ of Michigan; Ann Arbor VA Med Ctr, Ann Arbor, Mich)
Ann Intern Med 106:687–691, May 1987

Many enterococci isolated from clinical specimens are resistant to gentamicin, and there is evidence that patient-to-patient transmission of these strains may occur. A prospective study was carried out in 100 patients hospitalized on surgical and thoracic intensive care units and a general medical floor at a VA center. The patients, 98 men and 2 women, had a mean age of 61 years.

Colonies of enterococci with high-level gentamicin resistance were found in 43 cases. Usually these were isolated from rectal and perineal samples. In 33 of the 43 patients, the initial cultures yielded gentamicin-resistant enterococci; in 10 of the 43 patients, resistant enterococci were first cultured after the patients were admitted to the study units. All 33 patients whose initial cultures were positive had been hospitalized for longer than 72 hours before admission to the intensive care unit (ICU) or medical floor. Eight of the 17 patients on the medical floor had been transferred from a nursing home unit. Seven patients with initial colonies of resistant enterococci in the rectal or perineal region developed urinary tract or wound infection. Three deaths were related to enterococcal infection. All isolates were identified as *Streptococcus faecalis*.

Gentamicin-resistant enterococci were isolated from hand swabs in 4 of 28 personnel and were found on 30% of the environmental surfaces examined, most often in the surgical ICU. Patients whose cultures were positive after admission to intensive care were in adjacent beds and were associated by time of hospitalization. However, patients with resistant strains were not clustered on the medical floor.

Streptococcus faecalis is among those pathogens that are spread between hospital patients. It therefore is necessary to find effective means of preventing the spread of gentamicin-resistant strains among patients and hospitals.

▶ The enterococcus appears to be making yet another comeback. The increasing use of the cephalosporins, which have little activity against the enterococcus, has probably contributed to the emergence or reemergence of the enterococcus as a pathogen (see Dougherty SH, Flohr AB, Simmons RL: Breakthrough enterococcal septicemia in surgical patients: 19 cases and a review of the literature. *Arch Surg* 118:232–238, 1983). There has also been an upsurge of interest in the enterococcus as a pathogen in gynecologic infections. This study adds a new wrinkle by suggesting that aminoglycoside-resistant strains may be spread from patient to patient within the hospital.—M.J. Barza, M.D.

10 Pediatric Infections

Perinatal Infections

Coagulase-Negative Staphylococcal Bacteremia in the Changing Neonatal Intensive Care Unit Population: Is There an Epidemic?
Freeman J, Platt R, Sidebottom DG, Leclair JM, Epstein MF, Goldmann DA (Brigham and Women's Hosp, Brockton/West Roxbury VA Hosp, Children's Hosp, Boston)
JAMA 258:2548–2552, Nov 13, 1987   10–1

Beginning in 1981 there was a change in the organisms isolated from infant blood cultures in neonatal intensive care units (NICUs) in that coagulase-negative staphylococci were being recovered much more frequently. To determine whether this increased incidence is real, the records from the NICU at Children's Hospital, Boston, were investigated in 1975 and 1982.

The number of blood cultures was similar in these 2 years. The number of cultures reported to be positive for coagulase-negative staphylococci was similar in these 2 years. However, in 1982 there was a significant increase in probability that a positive blood culture would be interpreted as bacteremia rather than contamination. From 1975 to 1982 there was a 62.3% increase in occupancy of the NICU by very-low-birth-weight infants. In both years, positive cultures of blood from these infants were 3.8 times as likely to be considered clinically significant. The increase in occupancy of the NICU by very-low-birth-weight infants and the increased likelihood that positive cultures of blood from these infants will be interpreted as bacteremia may explain the reported increase in nosocomial coagulase-negative staphylococcal bacteremia in NICUs.

Buffy Coat Transfusions in Neutropenic Neonates With Presumed Sepsis: A Prospective, Randomized Trial
Baley JE, Stork EK, Warkentin PI, Shurin SB (Rainbow Babies and Childrens Hosp, Cleveland; Case Western Reserve Univ)
Pediatrics 80:712–720, Nov 5, 1987   10–2

Neonatal sepsis with neutropenia is associated with high mortality. To determine whether granulocyte transfusions are effective in these infants, 25 neutropenic, septic infants matched for birth weight were prospectively randomized to receive either buffy coat transfusion or no transfusion. Transfusions were given daily until the neutrophil count increased to greater than $1,500/\mu l$.

Only 5 infants with necrotizing enterocolitis required more than 1 transfusion. A circulating immature-to-total-neutrophil ratio (I:T) of greater than 0.80 was not predictive of a neutrophil storage pool of less than 7% in these infants. Neither I:T less than 0.80 nor a neutrophil storage pool of greater than 7% was predictive of survival. Granulocyte transfusions did not improve survival of the group as a whole, of those with positive cultures, of those with I:T ratios ≥ 0.80, or of those with a neutrophil storage pool ≤ 7%.

Granulocyte transfusion, administered as a buffy coat preparation, was without benefit to critically ill neutropenic neonates. The efficacy of buffy coat transfusions remains questionable. Additional studies should be performed prior to recommendation for clinical use.

Respiratory Tract

Pneumonia in Pediatric Outpatients: Cause and Clinical Manifestations
Turner RB, Lande AE, Chase P, Hilton N, Weinberg D (Univ of Utah School of Medicine; Children's Hosp Med Ctr of Northern California, Oakland)
J Pediatr 111:194–200, August 1987   10–3

In a previous study, only 13% of children with a diagnosis of bacterial pneumonia had positive blood cultures, as confirmed by lung puncture. However, lung puncture is far too invasive for routine use, and although antigen detection in sputum, serum, and urine of patients with bacterial pneumonia is more sensitive than blood cultures, its absolute sensitivity is unknown. The cause and clinical manifestations of radiographically confirmed pneumonia were examined in 98 pediatric outpatients, 61% of whom were younger than 2 years. Antigen detection was used for diagnosing bacterial infection, and virus isolation, antigen detection, and serologic studies were used to diagnose viral infection. Urine and viral cul-

Etiologic Diagnoses in 98 Children With Pneumonia		
	n	%
Viral infection	38	39
Respiratory syncytial virus	27	28
Parainfluenza	5	5
Rhinovirus	2	2
Influenza	2	2
Enterovirus	2	2
Adenovirus	1	1
Coronavirus 229E	1	1
Bacterial infection	19	19
Pneumococcus	17	17
Haemophilus influenzae	2	2
No etiologic diagnosis	51	52

(Courtesy of Turner RB, Lande AE, Chase P, et al: *J Pediatr* 111:194–200, August 1987.)

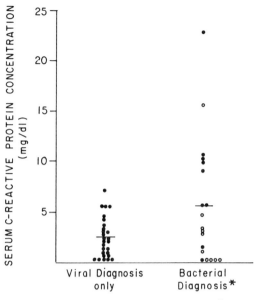

Fig 10–1.—Serum CRP level in patients with viral pneumonia alone and in patients with bacterial pneumonia either alone or associated with viral infection. (Courtesy of Turner RB, Lande AE, Chase P, et al: *J Pediatr* 111:194–200, August 1987.)

ture specimens were obtained from all patients, blood cultures were done for 75 (77%), and paired sera were obtained from 50 (51%) children.

Pneumonia was caused by viral infection in 38 children (39%) and by bacterial infection in 19 (19%) (table). Of the latter 19 patients, 10 (53%) had concurrent viral infection. No etiologic diagnosis was established for the other 51 (52%) patients. Of 38 viral infections, 25 (66%) were diagnosed by virus isolation or antigen detection only, 5 (13%) by serologic study only, and 8 (21%) by both serologic study and either virus isolation or antigen detection. Twenty-seven (71%) of 38 viral infections were caused by respiratory syncytial virus.

Neither clinical, laboratory, nor radiographic findings were indicative of viral or bacterial infection. Measurement of C-reative protein (CRP) levels in 97 (99%) patients showed that 15 (56%) of 27 with viral infection and 12 (63%) of 19 with bacterial infection had positive CRP reactions, but the difference between the 2 groups was not statistically significant (Fig 10–1). Bacterial pneumonia may be more common in pediatric outpatients than previously reported. It appears to be indistinguishable from viral pneumonia on clinical, laboratory, and radiographic parameters.

▶ The key clinical issues are whether to treat or not, and with what. In this study, half the patients with radiographically documented pneumonia were etiologically undiagnosed. Of the remainder, 80% were due to a virus, respiratory syncytial virus being the most common; approximately 10% had concomitant bacterial pneumonia; and another 10% had only bacterial pneumonia (Streptococcus pneumoniae was the isolate in 17 of 19 cases). Unfortunately, no test clearly distinguished those needing antibiotics from those who did not, except perhaps the presence of high CRP levels (<5 mg/dl). The authors conclude that this decision must rest on "overall assessment of the patient." This is not a very clear guideline and is why almost all of these children will be treated. We still need a simple, or at least a quick, and hopefully cheap test for this differential.— G.T. Keusch, M.D.

Role of *Chlamydia trachomatis* and *Mycoplasma pneumoniae* in Acute Pharyngitis in Children

Gerber MA, Randolph MF, Chanatry J, Mayo DR, Schachter J, Tilton RC (Univ of Connecticut, School of Medicine; State Dept of Health Services, Hartford, Conn; Univ of California Med Ctr, San Francisco)
Diagn Microbiol Infect Dis 6:263–265, March 1987   10–4

A recent study suggested that *Chlamydia trachomatis* and *Mycoplasma pneumoniae* may be common causes of acute pharyngitis in adults. To evaluate the contribution of infection by these same species in children, throat swabs were examined from 236 children, aged 2–24 years.

Blood agar plates were negative for group A β-hemolytic streptococci in 48 patients. Of these patients, 42 were examined microbiologically and serologically for evidence of *C. trachomatis* infection. None was positive for *C. trachomatis* infection. Of the 48 patients, 43 were examined serologically for *Mycoplasma* infection. Two patients were observed to have a fourfold increase in complement-fixing antibodies to *M. pneumoniae*. Neither *C. trachomatis* nor *M. pneumoniae* appears to be a common cause of acute pharyngitis in children.

▶ Several groups, including this one, have been unable to confirm the finding by Komaroff et al. (1983) that *C. trachomatis* was a fairly common cause of acute pharyngitis. With respect to *M. pneumoniae,* also reported to be a fairly common cause of acute pharyngitis by Komaroff et al., the prevalence in various studies has depended upon the age of the patients, being lowest among young children and highest among college students.— M. J. Barza, M.D.

IgG Subclass Deficiency in Children With IgA Deficiency Presenting With Recurrent or Severe Respiratory Infections

Beard LJ, Ferrante A, Oxelius V-A, Maxwell GM (Univ of Adelaide, Adelaide Children's Hosp, Australia; Univ Hosp, Lund, Sweden)
Pediatr Res 20:937–942, October 1987   10–5

Selective IgA deficiency is not uncommon. To determine whether children with selective IgA deficiency also have IgG subclass deficiencies, 22

Summary of Clinical and Immunologic Presentations*

Patient (P)	Clinical problems	Immunological abnormalities
1	URTIS, salmonella infection, UTI	↓IgG4, ↓neutrophil bactericidal activity
2	LRTIS	↓↓IgA, ↓IgG4
3	LRTIS (shunted hydrocephalus)	↓↓IgA, ↓IgG2, ↓IgG4
4	LRTIS	↓IgG1, ↓IgG4
5	LRTI, salmonella and monilia infections	↓IgG4, ↓chemotaxis
6	LRTIS, URTIS, asthma	↓IgG4, ↓C$_4$
7	URTIS, PUO	↓↓IgA, ↓IgG4
8	LRTIS, URTIS	↑IgE
9	URTIS	↓IgG1
10	URTIS	↓C$_4$, IgG2 level close to lower limit
11	URTIS, LRTIS, pneumococcal meningitis	↓IgG1, ↓IgG4, ↑IgE
12	LRTIS, URTIS	↓IgG1, ↓chemotaxis
13	URTIS, herpes simplex	↓↓IgA
14	LRTIS, URTIS	↓IgG4
15	URTIS, asthma	↓IgG1
16	URTIS	↓↓IgA
17	LRTIS, URTIS, haemophilus meningitis	↓IgG2, ↓chemotaxis
18	LRTIS, URTIS, hay fever	↓IgG1, ↓IgG2, ↑IgE, ↓bactericidal activity ↓C$_4$
19	LRTIS (bronchiectasis), URTIS	↓↓IgA, ↑IgE
20	URTIS, "infectious mononucleosis," UTI	↓IgG2, ↓IgG3
21	LRTIS, URTIS	↓↓IgA
22	URTIS, asthma, herpes zoster	↓↓IgA, ↑IgE

*URTIS, upper respiratory tract infections; UTI, urinary tract infection; LRTIS, lower respiratory tract infections; ↓, decreased; ↑, increased; ↓ IgG4 indicates an IgG$_4$ level of less than 1 mg/dl; ↓↓ IgA indicates a level of no more than 6 mg/dl.

(Courtesy of Beard LJ, Ferrante A, Oxelius V-A, et al: *Pediatr Res* 20:937–942, October 1987.)

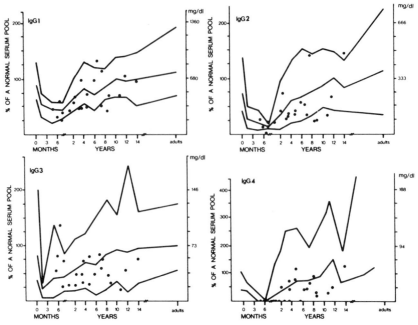

Fig 10-2.—Serum IgG subclass levels in patients with recurrent or severe respiratory infections, or both. *Solid lines* represent mean and normal range for age for IgG_1, IgG_2, and IgG_3, and mean plus upper limit of range for IgG_4. *Circles* represent serum levels in patients, and *semicircles* represent levels that were less than 1 mg/dl. (Courtesy of Beard LJ, Ferrante A, Oxelius V-A, et al: *Pediatr Res* 20:937–942, October 1987.)

children aged from infancy to about 14 years with selective IgA deficiency and severe respiratory infections were examined.

Most had IgG subclass levels below the mean for their age. Nine children had definite IgG subclass deficiency, and 2 had deficiencies in more than one IgG subclass (table). The major deficiency was in subclass IgG_1 (Fig 10–2). The patients with the lowest level of IgA did not have IgG subclass deficiencies. The IgG subclass deficiencies were common among those with IgA levels that were approximately 2 SD below the age-specific mean; 9 of these children had total IgG levels that were 2 SD below the age-specific mean. Six children had IgG subclass deficiency.

In patients with selective IgA deficiency and histories of recurrent or severe respiratory tract infections, those with the lowest levels of IgA did not have IgG subclass deficiencies, whereas those with IgA levels approximately 2 SD below the age-specific mean often had IgG subclass deficiencies. This IgG deficit may be involved in an increased incidence of infection. Immunoglobin prophylaxis may avoid the development of infection in these children.

▶ I found this report to be in marked contrast to other reports detailing recurrent respiratory infections in patients with "selective" IgA or IgG subclass deficiency. For example, most of the patients with IgG subclass deficiency had total IgG levels that were nearly 2 SD below the historical controls. In a previous report (Umetsu DT et al: *N Engl J Med* 313:1247–1251, 1985; see the 1987 YEAR BOOK, pp 225–227), only 3 of 20 IgG subclass-deficient patients were close to the lower limit of normal for total IgG and many were above the mean. The most common IgG subclass deficiency in this cohort was IgG_1, whereas IgG_2 and IgG_3 were deficient in the previous report and none of the patients had IgG_1 subclass deficiency.

Because antipolysaccharide antibodies are usually of the IgG_2 subclass, recurrent infections with encapsulated respiratory pathogens is easier to understand in patients deficient in this subclass. A more detailed description of the frequency and nature of the recurrent infections might have clarified this point. Because IgA deficiency is relatively common (1 in about 500–700 people in the general population and even more common among atopic patients attending allergy clinics) and because most of these people do not have recurrent infections, I would be reluctant to support the authors' suggestion that immunoglobulin prophylaxis be given to patients with IgG/A deficiency associated with the degree of low IgG subclasses demonstrated in their patients.—M.S. Klempner, M.D.

Central Nervous System

Difference Between Herpes Simplex Virus Type I and Type 2 Neonatal Encephalitis in Neurological Outcome
Corey L, Whitley RJ, Stone EF, Mohan K (Univ of Washington; Children's Hosp and Med Ctr, Seattle; Univ of Alabama in Birmingham)
Lancet 1:1–4, January 2–9, 1988   10–6

In a long-term study of patients with neonatal herpes simplex virus (HSV) infections treated with antiviral chemotherapy, patients with HSV-1 encephalitis fared much better neurologically than those with HSV-2 encephalitis. Twenty-four infants consecutively treated with acyclovir or vidarabine for neonatal HSV encephalitis were followed for 19.5 months on average (range, 6–35) to assess neurologic and developmental outcome. Nine patients had HSV-1 and 15 had HSV-2 encephalitis.

Infants with HSV-2 encephalitis presented with a higher frequency of lethargy and seizures, a greater degree of cerebrospinal fluid (CSF) pleocytosis, CSF protein elevations, and a higher frequency of structural CNS damage on computerized tomography than patients with HSV-1 encephalitis. One patient with HSV-2 infection died of the disease. At follow-up, all patients with HSV-1 encephalitis were normal neurologically and developmentally compared with 4 of the 14 (23%) surviving HSV-2 infected infants. Half the infants with HSV-2 encephalitis became microcephalic, 57% had persistent seizure disorders, 64% had ophthalmologic defects, 64% had cerebral palsy, and 57% had mental retardation.

Long-term prognosis is excellent for infants with neonatal HSV-1 encephalitis treated early with systemic antiviral chemotherapy. However, neurologic outcome with HSV-2 encephalitis is still poor.

Evaluation of Routine Lumbar Punctures in Newborn Infants With Respiratory Distress Syndrome

Eldadah M, Frenkel LD, Hiatt IM, Hegyi T (Univ of Medicine/Dentistry of New Jersey–Robert Wood Johnson Med School; St Peter's Med Ctr, New Brunswick, NJ)
Pediatr Infect Dis J 6:243–245, March 1987

It is often difficult to detect bacterial sepsis in the premature neonate because clinical features are variable and frequently nonspecific. Some infected infants resemble those with respiratory distress syndrome clinically. Cerebrospinal fluid (CSF) examination was assessed in a series of 238 consecutive infants presenting in the first 24 hours of life with clinical signs of respiratory distress syndrome. There were 38 infants weighing less than 1,000 gm in the series.

Blood cultures were positive in 17 infants and in 14 of the 203 who also had lumbar puncture (table). None of the CSF cultures was positive. Cerebrospinal fluid protein and glucose concentrations did not differ significantly between the septic and nonseptic infants. Neonatal infection was associated with low gestational age, low birth weight, prolonged rupture of membranes, thrombocytopenia, and leukopenia. Four infants with sepsis died, 3 from streptococcal infection.

Routine lumbar puncture for CSF culture is not indicated for neonates with signs of respiratory distress syndrome. The study may be reserved for infants having risk factors for CNS infection, such as hypothermia, poor feeding, or clinical features such as obtundation or seizures. Lumbar puncture also is appropriate if blood cultures are positive.

Clinical Characteristics of Infants With Positive Blood Cultures

Infant	Birth Weight (g)	Gestational Age (Weeks)	Apgar Score (at 1 Min)	Type of Respiratory Support	Blood Culture
1	2075	36	9	O	Staphylococcus epidermidis
2*	1165	28	1	V	Streptococcus
3	1505	27	4	V	Viridans streptococcus
4	660	25	1	V	GBS†
5*	870	26	3	V	GBS
6	3636	40	8	N	GBS
7	4640	40	4	O	GBS
8	1760	32	9	V	Bacillus subtilis
9	730	25	3	V	Haemophilus influenzae
10	980	32	4	V	Haemophilus influenzae
11	1400	32	3	V	Haemophilus influenzae
12	1535	32	2	V	S. capitis
13*	680	23	1	V	Diphtheroids†
14	1555	32	9	V	Staphylococcus epidermidis
15	2030	34	7	V	Staphylococcus epidermidis
16	1610	30	4	N	Staphylococcus epidermidis
17*	460	23	1	V	GBS†

*Died.
†CSF culture not done. V, ventilator; O, oxyhood; N, none; GBS, Group B Streptococcus.
(Courtesy of Eldadah M, Frenkel LD, Hiatt IM, et al: Pediatr Infect Dis J 6:243–245, March 1987.)

▶ Considering some of the histories I have obtained, I have always been secretly jealous of our colleagues treating pediatric infectious diseases, who often do without any history at all. Since signs of infection in newborns are often minimal, aggressive diagnosis and treatment of suspected sepsis is the rule. Blood cultures and lumbar puncture are usually included. This paper suggests that lumbar puncture doesn't add much and is not worth the pain or risk in the newborn with acute respiratory distress syndrome, since it adds little. It is good to see folklore explored and the risks and benefits defined for things we have come to do routinely.—G.T. Keusch, M.D.

Miscellaneous Topics

Invasive Bacterial Disease in Childhood: Efficacy of Oral Antibiotic Therapy Following Short Course Parenteral Therapy in Non-Central Nervous System Infections

Bradley JS, Ching DK, Hart CL (Oregon Children's Med Ctr, Portland)
Pediatr Infect Dis J 6:821–825, September 1987   10–8

The duration of parenteral therapy for common bacterial infections in children varies widely. To assess the efficacy of the current standard practice by private pediatricians in Portland, hospital records for 1981–1984 were reviewed for information on the treatment of children older than 6 months with noncentral nervous system disease due to *Haemophilus influenzae* type b, *Streptococcus pneumoniae*, *Neisseria meningitidis*, or group A *Streptococcus*.

The diagnoses were 21 cases of cellulitis, 17 cases of unfocused bacteremia, 13 cases of epiglottitis, 7 cases of pneumonia, and 4 other cases. The duration of fever was 0.5–21 days. The type of therapy used is listed in Table 1. The average duration of parenteral therapy was 2.9 days and that of oral therapy was 9.5 days (Table 2). There were no indications of inadequate therapy.

This review suggests that, for private practice patients where access to medical care and compliance are good, parenteral therapy for noncentral nervous system bacterial disease needs to be continued only until the child is without fever for 24–48 hours. Outpatient oral therapy can be used to complete the antibiotic course.

▶ We still do not know the optimal duration of therapy for most infections, now 4 decades after penicillin first became widely available. We also don't know how long we should give parenteral antibiotics to minimize hospital stay without sacrificing efficacy. This study is a retrospective evaluation of bacteremic children without CNS involvement who were treated initially with parenteral antibiotics and then switched to oral drugs, the majority after 1–2 days without fever. Most, but not all, were seen for follow-up within 4 weeks. No complications were noted, and though the results are considered excellent by the authors, there was no control group to compare with. The fate of the non-followed 6% is uncertain, but they at least did not turn up with recurrent bac-

TABLE 1.—Antibiotic Therapy of Bacteremia (1981 to 1984)*

| | Parenteral | | | | | Oral | | | |
| | Antibiotic | | | | Av. duration (days) | Antibiotic | | | Av. duration (days) |
	A/C	PCN	CTR	Other	None		AMX	CHL	PNV	
Haemophilus influenzae (35)†	20	0	9	5	1	2.7 (0–5)‡	28	7	0	10 (4–14)‡
Streptococcus pneumoniae (24)	11	0	1	4	8	1.8 (0–5)	16	0	8	10 (7–14)
Neisseria meningitidis (1)	0	1	0	0	0	0.5	0	0	1	10
Group A *Streptococcus* (2)	0	1	0	1	0	2.8 (2–3.5)	0	0	2	26 (10–42)

*A/C, ampicillin/choramphenicol; PCN, penicillin G; CTR, ceftriaxone; AMX, amoxacillin/ampicillin; CHL, chloramphenicol; PNV, penicillin V.
†Numbers in parentheses: number of isolates.
‡Numbers in parentheses: range.
(Courtesy of Bradley, JS, Ching DK, Hart CL, et al: *Pediatr Infect Dis J* 6:821–825, September 1987.)

TABLE 2.—Days Afebrile When Changed to Oral Therapy

Days Afebrile	Patients (n = 50)	Cumulative %
<1	7	14
1-2	29	72
2-3	7	86
3-4	4	94
4-5	1	96
5-6	1	98
6-7	1	100

(Courtesy of Bradley JS, Ching DK, Hart CL, et al: *Pediatr Infect Dis J* 6:821–825, September 1987.)

teremia at either of the 2 major pediatric hospitals in town, as determined by a search of the microbiology lab reports.

While this study suggests that it is safe to switch from parenteral to oral antibiotics when the patient becomes afebrile to complete therapy for simple bacteremia or bacteremia associated with cellulitis, epiglottitis, or pneumonia, it does not address the question of whether it is *necessary* to add oral drugs to "complete the course" or whether the parenteral-oral combination is as effective as a full course of parenteral drug. I was taught that illness considered serious enough to hospitalize the patient was serious enough to use parenteral drugs, because you knew what went into the bloodstream. Times have changed, and it is desirable for many reasons to get people out of the hospital sooner. More work remains on the very simple but bread-and-butter issues of how long to treat, with what, and by which route.—G.T. Keusch, M.D.

Nursery School Children's Views on the Causality of Illness
Wilkinson SR (Psykiatrisk Poliklinikk for Follo, Jernbaneveien, Norway)
Clin Pediatr (Phila) 26:465–469, September 1987   10–9

A study was undertaken to explore views that children might have about illness and how these views might change as they grow older. Sixteen Scottish nursery school children (3–5 years old) were interviewed at school and at home in an attempt to understand their outlooks, to respond more helpfully, and to minimize the chance of a clash of perspectives in the clinical situation. Methods used elicited the full breadth of their views rather than using a large sample to quantify the results.

If an event affects an important dimension of the child's relation with a person significant to him or her, it is considered illness. For 1 child, the fact that his father was sick and could not work did not mean his father was sick, for his father still read to him at bedtime. Often a cold was not seen as an illness because the child still went to nursery school and there was no difference in the child's routine.

Children at this age do not appear to feel guilty about precipitating illness. Germs are used to explain to the children how to avoid what might happen rather than to explain what has happened to them. For example, children are told to wash their hands after going to the toilet so they will not catch germs. One mother asked her child why he was made to wash his hands before eating; he answered that it was so he would not get his plate dirty.

The children believed they became vulnerable to illness when people they were close to were away, for example, at nighttime or when their eyes were closed. Adults cultivate the latter two views, for that is the time when Santa Claus and tooth fairies come. Being close to an ill person is clearly seen as increasing the chance of becoming ill.

Interchanging the word *germ* with *bug* compounds the semantic confusion experienced by children of this age. The predominant view of these children was that germs were blue and between 1 and 9 inches in diameter, and they thought they would see one some day. They had received a lot of information from dental health workers about the value of eating certain foods and avoiding others. There are implications for the medical profession in that links are made between the food eaten and the encouragement that certain foods give to bacteria or germs on the teeth. They said doctors are silly and know nothing about health because they were given sugar lumps by them.

The children do not easily distinguish fantasy from reality, and this is compounded by conflicts inherent in differing advice they are given. The children are learning to feel guilty about precipitating their illnesses through lapses in preventive strategies, although at their current age they do not appear to be totally aware of this. Caring relationships seem to provide protective influences. At this age, adults' actions are what predominantly determine the child's behavior in health and illness.

▶ This paper was both informative and alarming. Internists can probably extrapolate to the views adults have on causality, which I suspect would be a little closer to scientific truth than those of the kids but not half so creative.—G.T. Keusch, M.D.

Pseudomonas aeruginosa as a Primary Pathogen in Children With Bacterial Peritonitis
Aronoff SC, Olson MM, Gauderer MWL, Jacobs MR, Blumer JL, Izant RJ Jr (Case Western Reserve Univ School of Medicine; Rainbow Babies and Children's Hosp, Cleveland)
J Pediatr Surg 22:861–864, September 1987   10–10

Bacterial peritonitis following appendicitis or intestinal perforation often involves *Escherichia coli* and *Bacteroides fragilis*, some strains of which produce β-lactam hydrolyzing enzymes. Sulbactam is a β-lactamase inhibitor synergistic with ampicillin against β-lactamase-producing strains of these pathogens. The authors compared sulbactam/ampicillin and clindamycin/gentamicin therapy in a blinded study of 29 children with bacterial peritonitis. Initial doses of clindamycin and gentamicin were 10 mg/kg every 6 hours and 2.5 mg/kg every 8 hours, respectively. A 50-mg/kg dose of ampicillin was combined with 12.5 mg/kg of sulbactam on a 6-hour schedule.

Among the 17 evaluable patients with positive cultures of peritoneal fluid *E. coli* and *B. fragilis* were the most frequent isolates. The mean number of isolates per patient was 3.6. *Pseudomonas aeruginosa* was recovered from the peritoneal fluid in 41% of cases. Six of 7 isolates were susceptible to gentamicin. There was 1 clinical failure of ampicillin/sulbactam therapy. Both regimens were well tolerated.

Initial antimicrobial therapy for children with peritonitis should include drugs active against *P. aeruginosa*. Organisms of this species were isolated in more than 40% of the children with bacterial peritonitis.

▶ This study was undertaken to compare 2 regimens with in vitro efficacy against the 2 leading bacterial isolates from children with bacterial peritonitis secondary to appendicitis, namely *E. coli* and *B. fragilis*. Surprisingly, over 40% of the children had *P. aeruginosa* identified in the peritoneal fluid, and the 1 therapeutic "failure" (defined as prolonged fever, subsequently shown to be due to a subphrenic abscess that was sterile when drained surgically) occurred in a patient receiving a regimen with no *Pseudomonas* coverage, sulbactam plus ampicillin. This patient grew *B. fragilis, E. coli, Streptococcus pneumoniae,* and *P. aeruginosa* from the peritoneal fluid.

The authors recommend that therapy for bacterial peritonitis in children cover *Pseudomonas* but I don't think this study justifies the conclusion just yet. The series is, first of all, too small, and the number of failures not significant enough to choose between the clindamycin/gentamicin and sulbactam/ampicillin regimens. Growing an organism from a complex polymicrobial infection does not prove it is clinically important in that setting. The study does suggest that we should certainly look for *Pseudomonas* in postappendicitis peritonitis.

Should it be treated if isolated when the initial antibiotics do not cover it? Clearly, this should be considered if the patient does not do well. What about a situation such as the failure described in this paper, that is, prolonged and otherwise unexplained fever? The answer here is not so clear, because the most likely cause, abscess formation, has been shown by the pioneering experimental studies of Bartlett, Gorbach, and Onderdonk to be related to the anaerobes and not the facultatives in the inoculum.—G.T. Keusch, M.D.

Antibiotic Administration to Treat Possible Occult Bacteremia in Febrile Children
Jaffe DM, Tanz RR, Davis AT, Henretig F, Fleisher G (Northwestern Univ Med School; Children's Mem Hosp, Chicago; Univ of Pennsylvania; Children's Hosp of Philadelphia; Harvard Med School; Children's Hosp, Boston)
N Engl J Med 317:1175–1180, Nov 5, 1987   10–11

As many as 15% of febrile infants and children may have bacteremic infection, and the clinical state in many instances is indistinguishable

TABLE 1.—Pathogenic Bacteria Identified in the Study Groups

Study Group	S. PNEUMONIAE	H. INFLUENZAE TYPE b	SALMONELLA	TOTAL
	number of patients			
Randomized, antibiotic	16	1	2	19
Randomized, placebo	7	1	0	8
Total	23	2	2	27
Nonrandomized, antibiotic	4	0	0	4
Nonrandomized, not treated	9	1	1	11
Total	13	1	1	15

(Courtesy of Jaffe DM, Tanz RR, Davis AT, et al: N Engl J Med 317:1175–1180, Nov 5, 1987.)

from viral illness. Children with occult bacteremia may have serious complications such as pneumonia, septic shock, and meningitis. Expectant oral antibiotic therapy was evaluated in a prospective, double-blind trial in 955 children, aged 3–36 months, who presented with a rectal temperature of 39C or higher and no focal bacterial infection. The patients were assigned to receive amoxicillin in an orally given dose of 250 mg 3 times daily or 125 mg for those weighing 10 kg or less, or to placebo and were reassessed after 48 hours. Another 228 children were not randomly assigned.

In the randomized sample, 2.8% of children had bacteremic infection with pathogenic species (Table 1). Its prevalence was not closely related to age (Table 2). Major infectious morbidity occurred in 3 of the 27 bacteremic patients (Table 3). Major infectious morbidity was similarly frequent in the antibiotic and placebo groups, but antibiotics lowered fever and improved the clinical picture in bacteremic patients. Diarrhea tended to be more frequent in patients treated with amoxicillin.

TABLE 2.—Prevalence of Bacteremia, According to Age of Randomly Assigned Patients

Age	No. with Positive Culture	No. Enrolled	Percent Positive
mo			
3–6	0	53	0
7–12	9	309	2.9
13–18	7	211	3.3
19–24	3	184	1.6
25–30	4	113	3.5
31–36	4	85	4.7
Total	27	955	2.8

(Courtesy of Jaffe DM, Tanz RR, Davis AT, et al: N Engl J Med 317:1175–1180, Nov 5, 1987.)

TABLE 3.—Infectious Morbidity Associated with Bacteremia, According to Study Group*

	RANDOMIZED		NONRANDOMIZED	
	ANTIBIOTIC (DISORDER)	PLACEBO (DISORDER)	ANTIBIOTIC	NO ANTIBIOTIC (DISORDER)
		number of subjects		
Subjects with major morbidity				
S. pneumoniae	1 (with PO)	1 (with PB)	0	0
H. influenzae	0	0	0	0
Salmonella	1 (with PB and GE)	0	0	0
Total	2	1	0	0
Subjects with minor morbidity				
S. pneumoniae	4 (2 with F, 2 with OM)	3 (2 with F, 1 with F and OM)	0	4 (2 with F, 2 with F and OM)
H. influenzae	0	0	0	0
Salmonella	1 (with GE)	0	0	1 (1 with F and GE)
Total	5	3	0	5
Well subjects				
S. pneumoniae	11	3	4	5
H. influenzae	1	1	0	1
Salmonella	0	0	0	0
Total	12	4	4	6

*F, fever; GE, gastroenteritis; OM, otitis media; PB, persistent bacteremia; PO, periorbital cellulitis.
(Courtesy of Jaffe DM, Tanz RR, Davis AT, et al: N Engl J Med 317:1175–1180, Nov 5, 1987.)

Expectant antibiotic treatment did not lower the rate of major infectious morbidity associated with bacteremia in these pediatric patients, but it did tend to produce a better clinical appearance and lower fever. The findings fail to support the routine use of standard orally given doses of amoxicillin in febrile children lacking evidence of focal bacterial disease.

▶ This is an important study that looked at the efficacy of empiric administration of oral amoxicillin to a large group of very young children (3–36 months) who presented to the emergency room with high fever and no localizing findings. The major conclusions were that oral antibiotics hastened the symptomatic recovery of the small percentage of febrile children who had bacteremia but produced no benefit in those who did not and that the rare occurrence of major morbidity associated with bacteremia was not prevented by the administration of amoxicillin. Diarrhea occurred in 15.2% of the children who received amoxicillin and in 11.2% of those who received the placebo: a difference that approached significance.

There are other important data in this paper that deserve comment. As the authors point out, they observed an unexpectedly low rate of major infectious morbidity in the bacteremic patients. That is, only 12.5% of bacteremic patients who received placebo developed any major infectious complication. The literature states an incidence of 40% to 50% among patients who have *Strep-*

tococcus pneumoniae bacteremia or Hemophilus influenzae bacteremia, respectively. This low incidence would have markedly reduced the power to detect a major therapeutic advantage for oral amoxicillin, even in a sample size as large as this one.

It is also noteworthy that at the time this study was designed, a long-acting parenteral agent active against the major pathogens of concern (S. pneumoniae, H. influenzae, and Neisseria meningitidis) was not available. Ceftriaxone, which has a long half-life and is active against these organisms, would provide an alternative in which noncompliance would not be an issue and adequate time for blood culture results to return would be available. It will be interesting to poll our pediatric colleagues as to whether this study will have a major impact on their emergency room practices over the coming years.—M.S. Klempner, M.D.

Transmission of Invasive *Haemophilus influenzae* Type b Disease in Day Care Settings
Makintubee S, Istre GR, Ward JI (Oklahoma State Dept of Health, Oklahoma City; Univ of California, Los Angeles, at Torrance)
J Pediatr 111:180–186, August 1987

Children in day care facilities are at increased risk of invasive *Hemophilus influenzae* type b disease, but the risk of secondary transmission of infection is uncertain. The authors assessed this risk in day care contacts in Oklahoma over a 2-year period in a statewide prospective study. Four hundred nine cases of *H. influenzae* invasive disease in children, aged 12 years and younger, were reviewed.

Two thirds of affected children had meningitis. More than one third of evaluable children attended day care facilities. The median number of classroom contacts per case was 13, and 7 secondary cases were identified among contacts younger than age 4 years. None was a sibling or household contact of a primary case. The mean interval between onset of disease in the index and secondary cases was 15 days. Secondary disease rates were 10-fold higher for both children and adults not given rifampin. No secondary cases occurred among children who were vaccinated before or at the time of exposure and received rifampin.

The risk of secondary *H. influenzae* b disease in day care settings is important in many areas. Rifampin prophylaxis lowers the risk of secondary disease. However, secondary disease accounts for only about 2% to 4% of all infections, and prevention of primary disease will have a much greater impact on public health.

▶ The results of this prospective study, which showed an appreciable rate of secondary cases of *H. influenzae* type b infection among young contacts of infected children in day care centers, disagrees with the results of 2 other recent prospective studies that failed to show an increased risk of infection among contacts. Reasons for the disagreement are not clear, although many possible explanations can be postulated. However, even in this study, there were no cases among contacts over 36 months of age. Therefore, even if what to do with younger children is problematic, there seems to be no reason to give prophylaxis to contacts who are older than 36 months.—M.J. Barza, M.D.

Enteritis Necroticans Among Khmer Children at an Evacuation Site in Thailand
Johnson S, Echeverria P, Taylor DN, Paul SR, Coninx R, Sakurai J, Eampokalap B, Jimakorn P, Cooke RA, Lawrence GW, Walker PD (Armed Forces Research Inst of Med Science, Bangkok, Thailand; Catholic Relief Services, Surin, Thailand; United Nations Relief Operation, Bangkok; Tokushima Bunri Univ, Tokushima, Japan; Bamrasnaradura Hosp, Bangkok; et al)
Lancet 2:496–500, Aug 29, 1987
10–13

From July 1985 to July 1986, a severe illness characterized by bloody diarrhea and intestinal dysfunction was recognized in 62 Khmer children in an evacuation site on the Thai–Kampuchean border. The clinical and microbiologic features of this illness are presented.

The illness occurred in children aged 10 months to 10 years (mean, 4 years) beginning, in most cases, with mild fever and diarrhea. During the course of the illness, 94% of children had bloody diarrhea, 90% had fever, 73% had vomiting, and 78% had abdominal pain. Of 44 children with dietary histories, 36% had eaten pork a week prior to illness. Radiographs of the intestine showed ileus and edematous small intestine. Intestinal parasites were detected in 95% of cases, and the rate of infestation was higher than that of other children in the camp.

Overall case-fatality rate was 58%. Necropsies were performed in 16 children, and lesions varied from hyperemia through focal jejunal necrosis to full-thickness necrosis of small intestinal wall similar to those described in cases of enteritis necroticans (pigbel) in Papua, New Guinea. Beta-toxin-producing *Clostridium perfringens* type C was isolated from 2 of 23 patients from whom anaerobic cultures were obtained. Antibodies to beta toxin were detected in 5 of 9 survivors but not in 10 age-matched healthy controls. Enteritis necroticans (pigbel) first reported in Papua, New Guinea, can cause substantial morbidity and mortality elsewhere.

▶ A good laboratory-based epidemiologic study on pigbel. The investigators made the connection between the clinical story being reported and descriptions of Papua New Guinea enteritis necroticans and found microbiologic evidence to support it. As a result, an immunization program was begun. We may never know whether it is effective, given the political and social instability in these refugee settlements.—G.T. Keusch, M.D.

Trial of an Attenuated Bovine Rotavirus Vaccine (RIT 4237) in Gambian Infants

Hanlon P, Hamlon L, Marsh V, Byass P, Shenton F, Hassam-King M, Jobe O, Sillah H, Hayes R, M'Boge BH, Whittle HC, Greenwood BM (Med Res Council Labs, Med and Health Dept, Banjul, Gambia; London School of Hygiene and Tropical Medicine)
Lancet 1:1342–1345, June 13, 1987

A randomized, controlled trial of an attenuated bovine rotavirus vaccine, RIT 4237, was undertaken with 444 Gambian infants to measure vaccine efficiency in a developing country. Three doses of virus were given concurrently with oral or killed polio vaccine.

Prevention rotavirus antibody levels were high. After the vaccine was given, an increase in neutralizing antibody occurred in 45% of the infants. Only 22% of the unvaccinated infants had increased titers of neutralizing antibodies. Rotavirus infection occurred in 31% of the children given RIT 4237/oral polio vaccine, in 41% of those given placebo/oral polio vaccine, and in 25% of those given RIT 4237/killed polio vaccine. The overall vaccine efficacy was 33%; it did not appear to reduce the severity of infection.

Little protection was provided by the attenuated bovine rotavirus vaccine RIT 4237 in Gambian infants. Therefore, RIT 4237 does not appear effective in the Third-World environment. However, trials of other rotavirus vaccines remain justified.

▶ The vaccine RIT 4237 appears to work in Finnish babies, even when given in the first week of life, resulting in attenuated disease (see Vesckari et al: *Lancet* 1:977–981, 1984; Vesckari et al: *Pediatr Infect Dis J* 6:164–169, 1987), but it does not have much effect on babies in developing countries. A rhesus rotavirus vaccine (MMU-18006) has been under development and has been found to be effective in Nashville and Caracas (Wright et al: *Pediatrics* 80:473–480, 1987; Flores et al: *Lancet* 1:882–884, 1987). Bob Edelman recently reviewed the state of the art on rotavirus vaccines (see *Pediatr Infect Dis J* 6:704–710, 1987), a worthwhile perspective.—G.T. Keusch, M.D.

11 Miscellaneous Topics

Adult Kawasaki Syndrome
Butler DF, Hough DR, Friedman SJ, Davis HE (William Beaumont Army Med Ctr, El Paso, Tex)
Arch Dermatol 123:1356–1361, October 1987   11–1

Kawasaki syndrome (KS) is an idiopathic, acute, febrile, exanthematous illness that affects primarily infants and children. The case of a young woman whose condition fulfilled the clinical criteria for the diagnosis of KS and excluded other possible causes is described. The epidemiologic, clinical, laboratory, and pathologic features of 11 cases representing adult KS are also discussed.

CASE.—Woman, 20, presented with 12-day history of fever, fatigue, anorexia, pharyngitis, rhinorrhea, and arthralgias. A scarlatiniform rash developed on the distal extremities and spread centripetally over her trunk and face. Physcial examination showed inflamed palpebral and scleral conjunctiva; dry and fissured lips and accentuated tongue papillae; erythematous pharynx; cervical lymphadenopathy; diffuse erythematous skin rash; and marked desquamation of the palms, periungual regions, and soles. A grade 2/6 systolic ejection murmur was heard at the base.

The white cell and platelet counts were increased, and liver profile studies were slightly increased. Serologic studies were negative or nonreactive, and bacterial cultures were negative. Viral cultures of the erosions on the labia majora showed herpes simplex.

The patient remained febrile despite erythromycin therapy. A third heart sound was noted, and the patient was started on aspirin therapy. She became afebrile by the second week of hospitalization and showed gradual improvement. Echocardiography showed no evidence of coronary aneurysm. One month after discharge, Beau's lines were noted on her fingernails (Fig 11–1), and the ECG had returned to normal.

A total of 11 cases representing adult KS have been reported (Table 1). The male-to-female ratio was 2.7:1. The mean age of patients was 25.6 years (range, 18–40), and 8 (72%) cases occurred before age 29 years. The frequencies of elevated sedimentation rate, leukocytosis, and neurologic and cardiac abnormalities were similar to those noted in children with KS (Table 2). Thrombocytosis occurred in 5 adults, and the counts were normal in 3. Ten patients had mild elevation of liver enzymes, and 4 had elevated bilirubin levels. Histopathologic studies of skin and lymph nodes showed nonspecfic changes. Cardiac abnormalities were found in 7 patients, and most were asymptomatic. Congestive heart failure was doc-

TABLE 1.—Clinical Features of Adult Kawasaki Syndrome*

Patient No.	Source, y	Age, y/Sex/Race	Fever	Conjunctival Congestion	Oropharyngeal Inflammation	Diffuse Rash	Inflammation Distal	Adenopathy (Size), cm	Arthralgias (Arthritis)	Gastroenteritis	Neurologic Abnormalities	Cardiac Findings
1	Burnstein et al,[6] 1984	20/M/NR	+	+	+	+	+	6 × 8	+	+	NR	Normal ECG; normal echo
2	Keim and Celtner,[7] 1985	34/F/NR	+	+	+	+	+	3 × 1.5	NR	NR	NR	Normal echo
3	Marcella et al,[8] 1983	26/M/W	+	+	+	+	+	1 × 2	NR	+	NR	ECG changes; congestive heart failure
4	Takagi et al,[9] 1981	18/F/J	+	+	+	NR	+	(?) +	NR	+	Nystagmus; tremor; ataxia	ECG changes; coronary artery aneurysms
5	Hicks et al,[10] 1982	40/M/B	+	+	+	+	+	(?) +	(Swelling MP joints)	NR	Peripheral neuropathy	NR
6	Saxe et al,[11] 1980	18/M/W	+	+	+	+	+	(?) +	+	+	Meningismus; CSF pleocytosis	S3 gallop; ECG: right axis deviation
7	Liebmann et al,[12] 1982	25/M/NR	+	+	+	+	+	1	+	(Hydrops of gallbladder)	NR	ECG: left ventricular hypertrophy
8	Gomberg et al,[13] 1981	22/M/NR	+	+	+	+	+	(?) +	+	+	NR	Nonspecific ECG ST-T wave changes
9	Glanzer et al,[14] 1980	28/M/NR	+	+	+	+	+	(?) +	+	+	NR	Normal ECG
10	Takamoto et al,[15] 1982	31/M/J	+	+	+	+	+	(?) +	NR	NR	NR	ECG changes; coronary artery aneurysms
11	Present study	20/F/B	+	+	+	+	+	1	+	NR	NR	S3 gallop; first-degree heart block; normal echo

*W, white; B, black; J, Japanese; plus sign, presence of sign or symptom; question mark, size not reported; NR, not reported; MP, metacarpophalangeal; ECG, electrocardiogram; CSF, cerebrospinal fluid; echo, echocardiogram.
(Courtesy of Butler DF, Hough DR, Friedman SJ, et al: Arch Dermatol 123:1356–1361, October 1987.)

TABLE 2.—Laboratory Features of Adult Kawasaki Syndrome*

Patient No.	Source, y	WBC Count	Platelet Count	Sedimentation Rate	Liver Enzymes	Bilirubin	Sterile Pyuria	ANA	Throat Culture	Blood Culture	Urine Culture	Vaginal Culture	Sputum Culture	Viral Culture	Leptospira Agglutinins
1	Burnstein et al,[6] 1984	E	E	NR	E	E	NR	Negative	Negative	Negative	NR	NA	NR	NR	NR
2	Keim and Cellner,[7] 1985	E	E	E	E	E	NR	NR	Negative	Negative	NR	NR	NR	NR	Negative
3	Marcella et al,[8] 1983	E	E	E	E	E	P	Negative	NR	Negative	Negative	NA	NR	Negative	Negative
4	Takagi et al,[9] 1981	NR	NR	NR	N	E	NR	NR	NR	NR	NR	NR	NR	NR	NR
5	Hicks et al,[10] 1982	N	N	N	E	E	A	Negative	Negative	Negative	Negative	NA	NR	NR	NR
6	Saxe et al,[11] 1980	E	NR	E	E	NR	A	Negative	Negative	Negative	Negative	NA	Negative	Negative	Negative
7	Liebmann et al,[12] 1982	E	N	NR	E	E	NR	Negative	Negative	Negative	NR	NA	NR	NR	NR
8	Gomberg et al,[13] 1981	LS	E	E	E	E	A	NR	Negative	Negative	Negative	NA	NR	NR	NR
9	Glanzer et al,[14] 1980	E	N	E	E	E	P	Negative	Negative	Negative	Negative	NA	NR	NR	Negative
10	Takamoto et al,[15] 1982	LS	NR	E	E	E	A	NR	NR	NR	NR	NA	NR	NR	NR
11	Present study	E	E	E	E	N	P	Negative	Negative	Negative	Negative	Negative	Negative	NR	NR

*E, elevated; N, normal; LS, left shift; A, absent; P, present; NR, not reported; NA, not applicable; WBC, white blood cells; ANA, antinuclear antibodies. (Courtesy of Butler DF, Hough DR, Friedman SJ, et al: Arch Dermatol 123:1356–1361, October 1987.)

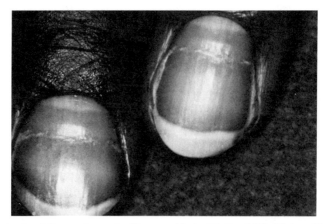

Fig 11–1.—Beau's lines on fingernails. (Courtesy of Butler DF, Hough DR, Friedman SJ, et al: *Arch Dermatol* 123:1356–1361, October 1987.)

umented in 1 patient, and coronary artery aneurysms were documented in 2.

Although the initial reports of adult KS in the United States may have actually represented toxic shock syndrome (TSS), the occurence of KS in adults should be acknowledged. Treatment consists of high-dose salicylates during the initial phase of the illness, while low-dose salicylate therapy may help prevent coronary artery thrombosis during the convalescent phase. Recent studies have shown that early administration of high-dose intravenous gammaglobulin plus aspirin will reduce the prevalence of coronary artery aneurysms and thrombosis to a greater degree than with aspirin alone.

▶ The lines between childhood, adolescence, and adulthood are fuzzy, to say the least. Age is one definition but has only a general relationship to maturity. Kawasaki syndrome is a disease of infants and children, peaking in the second year of life. This paper reports a case in a 20-year-old that has to be called Kawasaki (it's a syndrome, after all) and reviews 10 other adult patients (aged 18–40 years) in the literature. Diagnosis depends on meeting criteria for Kawasaki disease and exclusion of scarlet fever, TSS, leptospirosis, Stevens-Johnson syndrome, collagen-vascular disease, or mercury poisoning.—G.T. Keusch, M.D.

Unexplained Febrile Illnesses After Exposure to Ticks: Infection With an Ehrlichia?
Fishbein DB, Sawyer LA, Holland CJ, Hayes EB, Okoroanyanwu W, Williams D, Sikes RK, Ristic M, McDade JE (Ctrs for Disease Control, Atlanta; College of Veterinary Pathology, Univ of Illinois; Morehouse School of Medicine, Atlanta; Georgia Dept of Human Resources, Atlanta)
JAMA 257:3100–3104, June 12, 1987

Antibody Titers to *Ehrlichia canis*, Other Rickettsiae, and Tick-Borne Agents in 6 Patients

Patient No.	Days After Onset of Illness	Indirect Fluorescent Antibody Titer					ELISA†
		Ehrlichia canis (≥80)*	*Rickettsia rickettsii* (≥64)*	*Rickettsia typhi* (≥64)*	*Coxiella burnetii* (≥128)*	*Francisella tularensis* (≥160)‡	*Borrelia burgdorferi* (≥0.20)‡
1	10	160	<16	<16	≤64	<20	0.04
	19	1280	<16	<16	≤64	20	0.04
	44	2560	<16	<16	≤64	<20	0.03
	109	160	<16	<16	≤64	NT	NT
2	13	640	<16	<16	≤64	QNS	QNS
	155	40	<16	<16	≤64	<20	0.03
3	27	80	<16	<16	≤64	20	0.03
	152	20	32	32	≤64	<20	0.01
4	11	<10	64	<16	≤64	<20	0.01
	37	80	64	<16	≤64	20	0.02
	153	20	64	32	≤64	20	0.02
5	1	20	<16	<16	≤64	QNS	QNS
	22	80	<16	<16	≤64	QNS	QNS
6	5	20	32	<16	≤64	<20	0.05
	26	640	16	16	≤64	<20	0.05
	178	320	16	16	≤64	<20	0.05

*Values in parentheses indicate positive titer.
†Enzyme-linked immunosorbent assay (ELISA) expressed as an optical density ratio.
‡NT, not tested; QNS, insufficient quantity.
(Courtesy of Fishbein DB, Sawyer LA, Holland CJ, et al: *JAMA* 257:3100–3104, June 12, 1987.)

Ehrlichiae are obligate intracellular bacteria that infect circulating white blood cells of domestic and wild animals. In the United States, *Ehrlichia canis* was thought to cause infection only in dogs, most commonly in the southern states. The clinical, epidemiologic, and laboratory findings in 6 patients who had serologic evidence of a recent *E. canis* infection are reported.

Five men and 1 woman, aged 26 to 59 years, became ill after exposure to ticks during outdoor activities (table). Only 2 of the 6 patients had had contact with dogs in the 2 weeks before the onset of illness. Four patients required hospitalization. Clinical symptoms included nausea and vomiting, sudden onset of fever, myalgia, headache, anorexia, and rigors. Four patients were exposed in Georgia; 1 patient, in South Carolina; and 1 patient did not know where he had been exposed.

Laboratory findings included absolute lymphopenia in all 6 patients and thrombocytopenia in 4 patients. Four of the patients had abnormal liver function test results, and 3 patients were anemic. Five patients were treated with tetracycline, and 1 patient was not treated. The median duration of hospitalization was 7 days. All patients recovered completely. *Ehrlichia* infection should be considered for patients presenting with unexplained fever following exposure to ticks.

▶ Ticks are a nuisance in and of themselves. In addition, they transmit a number of infectious diseases to humans. Although Rocky Mountain spotted fever is the classic tick-borne disease in the United States, it has been overshadowed in both incidence and interest by the deer-tick-transmitted Lyme disease (caused by *B. burgdorferi*), and to a lesser extent by babesiosis, transmitted by the same insect. Ticks also transmit tularemia and relapsing fever and are the vectors of Crimean-Congo hemorrhagic fever (not too common a disease in this country). This report provides serologic and historical evidence that another agent may have a place on this list. The organism *Ehrlichia canis* is classified in the family Rickettsiaceae and is an obligate intracellular parasite of leukocytes. Whereas the evidence for human disease due to *E. canis* presented in this paper is not conclusive, it is provocative. In the search for a cause of tick-related febrile illnesses it seems reasonable to suggest that *E. canis* be looked for, especially in the presence of lymphopenia (with or without intraleukocytic inclusion bodies) and abnormal liver function tests.—G.T. Keusch, M.D.

Tobacco Smokers' Neutrophils Are Desensitized to Chemotactic Peptide-Stimulated Oxygen Uptake
Codd EE, Swim AT, Bridges RB (Univ of Kentucky Med Ctr)
J Lab Clin Med 110:648–652, November 1987
11–3

Polymorphonuclear leukocytes (PMNs) are the body's primary defenders against acute bacterial infections. Since tobacco smokers have more respiratory infections than nonsmokers, researchers have studied the potential influence of chronic exposure to smoke components on PMN function. Oxygen uptake in PMNs in response to the peptide

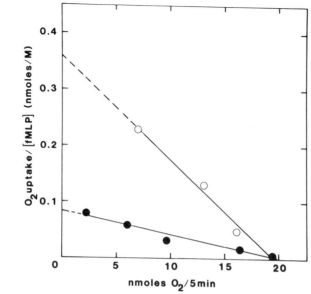

Fig 11–2.—Eadie-Hofstee plot of formyl-methionyl-leucyl-phenylalanine (FMLP) stimulation of O_2 uptake by PMNs from a tobacco smoker (*black dot*) and a nonsmoker (*white dot*). The x-intercept represents maximal rate of O_2 uptake. Negative reciprocal of slope represents ED_{50} or apparent K_m of FMLP in stimulation of uptake. (Courtesy of Codd EE, Swim AT, Bridges RB: *J Lab Clin Med* 110:648–652, November 1987.)

formyl-methionyl-leucylphenylalanine (FMLP) was investigated in tobacco smokers and nonsmokers.

Blood samples were drawn from 18 fasting male smokers and nonsmokers. Chemotactic peptide-stimulated oxygen uptake and superoxide release were measured in neutrophils and controls.

Cigarette smokers had elevated levels of plasma nicotine and cotinine. Smokers had a modest decrement in tests of lung function. Baseline values for unstimulated oxygen uptake showed no trend between groups. Stimulated oxygen uptake in smokers was less than that of nonsmokers. Decreased sensitivity to FMLP stimulation of oxygen was the result of an altered apparent K_m (Fig 11–2). There was a parallel decrement in superoxide release in smokers.

The findings suggest a modified response to FMLP in chronic smokers' neutrophils. Studies using other cell surface receptor-mediated stimuli should be undertaken to determine whether the changes in tobacco smokers' PMNs are found only in FMLP-stimulated responses or whether they are common to all receptor-mediated PMN events.

▶ As if we need more evidence that smoking is bad for you and is associated with an increased risk of respiratory infections, this study further documents that a major player in host defense against pulmonary infection, namely PMNs, don't respond normally to a chemotactic signal. We can add this to our ever-growing list to browbeat our patients into kicking the habit. I know there must be some patients out there who will cringe at this information, and this will be just what the doctor ordered to make them quit!—M.S. Klempner, M.D.

Functional Capacity of Marginated and Bone Marrow Reserve Granulocytes
Steele RW, Steele CR, Pilkington NS Jr, Charlton RK (Univ of Arkansas for Med Sciences; Arkansas Children's Hosp, Little Rock)
Infect Immunity 55:2359–2363, October 1987

11–4

Systemic bacterial infection is accompanied by leukocytosis, predominantly of granulocytes. The early additional circulating neutrophils come primarily from the marginated pool, whereas bone marrow reserves account for most cells during continued infection or during convalescence. To determine their functional capacity against bacterial pathogens, marginated and bone marrow reserve granulocytes were obtained from young healthy volunteers after subcutaneous administration of aqueous epinephrine or intravenous administration of hydrocortisone sodium succinate, respectively. Their abilities to adhere to surfaces, migrate in a random fashion, respond to chemoattractants, interact with autologous serum opsonins, and phagocytose and kill 5 common bacterial pathogens were compared to those of circulating granulocytes.

Whereas adherence, random migration, and chemotaxis of granulocytes did not differ between circulating and marginated leukocytes, enhanced phagocytosis and killing for some pathogens were greater for marginated cells. Bone marrow reserve cells showed significantly enhanced chemotaxis and phagocytosis than circulating cells, with 6% to 17% greater killing of the 5 common bacterial pathogens studied (table). Random migration and interaction with serum opsonins were unchanged in bone marrow granulocytes.

These enhanced functional properties of marginated and bone marrow reserve cells, which are outside the circulating pool, may represent important host defense mechanisms during bacterial infection.

▶ It may be surprising to recall that the peripheral blood contains fewer than 5% of the body's granulocytes. By far, the majority of cells are contained in the bone marrow and to a lesser extent in a pool of cells that are adherent to capillary endothelium (the marginated pool). One of the most interesting questions continues to be: what factors keep these various pools in the consistent equilibrium that we find clinically? We do know that agents such as epinephrine are capable of an early mobilization of the marginated pool, which consists almost entirely of mature granulocytes. The more immature forms, which are seen during the course of infection, come from the bone marrow and can be mobilized with slower kinetics after an injection of hydrocortisone. Unlike other peripheral blood cells like erythrocytes, the peripherally marginated cells are a less functional population but, as reported here, are at least as able as the peripheral blood neutrophil to get to and kill a microorganism. For that matter, the

Characteristics of Circulating and Bone Marrow Reserve Granulocytes*

Granulocyte	No. of granulocytes/mm³	Adherence	Random migration†	Chemotaxis†	Peak chemiluminescence response (cpm) with:		
					Zymosan	S. pneumoniae	S. aureus
Pre	2,464 ± 535	59 ± 4	473 ± 216	1,466 ± 293	317,964 ± 63,238	48,350 ± 9,211	85,439 ± 6,509
Post	7,317 ± 1,648	63 ± 6	531 ± 189	2,071 ± 214	364,052 ± 81,735	46,873 ± 7,752	89,031 ± 8,625

*Values are expressed as the mean of 10 samples ± the standard error of the mean. *Pre*, circulating granulocytes isolated before hydrocortisone treatment; *Post*, bone marrow reserve granulocytes isolated after hydrocortisone treatment. P values (Pre and Post) were as follows: number of granulocytes per cubic millimeter, < .001; chemotaxis, < .05. All other P values were not significant.
†Number of migrated cells in a single plane.
(Courtesy of Steele RW, Steele CR, Pilkington NS Jr, et al: *Infect Immunity* 55:2359–2363, October 1987.)

bone marrow contains a group of cells with an even greater ability to perform some of these functions.

These carefully done studies, along with a recent similar report (Heatherington: *Am J Hematol* 20:235–246, 1985), provide an excellent overview of the functional capacity of the various pools of neutrophils. It is perhaps because the much larger reserve pool has at least as good a functional capacity as the circulating neutrophil that our sampling such a small population accurately reflects the host's ability to deal with bacterial pathogens. What signals are involved in the actual release from the reserve pools and the adherence of cells in these pools remains an important question.—M.S. Klempner, M.D.

Pelagic Paralysis
Mills AR, Passmore R (Edinburgh)
Lancet 1:161–164, Jan 23, 1988   11–5

Poisoning of sea animals by toxins has been recognized since ancient times. The most frequently occurring form is ciguatera, seen in the Pacific and Caribbean islands. Puffer fish poisoning also is seen. Paralytic shellfish poisoning results from the ingestion of bivalve and gastropod mollusks and some crustaceans. The puffer fish toxin tetrodotoxin and the paralytic shellfish toxin saxitoxin block nerve conduction by lowering the conductance of sodium currents through membranes. Both fish and shellfish accumulate saxitoxin from dinoflagellates. Tetrodotoxin is one of the most poisonous nonprotein substances. Ciguatoxin remains to be well studied because it is present in such very small amounts.

Patients with one or another form of pelagic paralysis generally have an acute neurotoxic illness with paresthesias, ataxia, and muscle weakness. Feelings of electric shock are characteristic of ciguatera; hot objects may feel cold, and heavy objects, light. Symptoms are quite variable and idiosyncratic. Treatment should be supportive and symptomatic. An awareness of intoxication will help prevent the disorder. Fish that usually are toxic include red snapper, shark, and barracuda.

▶ If the readers of this excellent review have as much difficulty as I have in distinguishing the signs and symptoms of puffer fish poisoning from those of ciguatera or paralytic shellfish poisoning, they will be grateful for the authors' unification of these into a single entity that they have called "pelagic paralysis." In all 3 intoxications, the major manifestations are probably caused by the action of 1 or more of a closely related group of toxins on the autonomic innervation of the alimentary, genitourinary, and cardiovascular systems. Although there may be marked individual idiosyncrasy in the symptoms, paralysis is the most striking feature. An intriguing question is how puffer fish and salamanders survive with amounts of toxin in their bodies that are fatal to other animals.—M.J. Barza, M.D.

Stable Integration and Expression of a Bacterial Gene in the Mosquito Anopheles sambiae

Miller LH, Sakai RK, Romans P, Gwadz RW, Kantoff P, Coon HG (Natl Inst of Allergy and Infectious Diseases, Natl Heart, Lung, and Blood Inst, Natl Cancer Inst, Bethesda, Md)
Science 237:779–781, Aug 14, 1987

11-6

The method used to introduce DNA into the germline of the African malaria vector *Anopheles gambiae* was an adaptation of that used for fruitfly embryos. The eggs were covered with hydrated halocarbon oil and kept in a humid chamber. Because the eggs cannot be dechorionated, a 100-μm glass needle having a sharp, narrow tip of less than 3 μm is used for injection. An automatic injection device was used. The eggs are opaque. The injections consisted of DNA, 250–500 μg/ml of plasmid pUChsneo and 50–100 μg/ml of plasmid pUChsπ (Δ2–3)wc.

Of the injected eggs, 24% hatched; 145 female mosquitos and 175 male mosquitos survived to adulthood. They were mated, and the progeny (G_1 generation) were treated with G-418, a neomycin analogue, 200 ng/ml. By the third or fourth day, 99% of the control larvae had died and 9,283 of the G_1 generation survived. Of these, 28 males and 27 females reached adulthood and were mated. The plasmid was identified in the G_1 generation by Southern blotting. The Pst I fragments were identical, indicating a single integration event in a primordial germ cell. This same pattern of fragments has been maintained through 5 generations and appears to be stable. Heat shock increased the expression of the *neo* gene, indicating that the hsp70 promoter on the plasmid is functional (Fig 11–3).

DNA can be integrated stably into insects other than fruitflies. Genetic transformation can now be carried out in this medically important insect to allow study of the effects of introduced genes on the development of malarial parasites.

▶ Cloning genes into mosquitoes and transforming the insects in important ways may be reminiscent of Gregor's metamorphosis (see the original publication by Kafka F.) and in its own way as aesthetic scientifically as Kafka is in the literary sense. By defining the genes controlling development of parasites within their insect vectors, this study is a giant step toward the

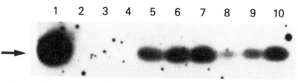

Fig 11–3.—Assay for neomycin phosphotransferase (NPT). The 29-kD NPT protein from *neo*-transformed cells was run as a control in lane 1. There is increased expression of NPT after exposure to heat shock (lanes 3, 4, 6, 7, 9, and 10). (Courtesy of Miller LH, Sakai RK, Romans P, et al: *Science* 237:779–781, Aug 14, 1987.)

ultimate goal of squashing malaria-vector mosquitoes one way or another.—
G.T. Keusch, M.D.

Chronic Recurrent Multifocal Osteomyelitis: A Follow-Up Study
Jurik AG, Helmig O, Ternowitz T, Møller BN (Univ of Aarhus, Denmark)
J Pediatr Orthop 8:49–58, January–February 1988 11–7

Thirteen children and adolescents and 2 young adults presented in a 16-year period with unifocal or multifocal nonpyogenic inflammatory bone lesions and received diagnoses of chronic recurrent multifocal osteomyelitis (CRMO). Four patients had histories of trauma, and 2 had had infectious disease. The onset was insidious, and the course was prolonged during a mean follow-up of 5½ years. Seven patients had attacks of severe pain that usually lasted 1 to 4 weeks and occurred at 1- to 3-month intervals. Pain and swelling corresponded to the areas of involvement. Seven patients had pustulosis palmoplantaris.

The sedimentation rate usually was elevated during exacerbations. The chemotactic activity of polymorphs was higher than in healthy adults. Nine patients had multifocal lesions. Most metaphyseal lesions began as areas of lytic destruction surrounded by sclerosis; they were close to the epiphyseal cartilage. Spread to the diaphysis was not infrequent. After repeated episodes, progressive hyperostosis and sclerosis were evident. Bone scan activity was distinctly increased. Biopsies failed to show evidence of suppurative infection or sequestration. The infiltrates consisted chiefly of lymphocytes. Antibiotics were not effective, but 2 patients responded to colchicine therapy. Nonsteroidal anti-inflammatory drugs relieved symptoms in the other patients.

This skeletal disorder may be a form of pustulotic arthro-osteitis. Although CRMO follows a prolonged and unpredictable course, the long-term outlook for function is good. Growth disturbance is a rare complication.

▶ This illness resembles chronic infective osteomyelitis. However, the authors of this article present evidence that the disease is not likely to be infectious. For example, the distribution of lesions differs from that in hematogenous osteomyelitis, often involving the clavicle in these patients but not in pyogenic osteomyelitis.

Recently, Hummell et al. wrote a letter to the editor of the *New England Journal of Medicine* (Hummell DS, Anderson SJ, Wright PF, et al 317:510–511, 1987) reporting isolation of *Mycoplasma hominis* from a biopsy specimen of the right radius of a young girl who apparently had this disorder. The patient was treated with intravenous clindamycin and doxycycline followed by long-term oral tetracycline. Her pain was relieved and her erythrocyte sedimentation rate fell from 54 ml/hour to 22 ml/hour. She had radiographic healing of the bone lesions and no new lesions since the beginning of treatment. This means that *M. hominis* may be involved in this disease.—M.J. Barza, M.D.

Inability to Predict Diagnosis in Febrile Intravenous Drug Abusers
Marantz PR, Linzer M, Feiner CJ, Feinstein SA, Kozin AM, Friedland GH (Montefiore Med Ctr, North Central Bronx Hosp, Albert Einstein College of Medicine, New York)
Ann Intern Med 106:823–828, June 1987

Hospitalization is recommended for all febrile intravenous drug abusers. To determine the efficacy of diagnosis in these patients, admission data, laboratory findings, emergency room physician's diagnostic prediction, and final diagnosis were prospectively analyzed for 75 febrile intravenous drug abusers admitted to the emergency room.

The final diagnosis was pneumonia in 37.9%, trivial diagnosis in 26.4%, other conditions in 23.0%, and infective endocarditis in 12.6%. A final diagnosis of endocarditis was associated with pyuria on urinalysis, higher median temperature, and lower median serum levels of sodium and potassium. Prediction of endocarditis by the emergency room physician was not correlated with a final diagnosis of endocarditis. There was a significant association between a prediction of trivial illness and a final diagnosis of a trivial illness. However, no reliable algorithm could be derived.

Although distinguishing between those febrile intravenous drug abusers who require hospitalization and those with trivial illnesses would save time and resources, no reliable method could be derived from these data. Physicians' initial predictions were often wrong. Therefore, hospitalization of all febrile intravenous drug abusers should be continued.

▶ Although the authors have in fact shown that many febrile, intravenous-drug abusers who present to emergency rooms have serious illness (13%, endocarditis; 38%, pneumonia), there was an excellent correlation between the initial and discharge diagnosis of trivial illness (26% of patients). In large urban centers, where intravenous-drug abusers make up a significant proportion of patients, a decrease in admission of patients with trivial illness would represent significant surveys in all regards. It seems to me that careful evaluation and close outpatient follow-up of individuals with presumed trivial illnesses would be preferable to automatically admitting all febrile intravenous-drug abusers.—S.M. Wolff, M.D.

Subject Index

A

Abusers
  drug (see Drug, abusers)
Acid
  -vesicle function, intracellular pathogens, and action of chloroquine against *Plasmodium falciparum*, 123
Acquired immunodeficiency syndrome (see AIDS)
Actinomycotic
  mycetoma, amikacin and trimethoprim-sulfamethoxazole in, 33
Acyclovir
  leukoplakia regression after, oral hairy, 181
  for prevention of cytomegalovirus infection and disease after marrow transplant, 87
Adenine
  arabinoside monophosphate in hepatitis B, 75
Agranulocytosis
  Staphylococcus aureus bacteremia and, 141
AIDS
  AZT in (see AZT, in AIDS)
  cardiomyopathy in, congestive, 169
  in children, 150
    antibodies to HIV and, 149
    CNS in, 172
  health care workers exposed to, risk of transmitting HIV, CMV and HBV to, 147
  HIV antigenemia in, AZT in, 164
  HIV infection and oral hairy leukoplakia, 168
  HIV-2 infection and, in West Africa, 151
  myelopoiesis, effect of granulocyte-macrophage colony-stimulating factor on, 179
  neurologic manifestations of, 169
  Pneumocystis carinii pneumonia in
    mortality of, in-hospital, early predictors of, 173
    pentamidine for, aerosolized, 176
    trimetrexate for, 178
  -related complex
    AZT in (see AZT, in AIDS-related complex)
    health care workers exposed to, risk of transmitting HIV, CMV and HBV to, 147
  risk in homosexual men with persistent HIV antigenemia, 165
  risk in homosexual men with persistent HIV antigenemia, 165
  survival with, 159
  vaccine, potential, 182
Air
  -fluid levels, lung bullae with, 10
Amantadine
  for influenza type A in nursing homes, benefits and costs of, 95
American travelers
  to Kenya, malaria prophylaxis in, 112
Amikacin
  in mycetoma, actinomycotic, 33
Aminoglycosides
  auditory toxicity due to, 46
  clinical response to, 48
  nephrotoxicity of, cost of, 47
Amoxicillin
  prophylaxis of dental bacteremia, in children, 3
Amphotericin B
  in candiduria, in children, 109
  chills and fever due to, and prostaglandin synthesis, 107
  in fungal infections in neutropenic cancer patients, 137
  in meningitis, cryptococcal, 105
  nephrotoxicity after sodium supplements with ticarcillin or saline, 108
Ampicillin
  in renal infection, in women, 24
Anomalies
  congenital, temporal relations between maternal rubella and, 90
Anopheles sambiae
  mosquito, integration and expression of bacterial gene in, 235
Antacids
  nosocomial pneumonia in intubated patients after, 201
Antibiotics
  in bacteremia, occult, in febrile children, 219
  in bacterial disease, invasive, in children, 215
  penetration into nucleus pulposus (in rabbit), 57
Antibody(ies)
  anti-idiotypic, which mimic T4 (CD4) epitope, neutralization of HIV isolates by (in mice), 182
  to herpes simplex virus in CSF of herpes simplex encephalitis patients, 80
  to HIV

239

AIDS and, in children and their
  families, 149
 in blood samples, prevalence of, 154
 transfusions screened as negative for,
  HIV transmission by, 157
 IgA, secretory, after oral immunization
  with *Streptococcus mutans*, 35
 to p24 and gp41, in hemophilia, 158
 to sporozoites, naturally acquired, and
  malaria prevention, 117
Antigen
 Aspergillus fumigatus,
  radioimmunoassay for aspergillosis
  in hematologic malignancy, 100
 cyst, encystation and expression by
  Giardia lamblia in vitro (in mice),
  130
 hepatitis B surface, in blood samples,
  154
 HIV, in hemophilia, 158
Antigenemia
 HIV (*see* HIV, antigenemia)
Anti-idiotypic
 antibodies which mimic T4 (CD4)
  epitope, neutralization of HIV
  isolates by (in mice), 182
Antimicrobial
 -resistant salmonellosis due to
  pasteurized milk, 13
 therapy
  oral, for osteomyelitis or septic
   arthritis, 32
  for osteoarticular infections, acute
   suppurative, 31
Antiseptic
 benzalkonium chloride, and epidemic
  septic arthritis due to *Serratia
  marcescens*, 34
Arthritis
 of Lyme disease, clinical evolution, 59
 septic
  antimicrobial therapy for, oral, 32
  epidemic, due to *Serratia marcescens*
   and associated with benzalkonium
   chloride antiseptic, 34
Aspergillosis
 cutaneous, primary, Hickman
  intravenous catheter-associated,
  191
 invasive, in hematologic malignancy,
  serodiagnosis of, 100
Aspergillus fumigatus
 antigen radioimmunoassay for
  aspergillosis in hematologic
  malignancy, 100
Auditory
 toxicity of aminoglycosides, 46
Azidothymidine (*see* AZT)

AZT
 in AIDS
  bone marrow failure after, 176
  efficacy of, 174
  toxicity of, 175
 in AIDS-related complex
  efficacy of, 174
  toxicity of, 175
 in HIV antigenemia, 164
 in AIDS, 164

B

Babesiosis
 seasonal variation of transmission risk
  of, 59
Bacteremia
 catheter-related, central venous, in situ
  management of, 196
 coagulase-negative staphylococcal, in
  neonatal intensive care unit, 207
 dental, amoxicillin prophylaxis, in
  children, 3
 Haemophilus aegyptius, in Brazilian
  purpuric fever, 66
 occult, in febrile children, antibiotics in,
  219
 shigella, in adults, 5
 Staphylococcus aureus, in hematological
  malignancies and/or
  agranulocytosis, 141
Bacterial
 disease, invasive, in children, 215
 gene integration and expression in
  mosquito *Anopheles sambiae*, 235
 infections, mixed, *Campylobacter jejuni*
  in, 70
 peritonitis, *Pseudomonas aeruginosa* as
  primary pathogen in, in children,
  218
 pneumonia, acute, diagnosis by
  bronchoalveolar lavage, 140
 polysaccharide immune globulin
  preventing *Haemophilus influenzae*
  type b infections in high-risk
  infants, 38
 respiratory infection, diagnosis by
  bronchoalveolar lavage, 138
Bactericidal test
 standardized serum, in osteomyelitis, 28
Bacteriuria
 asymptomatic, in institutionalized
  elderly women, therapy vs. no
  therapy for, 20
 in elderly institutionalized men, 23
Bacteroides fragilis
 in diarrhea, 19

Benzalkonium
  chloride antiseptic, and epidemic septic arthritis due to *Serratia marcescens*, 34
Benzathine
  penicillin for secondary syphilis with HIV infection, neurologic relapse after, 167
Beta-hemolytic
  streptococcal pharyngitis, group A, immediate penicillin for, 52
Biliary
  drainage devices, transhepatic, causing infections, 199
Bisexual
  /homosexual men, HIV transmission reduction by, 157
Bismuth
  subsalicylate tablet for prevention of travelers' diarrhea, 18
Blastomycosis
  serological tests for, 99
Bleeding
  platelet-mediated, due to broad-spectrum penicillins, 57
Blood
  cell, white (*see* Leukocyte)
  samples, prevalence of antibodies to HIV and hepatitis B surface antigens in, 154
Bone
  infection, and pressure sores, 29
  marrow (*see* Marrow)
Bordetella pertussis
  infection, 8
Brain
  MRI in childhood herpesvirus infections, 81
Brazilian purpuric fever
  discussion of, 65
  Haemophilus aegyptius bacteremia in, 66
Breath
  test, ^{13}C-urea, detecting *Campylobacter pylori*, 15
Bronchoalveolar
  lavage diagnosis
    of bacterial pneumonia, acute, 140
    of bacterial respiratory infection, 138
Buffy coat transfusions
  in neutropenic neonates with presumed sepsis, 207
Bullae
  lung, with air-fluid levels, 10

Burned patients
  critically ill, *Clostridium difficile* diarrhea in, 143

C

Caffeine
  elimination after co-administration of 4-quinolones, 49
Campylobacter
  infections, enteric, in infant, 17
  jejuni in mixed bacterial infections, 70
  pylori, ^{13}C-urea breath test detecting, 15
Cancer
  hematologic
    aspergillosis in, invasive, serodiagnosis of, 100
    Staphylococcus aureus bacteremia and, 141
  patients, neutropenic, amphotericin B or ketoconazole for fungal infections in, 137
Candidiasis
  invasive, diagnosis of, 102
Candiduria
  amphotericin B in, in children, 109
Cardiomyopathy
  congestive, in AIDS, 169
Catheter
  central venous
    colonization with *Malassezia furfur*, 105
    -related bacteremia, in situ management of, 196
    -related sepsis, diagnosis of, 193
  intravenous
    fungemia due to *Malassezia furfur*, 190
    Hickman, causing primary cutaneous aspergillosis, 191
  sepsis, Isolator cultures in, 195
Causality of illness
  nursery school children's views on, 217
Ceftriaxone
  for chancroid, 186
Cell
  blood, white (*see* Leukocyte)
  intracellular pathogens, acid-vesicle function, and action of chloroquine against *Plasmodium falciparum*, 123
  T cell leukemia virus (*see* HTLV)
Central nervous system
  in AIDS and HIV infections, 172

Central venous catheter (see Catheter, central venous)
Cerebrospinal fluid
  in herpes simplex encephalitis, antibodies to herpes simplex virus in, 80
Cervical
  cytology, abnormal, papillomavirus infections in women with and without, 92
  intraepithelial neoplasia, papillomavirus-associated penile intraepithelial neoplasia in sexual partners of women with, 185
Chancroid
  ceftriaxone for, 186
Chemotactic
  peptide-stimulated oxygen uptake, and tobacco smokers' neutrophils, 230
Children
  AIDS in, 150
  antibodies to HIV and, 149
  bacterial disease in, invasive, 215
  Brazilian purpuric fever in (see Brazilian purpuric fever)
  candiduria in, amphotericin B for, 109
  in day care setting, transmission of *Hemophilus influenzae* type b disease in, 222
  dental bacteremia in, amoxicillin prophylaxis of, 3
  febrile, antibiotics for occult bacteremia in, 219
  herpesvirus infections in, MRI of brain in, 81
  IgA deficiency, respiratory infections, and IgG subclass deficiency in, 210
  infant (see Infant)
  Khmer, enteritis necroticans among, 223
  malaria in, clinical, 120
  newborn (see Newborn)
  nursery school, views on causality of illness, 217
  peritonitis in, bacterial, *Pseudomonas aeruginosa* as primary pathogen in, 218
  pharyngitis in, *Chlamydia trachomatis* and *Mycoplasma pneumoniae*, 210
  pneumonia in, cause and clinical manifestations, 208
  tuberculosis in, spinal, treatment, 131
  young, as source of maternal and congenital cytomegalovirus infection, 83
Chills
  amphotericin B causing, and prostaglandin synthesis, 107

Chlamydia trachomatis
  infection, and pregnancy outcome, 185
  pharyngitis, in children, 210
Chloroquine
  action against *Plasmodium falciparum*, and acid-vesicle function and intracellular pathogens, 123
Cilastatin
  -imipenem, in severe clinical infections, 50
Ciprofloxacin
  in clinical infections, severe, 50
Circumsporozoite
  protein, malaria, use of new T-helper epitope on (in mice), 115
Cirrhosis
  in hepatitis B, influence of hepatitis delta virus on, 74
Clinics
  sexually transmitted disease, HIV infection among patients attending, 153
Clonorchiasis
  praziquantel in, 111
Clostridium
  difficile diarrhea in critically ill burned patients, 143
Colds
  rhinovirus, kinins in, 96
Colistin
  inhalation therapy in cystic fibrosis patients with chronic *Pseudomonas aeruginosa* lung infection, 7
Colitis
  hemorrhagic, due to *Escherichia coli* 0157:H7, outbreak in nursing home, 12
Colony-stimulating factor
  granulocyte-macrophage, effect on myelopoiesis in AIDS, 179
Congenital defects
  temporal relations between maternal rubella and, 90
Conjunctivitis
  purulent, in Brazilian purpuric fever (see Brazilian purpuric fever)
Cornea
  transplant, HIV transmission by, 155
Cost
  -effectiveness of prenatal screening and immunization for hepatitis B virus, 79
  of influenza type A infection prevention and control in nursing homes, 95
  of intravenous therapy administration set replacement at 48- vs. 72-hour intervals, 189

of nephrotoxicity of aminoglycosides, 47
Cough
  persistent, due to *Bordetella pertussis* infection, 8
Critically ill
  burned patients, *Clostridium difficile* diarrhea in, 143
  emergency patients, unsuspected HIV in, 152
Cruzin
  similarity to high-density lipoprotein, 128
Cryptococcal
  meningitis, amphotericin B-flucytosine in, 105
Cultures
  Isolator, in catheter sepsis, 195
^{13}C-urea breath test
  detecting *Campylobacter pylori*, 15
Cutaneous (*see* Skin)
Cyst
  antigens, encystation and expression by *Giardia lamblia* in vitro (in mice), 130
Cystic fibrosis
  patients with chronic *Pseudomonas aeruginosa* lung infection, colistin inhalation therapy in, 7
Cytology
  cervical, abnormal, papillomavirus infections in women with and without, 92
Cytomegalovirus
  disease after transplant
    marrow, acyclovir preventing, 87
    renal, CMV immune globulin preventing, 85
  infection
    ganciclovir in, 88
    after marrow transplant, acyclovir preventing, 87
    maternal and congenital, young children as source of, 83
  retinopathy, ganciclovir in, 180
  transmission risk to health care workers exposed to AIDS and AIDS-related conditions, 147

D

Day care settings
  Hemophilus influenzae type b disease transmission in, 222
Delta
  virus (*see* Hepatitis, delta)

Dental
  bacteremia, amoxicillin prophylaxis, in children, 3
  professionals, risk of HIV infection among, 148
Dermatitis
  nosocomial, due to pigeon mite infestation, 204
Diarrhea
  Bacteroides fragilis in, 19
  Clostridium difficile, in critically ill burned patients, 143
  travelers', prevention with tablet form bismuth subsalicylate, 18
Diphtheria
  toxoid conjugate vaccine, *Haemophilus influenzae* type b polysaccharide-, efficacy, in infant, 37
DNA
  Plasmodium falciparum sporozoite vaccine, safety and efficacy of, 118
Doxycycline
  prophylaxis for falciparum malaria, 113
Drainage
  devices, transhepatic biliary, causing infections, 199
Drug
  abusers
    intravenous, febrile, inability to predict diagnosis in, 237
    parenteral, hepatitis delta and hepatitis B outbreak in, 73

E

Ehrlichia
  infection after tick exposure, 228
Elderly
  men, institutionalized, bacteriuria in, 23
  women, institutionalized, therapy vs. no therapy for asymptomatic bacteriuria in, 20
Emergency
  patients, critically ill, unsuspected HIV in, 152
Encephalitis
  herpes simplex
    antibodies to herpes simplex virus in CSF fluid in, 80
    type 1 and 2, neonatal, neurological outcome, 213
  toxoplasma, therapy for, 173
Encystation
  of cyst antigens by *Giardia lamblia* in vitro (in mice), 130

Endocarditis
   native valve, due to coagulase-negative
      staphylococci, 2
Endophthalmitis
   microbial, due to ocular trauma, 71
Enteric
   Campylobacter infections, in infant,
      17
Enteritis
   necroticans among Khmer children,
      223
Enterobacterial
   carriage, periurethral, preceding urinary
      infection, 22
Enterotoxigenic
   Bacteroides fragilis in diarrhea, 19
   Escherichia coli, oral challenge with,
      milk immunoglobulin concentrate
      for protection against, 11
Epitope
   new T-helper, use on malaria
      circumsporozoite protein (in mice),
      115
   T4 (CD4), anti-idiotypic antibodies
      mimicking, neutralization of HIV
      isolates by (in mice), 182
Escherichia coli
   enterotoxigenic, oral challenge with,
      milk immunoglobulin concentrate
      for protection against, 11
   0157:H7, outbreak in nursing home,
      12

F

Falciparum
   malaria (*see* Malaria, falciparum)
Families
   of children with AIDS and antibodies to
      HIV, 149
Febrile
   children, antibiotics for occult
      bacteremia in, 219
   illness, unexplained, after tick exposure,
      228
   intravenous drug abusers, inability to
      predict diagnosis in, 237
Fever
   amphotericin B causing, and
      prostaglandin synthesis, 107
   Brazilian purpuric (*see* Brazilian
      purpuric fever)
   Lassa, clinical diagnosis and course of,
      92
   outbreak due to *Streptobacillus
      moniliformis*, 58
   typhoid (*see* Typhoid)

Fibrosis
   cystic, chronic *Pseudomonas aeruginosa*
      lung infection and colistin
      inhalation therapy, 7
Flucytosine
   in meningitis, cryptococcal, 105
Fungal
   infections in neutropenic cancer
      patients, amphotericin B or
      ketoconazole for, 137
   sepsis prevention in prolonged
      neutropenic patients, 135
Fungemia
   Malassezia furfur
      catheter-associated, intravenous,
      190
   in infancy, 104

G

Ganciclovir
   in cytomegalovirus infection, 88
   in retinopathy, cytomegalovirus, 180
Gene
   bacterial, integration and expression in
      mosquito *Anopheles sambiae*,
      235
Genital
   herpes during pregnancy, effects on
      infants of first episode of, 84
Gentamicin
   -resistant *Streptococcus faecalis* causing
      nosocomial infection, 205
Gentian violet
   skin-marking solution, contaminated,
      causing *Mycobacterium chelonae*
      wound infections after plastic
      surgery, 132
Giardia lamblia
   encystation and expression of cyst
      antigens by, in vitro (in mice), 130
Globulin
   immune (*see* Immunoglobulin)
Glove and gown
   isolation precautions preventing
      nosocomial respiratory syncytial
      virus infections, 203
Glucocorticoids
   in sepsis, systemic, mortality after, 1
Glycine
   betaine isolation from urine, 26
Gown and glove
   isolation precautions preventing
      nosocomial respiratory syncytial
      virus infections, 203
gp41
   antibodies to, in hemophilia, 158

Granulocyte
-macrophage colony-stimulating factor, effect on myelopoiesis in AIDS, 179
marginated and marrow reserve, functional capacity of, 232

H

Haemophilus aegyptius
bacteremia in Brazilian purpuric fever, 66
Haemophilus influenzae
type b infection
in high-risk infant, prevention with BPIG, 38
second episodes after rifampin prophylaxis, 54
transmission in day care settings, 222
type b vaccine, in infant
capsular polysaccharide, immunogenicity of, 36
polysaccharide-diphtheria toxoid conjugate, efficacy of, 37
Hairy
leukoplakia (*see* Leukoplakia, oral hairy)
Hand
Mycobacterium marinum infection of, treatment results, 133
Health
care workers exposed to AIDS and AIDS-related conditions, risk of transmitting HIV, CMV and HBV to, 147
Hematologic
malignancy (*see* Cancer, hematologic)
Hemophilia
HIV antigen and antibodies to p24 and gp41 in, 158
Hemorrhagic
colitis due to *Escherichia coli* 0157:H7, outbreak in nursing home, 12
Hepatitis
B
chronic, adenine arabinoside monophosphate and interferon in, 75
chronic, influence of hepatitis delta virus infection on progression to cirrhosis in, 74
-hepatitis delta coinfection in drug abusers, 73
screening during pregnancy, 77
screening during pregnancy, cost-effectiveness of, 79
surface antigen in blood samples, prevalence of, 154

transmission risk to health care workers exposed to AIDS and AIDS-related conditions, 147
delta
-hepatitis B coinfection in drug abusers, 73
infection, and progression to cirrhosis in chronic hepatitis B, 74
post-vaccination, in 1942 epidemic in U.S. Army, follow-up, 76
Herpes
genital, during pregnancy, effects on infants of first episode of, 84
simplex virus
antibodies in CSF of herpes simplex encephalitis patients, 80
type 1 and type 2 neonatal encephalitis, neurological outcome, 213
virus infection, childhood, MRI of brain in, 81
Hickman
intravenous catheter-associated primary cutaneous aspergillosis, 191
Histamine
type 2 blockers, nosocomial pneumonia in intubated patients after, 201
HIV
antibodies to (*see* Antibodies, to HIV)
antigen in hemophilia, 158
antigenemia
AZT in, 164
AZT in, in AIDS, 164
in homosexual men, and risk of AIDS and AIDS-related complex, 165
HTLV-4 and, in West Africa, 151
infection
CNS in, 172
HIV-2, and AIDS, in West Africa, 151
in homosexuals, seronegative, with acute viral syndrome, 168
leukoplakia and, oral hairy, 168
in parturients, serosurvey of, 154
among patients attending clinics for sexually transmitted diseases, 153
risk among dental professionals, 148
sexually transmitted, long term latency preceding overt seroconversion in, 161
syphilis and, secondary, neurologic relapse after benzathine penicillin for, 167
isolates, neutralization by anti-idiotypic antibodies which mimic T4 (CD4) epitope (in mice), 182
Kaposi's sarcoma and seronegative secondary syphilis, 166

screening for, compulsory premarital, 163
transmission
by organ donation, 155
reduction among homosexual/bisexual men, 157
risk to health care workers exposed to AIDS and AIDS-related conditions, 147
by transfusions screened as negative for HIV antibody, 157
by transplantation, 156
unsuspected, in critically ill emergency patients, 152
Homosexual
/bisexual men, HIV transmission reduction among, 157
men, HIV antigenemia in, and risk of AIDS and AIDS-related complex, 165
seronegative, HIV infection and acute viral syndrome in, 168
HTLV
-1 infection in leukemia patients, 96
-4, and HIV, in West Africa, 151

I

Ig (see Immunoglobulin)
Illness
causality of, nursery school children's views on, 217
Imaging
indium-111 leukocyte, in musculoskeletal sepsis, 27
magnetic resonance (see Magnetic resonance imaging)
Imipenem
-cilastatin in severe clinical infections, 50
Immune
globulin (see Immunoglobulin)
Immunization
hepatitis B virus, in infant, cost-effectiveness of, 79
oral, with *Streptococcus mutans*, secretory IgA antibodies after, 35
Immunodeficiency
candidiasis diagnosis and, invasive, 102
syndrome, acquired (see AIDS)
virus, human (see HIV)
Immunogen
synthetic, construction of, for malaria vaccine (in mice), 115

Immunogenicity
of *Haemophilus influenzae* type b capsular polysaccharide vaccines, in infant, 36
of malaria vaccine, synthetic peptide, against *Plasmodium falciparum* sporozoites, 115
Immunoglobulin
A
antibodies, secretory, after oral immunization with *Streptococcus mutans*, 35
deficiency, IgG subclass deficiency, and respiratory infections, in children, 210
bacterial polysaccharide, preventing *Haemophilus influenzae* type b infections in high-risk infants, 38
concentrate, milk, for protection against oral challenge with enterotoxigenic *Escherichia coli*, 11
cytomegalovirus, for prevention of CMV disease after kidney transplant, 85
G subclass deficiency, IgA deficiency, and respiratory infections, in children, 210
Indium-111
leukocyte imaging in musculoskeletal sepsis, 27
Infant
Campylobacter infections in, enteric, 17
effects of first episode of genital herpes during pregnancy, 84
Haemophilus influenzae type b vaccine in (see *Haemophilus influenzae*, type b vaccine, in infant)
high-risk, BPIG preventing *Haemophilus influenzae* type b infections in, 38
Malassezia fufur fungemia in, 104
rotavirus vaccine in, 224
Infections
biliary drainage devices causing, transhepatic, 199
clinical, severe, ciprofloxacin vs. imipenem-cilastatin in, 50
after liver transplant, 144
Influenza
infections, type A, in nursing homes, 95
Intensive care
management, and tetanus prognosis, 68
unit, neonatal, coagulase-negative staphylococcal bacteremia in, 207
Interferon
leukocyte, in chronic hepatitis B, 75

Intracellular
  pathogens, acid-vesicle function, and action of chloroquine against *Plasmodium falciparum*, 123
Intravenous
  therapy, replacing administration sets at 48- vs. 72-hour intervals, 189
Intubated patients
  nosocomial pneumonia after sucralfate therapy in, 201
Isolation
  precautions, glove and gown, for prevention of nosocomial respiratory syncytial virus infections, 203
Isolator cultures
  in catheter sepsis, suspected, 195
Ivermectin
  in onchocerciasis, 111

K

Kaposi's sarcoma
  HIV and seronegative secondary syphilis, 166
Kawasaki syndrome
  adult, 225
Kenya
  malaria prophylaxis in American and Swiss travelers to, 112
Ketoconazole
  in fungal infections in neutropenic cancer patients, 137
  high-dose, pharmacology and toxicity of, 106
Khmer children
  enteritis necroticans among, 223
Kidney
  disease, autosomal dominant polycystic, renal infection in, 26
  infection
    acute, in women, treatment of, 24
    in polycystic kidney disease, autosomal dominant, 26
  transplantation (*see* Transplantation, kidney)
Kinins
  in rhinovirus colds, 96

L

Lassa fever
  clinical diagnosis and course of, 92
Lavage
  bronchoalveolar (*see* Bronchoalveolar, lavage)

Leptospirosis
  penicillin in, IV, 67
Leukemia
  patients, HTLV-1 infection in, 96
  virus, T cell (*see* HTLV)
Leukocyte
  imaging, indium-111, in musculoskeletal sepsis, 27
  interferon in chronic hepatitis B, 75
Leukoplakia
  oral hairy
    acyclovir in, 181
    HIV infection and AIDS, 168
Lipoprotein
  high-density, similarity of cruzin to, 128
Liver
  transplant, infections after, 144
Lumbar
  punctures in newborn with respiratory distress syndrome, 214
  spine tuberculosis, treatment of, 131
Lung
  bullae with air-fluid levels, 10
  disease due to *Mycobacterium malmoense*, 132
  infection, chronic *Pseudomonas aeruginosa*, in cystic fibrosis patients, and colistin inhalation therapy, 7
Lyme disease
  arthritis of, clinical evolution, 59
  neuropathy in, peripheral, 62
  seasonal variation of transmission risk of, 59
Lymphotropic
  virus, T-, human (*see* HTLV)

M

Macrophage
  -granulocyte colony-stimulating factor, effect on myelopoiesis in AIDS, 179
Magnetic resonance imaging
  of brain in childhood herpesvirus infections, 81
  of CNS involvement in AIDS and HIV infections, 172
Malaria
  circumsporozoite protein, use of new T-helper epitope on (in mice), 115
  clinical, in semi-immune children exposed to intense and perennial transmission, 120
  falciparum
    doxycycline prophylaxis for, 113
    splenic function during, 121

prevention, and naturally acquired
     antibodies to sporozoites,
     117
  prophylaxis in travelers to Kenya,
     efficacy of, 112
  vaccine, synthetic peptide, against
     Plasmodium falciparum
     sporozoites, safety and
     immunogenicity of, 115
Malassezia furfur
  catheter colonization with, central
     venous, 105
  fungemia (*see* Fungemia, *Malassezia furfur*)
Malignancy (*see* Cancer)
Marrow
  failure after AZT in AIDS, 176
  reserve granulocytes, functional capacity
     of, 232
  transplantation, acyclovir preventing
     CMV infection and disease after, 87
Maternal
  cytomegalovirus infection, young
     children as source of, 83
  rubella, temporal relations between
     congenital defects and, 90
Meningitis
  cryptococcal, amphotericin B-flucytosine
     in, 105
Menstrual
  toxic shock syndrome related to tampon
     characteristics, 68
Methylprednisolone
  in sepsis and septic shock, 1
Miconazole
  prophylaxis of fungal sepsis in
     prolonged neutropenia, 135
Microbial
  endophthalmitis due to ocular trauma, 71
Microbiology
  of endocarditis, native valve, due to
     coagulase-negative staphylococci, 2
Milk
  immunoglobulin concentrate for
     protection against oral challenge
     with enterotoxigenic *Escherichia coli*, 11
  pasteurized, causing
     antimicrobial-resistant
     salmonellosis, 13
Mite
  infestation, pigeon, causing nosocomial
     dermatitis and pruritis, 204
Monkeypox
  clinical features of, 93

Mortality
  in-hospital, for *Pneumocystis carinii*
     pneumonia in AIDS, early
     predictors of, 173
  of pneumonia, community-acquired, 6
  in sepsis, systemic, and glucocorticoids, 1
Mosquito
  Anopheles sambiae, integration and
     expression of bacterial gene in, 235
MRI (*see* Magnetic resonance imaging)
Musculoskeletal
  sepsis, indium-111 leukocyte imaging
     in, 27
Mycetoma
  actinomycotic, amikacin and
     trimethoprim-sulfamethoxazole in, 33
Mycobacterium
  chelonae wound infections after plastic
     surgery, 132
  malmoense causing pulmonary disease, 132
  marinum infection of hand and wrist,
     treatment results, 133
Mycoplasma pneumoniae
  pharyngitis, in children, 210
Myelopoiesis
  in AIDS, effect of
     granulocyte-macrophage
     colony-stimulating factor on, 179
Myocardial
  retrovirus, and congestive
     cardiomyopathy in AIDS, 169

N

nalidixic acid
  plasmid-resistance to, in *Shigella
     dysenteriae* type 1, 53
Neonate (*see* Newborn)
Neoplasia
  penile intraepithelial,
     papillomavirus-associated, in sexual
     partners of women with cervical
     intraepithelial neoplasia, 185
Nephrotoxicity
  aminoglycoside, cost of, 47
  amphotericin B, after sodium
     supplements with ticarcillin or
     saline, 108
Nervous system
  central, in AIDS and HIV infections, 172

Subject Index / 249

Neuraminidase
  inhibitor, *Trypanosoma cruzi*, cruzin as, similarity to high-density lipoprotein, 128
Neurologic
  manifestations of AIDS, 169
  outcome of encephalitis, neonatal herpes simplex type 1 and 2, 213
  relapse after benzathine penicillin for secondary syphilis in HIV infection, 167
Neuropathy
  peripheral, due to Lyme disease, 62
Neuropsychologic testing
  of CNS involvement in AIDS and HIV infections, 172
Neutropenia
  in cancer patients, amphotericin B or ketoconazole for fungal infections in, 137
  in newborn, with presumed sepsis, buffy coat transfusions in, 207
  prolonged, prevention of fungal sepsis in, 135
Neutrophils
  tobacco smokers', desensitized to chemotactic peptide-stimulated oxygen uptake, 230
Newborn
  encephalitis, herpes simplex virus type 1 and type 2, neurological outcome, 213
  intensive care unit, coagulase-negative staphylococcal bacteremia in, 207
  lumbar punctures in respiratory distress syndrome, 214
  neutropenic, with presumed sepsis, buffy coat transfusions in, 207
Nosocomial
  dermatitis due to pigeon mite infestation, 204
  pneumonia in intubated patients after sucralfate therapy, 201
  pruritis due to pigeon mite infestation, 204
  respiratory syncytial virus infections, prevention of, 203
  Streptococcus faecalis infection, gentamicin-resistant, 205
Nucleus pulposus
  antibiotic penetration into (in rabbit), 57
Nursery school
  children's views on causality of illness, 217

Nursing home
  Escherichia coli 0157:H7 outbreak in, 12
  influenza infections in, type A, 95

O

Ocular
  trauma causing microbial endophthalmitis, 71
Onchocerciasis
  ivermectin in, 111
Oral
  leukoplakia (*see* Leukoplakia, oral hairy)
Organ
  donation, HIV transmission by, 155
Osteoarticular
  infections, acute suppurative, antimicrobial therapy for, 31
Osteomyelitis
  antimicrobial therapy for, oral, 32
  bactericidal test in, standardized serum, 28
  chronic recurrent multifocal, follow-up, 236
Otitis
  malignant external, therapy of, 56
Oxygen
  uptake, chemotactic peptide-stimulated, and tobacco smokers' neutrophils, 230

P

Papillomavirus
  -associated penile intraepithelial neoplasia in sexual partners of women with cervical intraepithelial neoplasia, 185
  infections in women with and without abnormal cervical cytology, 92
Paralysis
  pelagic, discussion of, 234
Paralytic
  poliomyelitis, vaccine-associated, 94
Parturients
  HIV infection in, serosurvey of, 154
Pasteurized milk
  salmonellosis due to, antimicrobial-resistant, 13
Pathogens
  intracellular, acid-vesicle function, and action of chloroquiine against *Plasmodium falciparum*, 123
Pediatric (*see* Children)

Pelagic
  paralysis, discussion of, 234
Penicillin
  benzathine, for secondary syphilis with HIV infection, neurologic relapse after, 167
  broad-spectrum, causing platelet-mediated bleeding, 57
  immediate, for group A beta-hemolytic streptococcal pharyngitis, 52
  IV, in leptospirosis, 67
Penile
  intraepithelial neoplasia, papillomavirus-associated, in sexual partners of women with cervical intraepithelial neoplasia, 185
Pentamidine
  administration, torsade de pointes during, 126
  aerosolized, for *Pneumocystis carinii* pneumonia in AIDS, 176
  inhaled or reduced-dose intravenous, for *Pneumocystis carinii* pneumonia, 177
Peptide
  chemotactic, stimulating oxygen uptake, and tobacco smokers' neutrophils, 230
Peritonitis
  bacterial, *Pseudomonas aeruginosa* as primary pathogen in, in children, 218
Periurethral
  enterobacterial carriage preceding urinary infection, 22
Pharmacology
  of ketoconazole, high-dose, 106
Pharyngitis
  Chlamydia trachomatis and *Mycoplasma pneumoniae* causing, in children, 210
  streptococcal, group A beta-hemolytic, immediate penicillin for, 52
Pigeon
  mite infestation causing nosocomial dermatitis and pruritis, 204
Plasmid
  -mediated nalidixic acid resistance in *Shigella dysenteriae* type 1, 53
Plasmodium falciparum
  chloroquine action against, and acid-vesicle function and intracellular pathogens, 123
  malaria (*see* Malaria, falciparum)
  sporozoite vaccine
    DNA, safety and efficacy of, 118
    safety and immunogenicity of, 115

Plastic
  surgery, *Mycobacterium chelonae* wound infections after, 132
Platelet
  -mediated bleeding due to broad-spectrum penicillins, 57
Pneumocystis carinii
  pneumonia (*see* Pneumonia, *Pneumocystis carinii*)
Pneumonia
  bacterial, acute, diagnosis by bronchoalveolar lavage, 140
  in children, cause and clinical manifestations, 208
  community-acquired, survey of, 6
  nosocomial, in intubated patients after sucralfate therapy, 201
  Pneumocystis carinii
    in AIDS (*see* AIDS, *Pneumocystis carinii* pneumonia in)
    pentamidine in, inhaled or reduced-dose intravenous, 177
Poliomyelitis
  paralytic, vaccine-associated, 94
Polycystic
  kidney disease, autosomal dominant, renal infection in, 26
Polysaccharide
  Haemophilus influenzae type b, -diphtheria toxoid conjugate vaccine, efficacy, in infant, 37
  immune globulin, bacterial, preventing *Haemophilus influenzae* type b infections in high-risk infants, 38
  of *Salmonella typhi*, Vi capsular, preventing typhoid fever, 42
  vaccine
    Haemophilus influenzae type b, immunogenicity, in infant, 36
    Vi capsular, for typhoid fever, 44
Post-vaccination
  hepatitis in U.S. Army, 1942 epidemic, follow-up, 76
Praziquantel
  in clonorchiasis, 111
Pregnancy
  genital herpes during, effects on infants of first episode of, 84
  hepatitis B screening during, 77
    cost-effectiveness of, 79
  HIV testing programs during, 154
  outcome, and *Chlamydia trachomatis* infection, 185
Premarital
  screening for HIV, compulsory, 163
Prenatal screening
  for hepatitis B, 77
    cost-effectiveness of, 79

Pressure
  sores, and bone infection, 29
Proline
  betaine isolation from urine, 26
Prostaglandin
  synthesis, and chills and fever due to amphotericin B, 107
Protein
  malaria circumsporozoite, use of new T-helper epitope on (in mice), 115
Pruritis
  nosocomial, due to pigeon mite infestation, 204
Pseudomonas aeruginosa
  lung infection in cystic fibrosis, and colistin inhalation therapy, 7
  as primary pathogen in bacterial peritonitis, in children, 218
p24
  antibodies to, in hemophilia, 158
Pulmonary (*see* Lung)
Punctures
  lumbar, in newborn with respiratory distress syndrome, 214
Purpura
  fulminans in Brazilian purpuric fever (*see* Brazilian purpuric fever)
Purpuric
  fever, Brazilian (*see* Brazilian purpuric fever)

Q

4-Quinolones
  co-administration, caffeine elimination after, 49

R

Radioimmunoassay
  Aspergillus fumigatus antigen, for aspergillosis in hematologic malignancy, 100
Renal (*see* Kidney)
Respiratory
  distress syndrome, lumbar punctures in newborn with, 214
  infection
    bacterial, diagnosis by bronchoalveolar lavage, 138
    IgG subclass deficiency and IgA deficiency, in children, 210
    syncytial virus infections, nosocomial, prevention of, 203
Retinopathy
  cytomegalovirus, ganciclovir in, 180

Retrovirus
  myocardial, and congestive cardiomyopathy in AIDS, 169
Rhinovirus
  colds, kinins in, 96
Rifampin
  prophylaxis in *Hemophilus influenzae* type b disease, second episodes after, 54
Rotavirus
  vaccine (RIT 4237), in infant, 224
Rubella
  maternal, temporal relations between congenital defects and, 90

S

Saline
  IV, amphotericin B nephrotoxicity after, 108
Salmonella
  typhi Vi capsular polysaccharide preventing typhoid fever, 42
Salmonellosis
  antimicrobial-resistant, due to pasteurized milk, 13
Sarcoma
  Kaposi's, HIV and seronegative secondary syphilis, 166
Seasonal
  variation of transmission risk of Lyme disease and babesiosis, 59
Sepsis
  catheter-related
    central venous, diagnosis, 193
    Isolator cultures in, 195
  fungal, prevention in prolonged neutropenic patients, 135
  musculoskeletal, indium-111 leukocyte imaging in, 27
  presumed, in neutropenic neonates, buffy coat transfusions in, 207
  severe, methylprednisolone in, 1
  systemic, glucocorticoids in, mortality after, 1
Septic
  arthritis (*see* Arthritis, septic)
  shock, methylprednisolone in, 1
Serodiagnosis
  of invasive aspergillosis in hematologic malignancy, 100
Serological
  tests for blastomycosis, 99
Serratia
  marcescens causing septic arthritis, associated with benzalkonium chloride antiseptic, 34

Sexual
  partners of women with cervical intraepithelial neoplasia, papillomavirus-associated penile intraepithelial neoplasia in, 185
Sexually transmitted
  disease clinics, HIV infection among patients attending, 153
  infection, long term latency preceding overt seroconversion in, 161
Shigella
  bacteremia, in adults, 5
Shigella
  dysenteriae type 1, plasmid-resistance to nalidixic acid in, 53
Shock
  septic, methylprednisolone in, 1
  toxic shock syndrome, menstrual, related to tampon characteristics, 68
Skin
  aspergillosis, primary, Hickman intravenous catheter-associated, 191
  -marking solution, contaminated gentian violet, causing *Mycobacterium chelonae* wound infections after plastic surgery, 132
Smokers
  tobacco, neutrophils in, densensitized to chemotactic peptide-stimulated oxygen uptake, 230
Sodium
  supplements, amphotericin B nephrotoxicity after, 108
Sore
  pressure, and bone infection, 29
Spine
  tuberculosis, treatment, 131
Spleen
  function during falciparum malaria, 121
Sporozoites
  antibodies to, naturally acquired, and malaria prevention, 117
  Plasmodium falciparum (see *Plasmodium falciparum*, sporozoite vaccine)
Staphylococci
  coagulase-negative
    bacteremia due to, in neonatal intensive care unit, 207
    endocarditis due to, native valve, 2
    vancomycin resistance in, 51
Staphylococcus
  aureus bacteremia in hematological malignancies and/or agranulocytosis, 141

Streptobacillus
  moniliformis causing fever outbreak, 58
Streptococcal
  pharyngitis, group A beta-hemolytic, immediate penicillin for, 52
Streptococcus
  faecalis, gentamicin-resistant, causing nosocomial infection, 205
  mutans, oral immunization with, secretory IgA antibodies after, 35
Sucralfate
  in intubated patients, nosocomial pneumonia after, 201
Sulfamethoxazole (see Trimethoprim, -sulfamethoxazole)
Supraglottitis
  adult, 7
Surgery
  plastic, *Mycobacterium chelonae* wound infections after, 132
Swiss travelers
  to Kenya, malaria prophylaxis in, 112
Syphilis
  secondary
    HIV infection and, neurologic relapse after benzathine penicillin in, 167
    seronegative, in patient with HIV and Kaposi's sarcoma, 166

T

Tampon
  characteristics related to menstrual toxic shock syndrome, 68
T cell
  leukemia virus (see HTLV)
Temporal
  relations between maternal rubella and congenital defects, 90
Tetanus
  prognosis, and intensive care management, 68
T4 (CD4) epitope
  anti-idiotypic antibodies mimicking, neutralization of HIV isolates by (in mice), 182
T-helper
  epitope, new, use on malaria circumsporozoite protein (in mice), 115
Thoracic
  spine tuberculosis, treatment of, 131
Ticarcillin
  amphotericin B nephrotoxicity after, 108

Tick
 exposure, unexplained febrile illness after, 228
T-lymphotropic
 virus, human (see HTLV)
Tobacco
 smokers' neutrophils desensitized to chemotactic peptide-stimulated oxygen uptake, 230
Torsade de pointes
 during pentamidine administration, 126
Toxic
 shock syndrome, menstrual, related to tampon characteristics, 68
Toxicity
 auditory, of aminoglycosides, 46
 of AZT in AIDS and AIDS-related complex, 175
 of ketoconazole, high-dose, 106
 nephrotoxicity (see Nephrotoxicity)
Toxoplasma
 encephalitis, therapy for, 173
Toxoplasmosis
 in renal transplant recipients, 144
Transfusion
 buffy coat, in neutropenic neonates with presumed sepsis, 207
 screened as negative for HIV antibody, HIV transmission by, 157
Transplantation
 cornea, HIV transmission by, 155
 HIV transmission by, 156
 kidney
  cytomegalovirus disease in recipients after, cytomegalovirus immune globulin for prevention of, 85
  HIV transmission by, 155
  toxoplasmosis in recipients, 144
 liver, infections after, 144
 marrow, acyclovir preventing CMV infection and disease after, 87
Trauma
 ocular, causing microbial endophthalmitis, 71
Travelers
 diarrhea in, prevention with tablet form bismuth subsalicylate, 18
 to Kenya, efficacy of malaria prophylaxis in, 112
 -sulfamethoxazole
  in mycetoma, actinomycotic, 33
  in renal infection, in women, 24
Trimetrexate
 for *Pneumocystis carinii* pneumonia in AIDS, 178

Trypanosoma cruzi
 neuraminidase inhibitor, cruzin, similarity to high-density lipoprotein, 128
Tuberculosis
 of spine, treatment, 131
Typhoid
 prevention with Vi capsular polysasccharide of *Salmonella typhi*, 42
 vaccine
  Ty21a live oral, capsule form, 41
  Vi capsular polysasccharide, 44
Ty21a
 live oral typhoid vaccine in capsule form, 41

U

Urea
 ^{13}C-, breath test detecting *Campylobacter pylori*, 15
Urinary
 infection, periurethral enterobacterial carriage preceding, 22
Urine
 glycine betaine and proline betaine isolation from, 26

V

Vaccination
 for influenza type A in nursing homes, benefits and costs of, 95
 post-vaccination hepatitis in U.S. Army, 1942 epidemic, follow-up, 76
Vaccine
 AIDS, potential, 182
 -associated paralytic poliomyelitis, 94
 Haemophilus influenzae type b (see *Haemophilus influenzae*, type b vaccine)
 malaria, synthetic peptide, against *Plasmodium falciparum* sporozoites, safety and immunogencity of, 115
 Plasmodium falciparum sporozoite, DNA, safety and efficacy of, 118
 rotavirus (RIT 4237), in infant, 224
 typhoid (see Typhoid, vaccine)
Valve
 native, endocarditis due to coagulase-negative staphylococci, 2
Vancomycin
 resistance in coagulase-negative staphylococci, 51

Venous
  catheter (see Catheter, central venous)
Vesicle
  acid-, function, intracellular pathogens, and action of chloroquine against *Plasmodium falciparum*, 123
Vi
  capsular polysaccharide of *Salmonella typhi* preventing typhoid fever, 42
  capsular polysaccharide vaccine for typhoid fever, 44
Vidarabine
  phosphate in chronic hepatitis B, 75
Virus
  cytomegalovirus (see Cytomegalovirus)
  hepatitis (see Hepatitis)
  herpes (see Herpes)
  immunodeficiency, human (see HIV)
  papillomavirus (see Papillomavirus)
  respiratory syncytial, nosocomial infections, prevention of, 203
  retrovirus, myocardial, and congestive cardiomyopathy in AIDS, 169
  rhinovirus colds, kinins in, 96
  rotavirus vaccine, in infant, 224
  syndrome, acute, and HIV infection in seronegative homosexuals, 168
  T cell leukemia (see HTLV)
  T-lymphotropic, human (see HTLV)

W

White blood cell (see Leukocyte)
Wound
  infections, *Mycobacterium chelonae*, after plastic surgery, 132
Wrist
  Mycobacterium marinum infection in, treatment results, 133

Z

Zidovudine (see AZT)

Author Index

A

Ablashi DV, 181
Abrams DI, 168
Abrouk F, 193
Acharya IL, 42
Ackley A, 28
Affeldt JC, 71
Ahmed Zu, 53
Albaum M, 151
Alberti A, 74
Alberts WM, 132
Alford CA, 83
Allain J-P, 158, 161
Allegra CJ, 178
Allen JR, 157
Allo MD, 191
Almeido-Hill J, 38
Alpert G, 104
Alpert LC, 15
Alsip SG, 106
Ambrosino DM, 38
Amstutz HC, 27
Anderson RD, 81
Anderson RE, 157
Anderson RL, 34
Antonen J, 161
Araujo V, 46
Archer GL, 2
Arden NH, 95
Arevalo JA, 79
Armand J, 42, 44
Armstrong D, 96
Aronoff SC, 218
Aschner JL, 105
Ashe KM, 36
Ashton JJ, 57
Aspery KM, 38
Atherton S, 181
Atkinson JH, 172
Awe RJ, 10
Aziz MA, 111

B

Bagar S, 115
Baird B, 178
Baker AS, 7
Baker JL, 152
Bal JF Jr, 81
Baley JE, 207
Balfour HH Jr, 87
Balis F, 178
Balk RA, 1
Ballou WR, 118
Bander SJ, 26
Barin F, 151
Barrasso R, 185
Barrett FF, 196
Barry MJ, 163
Bart KJ, 94

Baughman RP, 140
Beard LJ, 210
Beebe GW, 76
Beer C, 49
Beier JC, 117
Bell LM, 104
Benedetti J, 84
Benson PM, 166
Berardi VP, 85
Beraud-Cassel AM, 17
Bergman AG, 205
Berkley SF, 68
Berry CD, 167
Berry S, 84
Berzofsky JA, 115
Bessette R, 73
Bissett J, 75
Bitsura JAM, 18
Bjornson J, 23
Blaauw B, 168
Black J, 32
Black RE, 41
Blackwelder WC, 105
Blake PA, 13
Bland LA, 132
Block CS, 5
Blumer JL, 218
Bodey GP, 137
Bone RC, 1
Bonet M, 46
Borczyk AA, 12
Borner K, 50
Boscaro S, 74
Bosser C, 158
Botticelli JT, 189
Boudreau EF, 113
Boutton TW, 15
Bowen PA II, 156
Bowles CA, 105
Bowmer MI, 186
Boye C, 151
Bradley JS, 215
Braine HG, 135
Branch RA, 108
Brandt AM, 163
Brandt JT, 57
Bridges RB, 230
Brighton CT, 57
Britt WJ, 83
Broome CV, 68
Brown BW Jr, 75
Brown ZA, 84
Bruckner HW, 199
Brumfitt W, 22
Brun-Buisson C, 193
Brunette EN, 176
Bryan L, 20
Bryant-LeBlanc CE, 147
Bryla DA, 42
Brynes RK, 176
Bryson RJ, 185
Bukholm G, 70
Bunnag D, 121
Burge G, 38

Burke RA, 201
Bush HL Jr, 85
Bush TJ, 150
Buskell-Bales Z, 76
Butler DF, 225
Byass P, 224

C

Cadoz M, 42, 44
Calabrese LH, 169
Calderwood SB, 2
Calubaquib C, 67
Campbell CH, 153
Campos JM, 104
Cannon RO, 153
Caputo GM, 2
Carlson JAK, 12
Carlson JR, 147
Carpenter CB, 85
Carson LA, 132
Carter AO, 12
Caruana RJ, 156
Cassidy R, 77
Castillo A, 68
Cates KL, 54
Causey D, 176
Cederberg DM, 88
Celli BR, 201
Chabner BA, 178
Chamaret S, 151
Chambers HF, 147
Chambers ST, 26
Champalimaud J-L, 151
Champlin RE, 180
Chanatry J, 210
Chandler KW, 132
Chanh TC, 182
Charlton RK, 232
Chase P, 208
Chatterjee S, 80
Chein N, 96
Cherry JD, 180
Chesney PJ, 109
Ching DK, 215
Cho SI, 85
Chow SP, 133
Chulay JD, 117, 118
Clarkson B, 96
Clarkson JG, 71
Clavel F, 151
Cleary PD, 163
Clemmer TP, 1
Cload P, 164
Cloud GA, 105, 106
Clyde DF, 115
Codd EE, 230
Cohen ML, 13
Cohn DL, 157
Collier AC, 167
Collins RJ, 133
Conant MA, 168

Coninx R, 223
Connell ML, 47
Connolly CK, 6
Conte JE Jr, 177
Cooke RA, 223
Coon HG, 235
Copelan EA, 57
Corey L, 84, 213
Corkery KJ, 176
Cornette JL, 115
Cortesia M, 115
Corvi G, 190
Counts GW, 24
Coutinho RA, 164, 165
Coyle PK, 62
Cramton T, 42
Craven DE, 201, 204
Craven PC, 105, 106
Critchley SE, 157
Critchlow CW, 84
Crocco JA, 173
Croissant O, 185
Croll L, 38
Crowley CM, 203
Cummings MJ, 154
Curtas S, 195
Cusick LB, 132

D

Dalgleish AG, 182
Dammin GJ, 59
Dandliker PS, 87
Dang Bui RH, 144
D'Anna SA, 111
Das S, 130
Dattwyler RJ, 62
Davis AT, 219
Davis HE, 225
Davis J, 115
Davis JP, 99
Davis JR, 157
Dawson NV, 77
D'Costa LJ, 186
De Brux J, 185
Debs RJ, 176
de Gans J, 164
de la Cabada FJ, 18
DeLeo MJ, 179
De Lerma C, 111
Demopulos PA, 126
Denis F, 151
Despotes JC, 164
de Villiers E-M, 92
de Wolf F, 164, 165
Diasio RB, 105
Dietz K, 96
Diggs CL, 118
DiNubile MJ, 2
Dismukes WE, 105, 106
Disney FA, 52
Douglas H, 130
Drake JC, 178

Drew WL, 147
Driks MR, 201
Drucker M, 5
Dummer JS, 143
Dunning RW, 153
DuPont HL, 18
DuPont MW, 18
Durack DT, 174, 175
Dylewski J, 186

E

Eampokalap B, 223
Eavey RD, 7
Echeverria P, 223
Eisenberg JM, 47
Eisenberg M, 75
Eismont FJ, 57
Eldadah M, 214
Elting L, 137
Emeson EE, 164
Endo T, 13
Epstein MF, 207
Ericsson CD, 18
Eron LJ, 88
Erttmann KD, 111
Eskola J, 37
Espaä J, 68
Espersen F, 141
Esquivel C, 143
Essex M, 151
Evans DG, 15
Evans DJ Jr, 15

F

Faber V, 141
Fainstein V, 137
Falk LA, 164, 168
Farber HW, 201
Farr BM, 6
Fass RJ, 57
Fattovich G, 74
Fauci AS, 153
Favier V, 151
Feiner CJ, 237
Feinstein SA, 237
Felix AM, 115
Fellows KW, 109
Ferran F, 46
Ferrante A, 210
Ferreccio C, 41
Fiddian AP, 164
Fields HA, 73
Filler SJ, 35
Fineberg HV, 163
Fischl MA, 174, 175
Fishbein DB, 228
Fisher CJ Jr, 1
Fisher JF, 105
Flaherty RJ, 19
Fleisher G, 219

Flournoy N, 87
Flynn HW Jr, 71
Flynn PM, 196
Forbes B, 195
Forster RK, 71
Foster S, 38
Frame PT, 140
Franchini G, 161
Francis AB, 52
Frank B, 181
Fransen L, 186
Frech K, 49
Freeman J, 203, 207
Freeman K, 148
Frenkel LD, 214
Frenkel LM, 180
Friedland GH, 148, 237
Friedman SJ, 225
Frimodt-Møller N, 141

G

Gabrilove J, 96
Galgiani JN, 106
Gallis HA, 105
Garcia CR, 190
Garcia G, 75
Gargan RA, 22
Garne S, 7
Garrett S, 38
Garvin GM, 201
Gatell JM, 46
Gauderer MWL, 218
Gault MJ, 130
Gazengel C, 158
Gee T, 96
George WL, 190
Georges AJ, 17
Georges-Courbot MC, 17
Gerber MA, 210
Gerberding JL, 147
Germanier R, 41
Gerson SL, 100
Gibson C, 13
Gigliotti F, 107
Gilbertson IT, 44
Gill PS, 176
Gillessen D, 115
Gilligan PH, 51
Gillin FD, 130
Glasser D, 153
Glick HA, 47
Godley PJ, 32
Gold JWM, 96
Goldberg H, 8
Golde DW, 179
Golden JA, 177
Goldman AL, 132
Goldman DA, 203, 207
Goldschlager N, 126
Gonzalez J, 33
Good MF, 115
Goodman RA, 95

Gordon DM, 118
Gordon LK, 37
Gostin L, 163
Gotlieb MS, 10, 174, 175, 180
Gouandjika I, 17
Goudsmit, 164, 165
Grady GF, 73, 85
Graham DY, 15
Grames GM, 144
Granoff DM, 54
Grant I, 172
Graybill JR, 106
Green JL, 52
Greene BM, 111
Greenspan D, 168
Greenspan JS, 168
Greenwood BM, 224
Gregg CR, 105
Gregory PB, 75
Gregory RL, 35
Grieco MH, 174, 175
Grogan TJ, 27
Groopman JE, 174, 175, 179
Grose C, 81
Grube BJ, 143
Guesry P, 11
Guetard D, 151
Gurubacharya VL, 42
Gurwitz A, 73
Gwadz RW, 235
Gwaltney JM, 96

H

Hadler SC, 73
Haider K, 53
Hakulinen M, 37
Halperin JJ, 62
Hamilton-Miller JMT, 22
Hamlon L, 224
Hampson M, 77
Handsfield HH, 154
Hanlon P, 224
Harder S, 49
Harding GKM, 23
Hardy D, 180
Hardy WD, 96
Hargrett-Bean NT, 13
Harinasuta T, 121
Harmon WE, 85
Harris RD, 144
Harrison BDW, 6
Hart CL, 215
Harvey B, 12
Hassam-King M, 224
Hawley HB, 28
Hayes EB, 228
Hayes R, 224
Hearst NG, 168
Hegyi T, 214
Heidemann H, 108

Heilmann C, 7
Heimbach DM, 143
Heimer EP, 115
Heinze-Lacey B, 85
Helmig O, 236
Henderson E, 23
Hendley JO, 36, 96
Henretig F, 219
Herbst JS, 181
Herrington DA, 115
Hertz R, 77
Hesselink JR, 172
Hiatt IM, 214
Hicks CB, 166
Hightower AW, 68
Hilpert H, 11
Hilton N, 208
Hinman AR, 94
Hirsch MS, 175
Hirschman SZ, 56, 199
Ho M, 121, 143
Ho WG, 180
Hoang Y, 11
Hobbs RE, 169
Hockin JC, 12
Hockmeyer WT, 118
Hoekelman RA, 52
Hoffer J, 96
Höffken G, 50
Hoffman F, 155
Hoffman SL, 117, 118
Høiby N, 7
Holland CJ, 228
Holland GN, 180
Hollander H, 168, 177
Hollingdale MR, 115, 117
Holman S, 154
Holmberg SD, 157
Holt R, 3
Holzel H, 90
Hoofnagle JH, 76
Hooijkaas C, 165
Hook EW III, 153
Hooton TM, 167
Hopewell PC, 176
Horwitz SN, 181
Hough DR, 225
House MA, 156
Huet Y, 193
Huminer D, 5
Humphries AL, 156
Hunt TL, 32
Hurwitz S, 100

I

Idelson B, 85
Ip FK, 133
Irvine WG, 73
Israel E, 153
Istre GR, 222

Iwatsuki S, 143
Izant RJ Jr, 218

J

Jackson EK, 108
Jackson GG, 164, 174, 175
Jacobs MR, 218
Jacqz E, 108
Jaffe DM, 219
Jaffe HW, 150, 157
Jarus GD, 71
Jarvie BH, 8
Jarvis WR, 132
Jensen T, 7
Jessen O, 141
Ježek Z, 93
Jimakorn P, 223
Jobe O, 224
Johnson KM, 92
Johnson PC, 18
Johnson S, 223
Johnston BL, 190
Jones G, 90
Jones JM, 138
Jurik AG, 236

K

Kagey-Sobotka A, 96
Kahlon J, 80
Kahn FW, 138
Kales CP, 173
Kanki PJ, 151
Kantoff P, 235
Kaplowitz LG, 105
Kaplowitz N, 76
Kapperud G, 70
Karanko V, 37
Karchmer AW, 2
Karmali MA, 12
Katz BZ, 149
Kauffman CA, 205
Kautman L, 105
Käyhty H, 37
Keating M, 137
Kela E, 37
Kelen GD, 152
Kennedy CJ, 172
Kennedy RC, 182
Kenney RT, 13
Kerkering TM, 105
Kersey JH, 87
Kessler HA, 168
Kew OM, 94
Keyvan-Karijani E, 111
Kiefer H, 77
Kim I, 131
King D, 174
King IJ, 92
King KC, 77
Kirkman RL, 85

Klahr S, 26
Klein BS, 99
Klein PD, 15
Klein RS, 148
Kleinman SH, 157
Kline RL, 153
Klugman KP, 44
Knigge M, 164
Koch C, 7
Koff RS, 76
Koffer H, 47
Kohn DB, 109
Koorhnof HJ, 44
Koplan JP, 95
Korn DA, 12
Kovacs JA, 178
Kozin AM, 237
Krause PJ, 54
Kreiger AE, 180
Krik LE, 87
Krishnan C, 12
Krogstad DJ, 123
Krohn K, 161
Krohn M, 161
Krugman S, 80
Kubitschek KR, 10
Kumar ML, 77
Kunches LM, 201
Kunin CM, 26
Kusne S, 143

L

Lack EE, 178
L'age-Stehr J, 155
Lakeman FD, 80
Landay A, 168
Lande AE, 208
Landers DV, 185
Landesman S, 154
Lane HC, 178
Lang W, 157
Lange JMA, 164, 165
Langkop CW, 13
Larabi S, 193
Larieu M-J, 158
Laskin OL, 88, 174, 175
Lastavica CC, 59
Lau JHK, 133
Laughlin LW, 67
Laurian Y, 158
Lawrence GW, 223
Leclair JM, 203, 207
Lee F, 80
Leedom JM, 174, 175
Leffell MS, 156
Legrand P, 193
Lenes BA, 157
LeRoy ML, 189
Leszczynski J, 85
Letson GW, 19
Lettau LA, 73
Leuther M, 158, 161

Levey AS, 85
Levey RH, 85
Levin JM, 85
Levine AM, 176
Levine MM, 11, 41, 115
Levy JA, 147, 157, 168
Lichtenstein LM, 96
Lietman PS, 48
Limsomwong N, 113
Lin ET, 176
Link H, 11
Linzer M, 237
Lior H, 12
Little BW, 62
Little EA, 83
Lobel HO, 112
Lobel SA, 156
Lode H, 50
LoGerfo F, 85
Looareesuwan S, 121
Losonsky G, 11, 115
Loss LE, 47
Lott L, 107
Loureiro C, 176
Lowe CU, 42
Luce JM, 176
Luk KDK, 133
Lukehart SA, 167
Lunde MN, 115
Lupton GP, 166
Lyman GH, 111

M

McArthur JC, 169
McCabe WR, 201
McCalla S, 154
McCarthy JG, 73
McCarthy MA, 34
McCormick JB, 92
McCredie KB, 137
McCullough AJ, 77
McCutchan JA, 172
McDade JE, 228
McDonald RC, 13
MacDonnell JA, 23
McDonnell PJ, 13
McEvoy MB, 58
McIntyre M, 23
McIver J, 85
Mack D, 164
Mackett MCT, 144
McKevitt M, 24
Mäkelä PH, 37
Maki DG, 189
Makintubee S, 222
Makowka L, 143
Maksymiuk A, 137
Malkovsky M, 182
Maloy WL, 115
Mandelbaum S, 71
Maniscalco WM, 105
Manning M, 201

Mansinho K, 151
Manzo A, 68
Marantz PR, 237
Margalit H, 115
Marlink R, 151
Marsh V, 224
Martin K, 149
Martin RJ, 13
Martone WJ, 34
Marvin JA, 143
Mason JC, 144
Mastre B, 75
Masur H, 178
Mather TN, 59
Matthew E, 32
Matuszak DL, 153
Maxwell GM, 210
Mayer K, 96
Mayer KH, 163
Mayer L, 13
Mayhew WJ, 20
Maynard JE, 73
Mayo DR, 210
M'Boge BH, 224
M'Boup S, 151
Medoff G, 105
Meguid MM, 195
Mendelson MH, 56, 199
Menegus MA, 105
Merigan TC, 75
Merz WG, 135
Metersky ML, 204
Metz CA, 1
Meusers P, 108
Meyers BR, 56
Meyers JD, 87
Michel MF, 102
Mieke S, 49
Mikesell TS, 205
Miklaw H, 92
Milberg J, 159
Mildvan D, 88, 174, 175
Milford EL, 85
Miller G, 149
Miller, J, 191
Miller LH, 115, 235
Mills AR, 234
Mills J, 88
Minamoto GY, 96
Minkoff H, 154
Mitsuyasu RT, 179
Mitty HA, 199
Moeschberger ML, 57
Mohan K, 213
Møller BN, 236
Montagnier L, 151
Montgomery AB, 176
Moon M-S, 131
Moore RD, 48
Morduchowicz G, 5
Morse LJ, 73
Morshed MG, 53
Mosca R, 195
Moss AR. 147
Moss B, 115

Author Index / 259

Moxon R, 38
Mugambi M, 117
Munro ND, 90
Munshi MH, 53
Murphy JR, 115
Murphy TV, 54
Murren JR, 173
Mutombo M, 93
Myers LL, 19

N

Naclerio RM, 96
Nahmias AJ, 80
Nair PV, 75, 80
Nakashima AK, 34
Nara A, 111
Nardin D, 115
Nelson JD, 31
Nelson K, 147
Neva FA, 118
Newland HS, 111
Newman FS, 19
Nickels MK, 13
Nicolle LE, 20, 23
Nina J, 151
Nkowane BM, 94
Noa MC, 150
Noah ND, 58
Norman JE, 76
Noventa F, 74
Nsanze H, 186
Nusinoff-Lehrman S, 175
Nussenzweig RS, 115
Nussenzweig V, 115

O

Ocampo J, 33
Oette DH, 179
Offermann G, 155
Ogata-Arakari D, 178
Ohnhaus EE, 108
Okoroanyanwu W, 228
Olson MM, 218
Opekun AR, 15
Ordelheide KS, 144
Ordovas JM, 128
Orenstein WA, 94
Orth G, 185
Osmond D, 147
Oster CN, 117
O'Sullivan R, 92
Ouzounian TJ, 27
Oxelius V-A, 210

P

Padian NS, 157
Padre LP, 67

Page P, 38
Paluku KM, 93
Pan L-Z, 168
Pang LW, 113
Papendick U, 92
Parisier SC, 56
Park Y-O, 131
Parker R, 159
Pass RF, 83
Passmore R, 234
Patriarca PA, 95
Paul DA, 158, 164, 165, 168
Paul SR, 223
Pedersen SS, 7
Peltola H, 37
Pereira MEA, 128
Peters JI, 10
Peters ME, 109
Petrini JL, Jr, 76
Phelan JA, 148
Pichichero ME, 52
Piesman J, 59
Pilkington NS Jr, 232
Pilsworth R, 58
Piot P, 186
Pitlik SD, 5
Platenkamp GJ, 102
Platt R, 207
Plowe CV, 117
Pollard RB, 75
Pornaro E, 74
Porsius JC, 102
Potter ME, 13
Prescott RJ, 6
Price DL, 111
Priehs C, 38
Prioli RP, 128
Proffitt MR, 169
Proud D, 96
Provencher M, 100
Pugh S, 6
Puhr ND, 13
Pun WK, 133
Punsalang A Jr, 105

Q

Quinet MC, 120
Quinn MG, 157
Quinn TC, 152, 153

R

Radford P, 3
Radivoyevitch M, 77
Rahaman MM, 53
Randolph MF, 210
Ranki A, 161
Ranoa CP, 67
Rapin M, 193
Rarick M, 176
Ratliff NB, 169

Ravenholt O, 157
Ray WA, 108
Realdi G, 74
Reed EC, 87
Reeve P, 118
Regan AM, 204
Reich L, 96
Reid R, 38
Reiner DS, 130
Reingold AL, 68
Rekola P, 37
Reller LB, 28
Resnick L, 181
Ricard D, 151
Richman DD, 172, 174, 175
Rissing JP, 156
Ristic M, 228
Robbins JB, 42, 44
Roberts GJ, 3
Roberts JM, 112
Robertson PW, 8
Robinson WS, 75
Rogers MF, 150
Roghmann KJ, 52
Romans P, 235
Rome-Lemonne J-L, 151
Ronald AR, 186
Rönnberg P-R, 37
Rosdahl VT, 141
Rosen L, 181
Rosenberg I, 128
Rosendal K, 141
Roskamp D, 75
Rosno S, 75
Rothenberg R, 159
Rothman RH, 57
Rubenis M, 164
Ruol A, 74
Ryan CA, 13

S

Sack DA, 53
Sack RB, 19
Safranek TJ, 132
Sakai RK, 235
Sakamoto MJ, 180
Sakurai J, 223
Sammelson JS, 37
Samuel M, 157
Samuelson JS, 36
Sande MA, 147
Sangare L, 151
SanMiguel JG, 46
Santiago E, 67
Santos-Ferreira M-O, 151
Santosham M, 38
Saral R, 135
Sauceda E, 33
Sauch JF, 130
Sawyer LA, 228
Schaberg DR, 205
Schable C, 148

Schachter J, 185, 210
Schaefer EJ, 128
Scheinberg DA, 96
Schellekens PTA, 164, 165
Schiff ER, 76
Schlesinger PH, 123
Schneerson R, 42, 44
Schneider A, 92
Schneider I, 118
Schoen RT, 59
Schonberger LB, 94
Schooley RT, 174
Schouten HJA, 102
Schröter GPJ, 85
Schulz D, 42, 44
Schwab SJ, 26
Schwalbe RS, 51
Schwarz A, 155
Seeff LB, 76
Selkon JB, 6
Sells CJ, 84
Senn D, 158
Shadomy S, 105
Shah PM, 49
Shapiro J, 7
Shapiro ME, 85
Shelhamer JH, 178
Shenep JL, 107, 196
Shenton F, 224
Shepp DH, 87
Sheppard S, 90
Sherwood JA, 118
Shoop DS, 19
Shorey J, 76
Shrestha MB, 42
Shurin SB, 207
Shusterman NH, 47
Siber GR, 38
Sidebottom DG, 207
Sidikaro Y, 180
Siegman-Igra Y, 5
Sijin O, 154
Sikes RK, 228
Silcox VA, 132
Sillah H, 224
Simmons JT, 178
Singh N, 143
Singharaj P, 113
Sivertson KT, 152
Slotman GJ, 1
Smith CI, 75
Smith CR, 48
Smith DD, 8
Smith ES, 92
Smith GL, 115
Smith MH, 73
Smithells RW, 90
Snydman DR, 85
So YC, 133
Solomon DA, 132
Somaini B, 112
Soong S-J, 105
Soriano E, 46
Sorrentino J, 96
Spear J, 168

Spector SA, 88, 172
Spielman A, 59
Stackhouse LL, 19
Stagno S, 83
Staib AH, 49
Stamm AM, 105
Stamm WE, 24
Staneck JL, 140
Stanley MM, 76
Stapleton JT, 51
Starcher ET, 150
Starzl TE, 143
Steele CR, 232
Steele RW, 232
Steere AC, 59
Steffen R, 112
Steigbigel NH, 148
Stein R, 108
Steinman T, 85
Stenico D, 74
Stevens CE, 80
Stevens DA, 106
Stille W, 49
Stokes DC, 196
Stone EF, 213
Stoneburner R, 159
Stork EK, 207
Stratton CW, 28
Strom BL, 47
Strom TB, 85
Stutman HR, 54
Sugar AM, 106
Sugarman B, 29
Sullivan BF, 203
Sweet RL, 185
Swenson JM, 132
Swenson PD, 154
Swim AT, 230
Syrogiannopoulos GA, 31
Szabo S, 199
Szczeniowski M, 93

T

Tacket CO, 11
Takala AK, 37
Talbot GH, 47, 100
Talpey WB, 52
Tan C, 191
Tanz RR, 219
Tavill AS, 77
Taylor DN, 223
Taylor E, 59
Taylor HR, 111
Taylor PE, 80
Tegzess AM, 155
Telford SR III, 59
Ternowitz T, 236
Thapa R, 42
Therasse PM, 205
Thielke TS, 189
Thomas ED, 87
Thomas PA, 150

Thompson L, 27
Thomson BF, 182
Thornquist M, 87
Thornton D, 107
Thorpe JE, 140
Thrasher TV, 144
Tilney NL, 85
Tilton RC, 210
Tong MJ, 75, 80
Tong TC, 92
Torres RA, 173
Townsend T, 191
Toy PT, 80
Tramont EC, 166
Transerra J, 46
Trape JF, 120
Travers K, 151
Trieger N, 148
Trippel S, 92
Trollfors B, 42
Trujillo MH, 68
Truman B, 159
Tuazon CU, 178
Tuazon ML, 67
Turner J, 176
Turner RB, 208
Tzakis AG, 143

U

Uehling DT, 109
Ukena T, 73

V

Valle S-L, 161
van der Noordaa J, 164
VanDuin AM, 102
Varkey B, 99
Vaughan WP, 135
Verroust F, 158
Vicary CA, 87
Volberding PA, 174, 175
Vontver LA, 84
Vyas GN, 80

W

Waggoner JG, 76
Wagner D, 92
Wagner J, 50
Wahrendorf J, 92
Walker C, 185
Walker LJ, 190
Walker PD, 223
Walker R, 178
Ward JI, 222
Ward JW, 157
Warkentin PI, 207
Warrell DA, 121

Washington AE, 79
Wasserman GF, 118
Wassilak SGF, 94
Waterman K, 75
Watt G, 67
Wattanagoon Y, 121
Webb PA, 92
Webber MM, 27
Wedel SA, 201
Weinberg D, 208
Weiner MH, 100
Weinstein MP, 28
Weissberg JI, 75
Weissman JV, 80
Welsh O, 33
Wenzel JG, 36
Werner BG, 85
Wesch H, 92
Wesseler TA, 140
Wharton JM, 126
White AT, 111
White NJ, 121

Whitley RJ, 80, 213
Whittle HC, 224
Whybin LR, 8
Wiesel SW, 57
Wiley JA, 157
Wiley R, 50
Wilkinson SR, 217
Williams D, 228
Williams PN, 111
Wingard JR, 135
Winkelstein W Jr, 157
Winston DJ, 180
Winters RE, 180
Woelfel M, 159
Wolfe PR, 180
Wolff MC, 38
Woo Y-K, 131
Woollett GR, 117
Writz RA, 117, 118
Wunderlich A, 130
Wyler DJ, 121

Y

Yango BG, 111
Yen-Lieberman B, 169
Young JR, 118

Z

Zacher B, 38
Zerpa R, 68
Zervos MJ, 205
Zimmerman CE II, 85
Zondervan PE, 102
Zoulani A, 120
Zuckerman E, 96
zur Hausen H, 92